Designing Exoskeletons

Designing Exoskeletons focuses on developing exoskeletons, following the lifecycle of an exoskeleton from design to manufacture. It demonstrates how modern technologies can be used at every stage of the process, such as design methodologies, CAD/CAE/CAM software, rapid prototyping, test benches, materials, heat and surface treatments, and manufacturing processes. Several case studies are presented to provide detailed considerations on developing specific topics.

Exoskeletons are designed to provide work-power, rehabilitation, and assistive training to sports and military applications. Beginning with a review of the history of exoskeletons from ancient to modern times, the book builds on this by mapping out recent innovations and state-of-the-art technologies that utilize advanced exoskeleton design. Presenting a comprehensive guide to computer design tools used by bioengineers, the book demonstrates the capabilities of modern software at all stages of the process, looking at computer-aided design, manufacturing, and engineering. It also details the materials used to create exoskeletons, notably steels, engineering polymers, composites, and emerging materials. Manufacturing processes, both conventional and unconventional are discussed—for example, casting, powder metallurgy, additive manufacturing, and heat and surface treatments.

This book is essential reading for those in the field of exoskeletons, such as designers, workers in research and development, engineering and design students, and those interested in robotics applied to medical devices.

Designing Exoskeletons

Luis Adrian Zuñiga-Aviles
Giorgio Mackenzie Cruz-Martinez

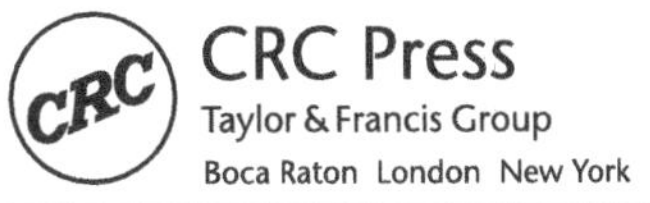

CRC Press
Taylor & Francis Group
Boca Raton London New York

CRC Press is an imprint of the
Taylor & Francis Group, an **informa** business

Designed cover image: Luis Adrian Zuñiga-Aviles

First edition published 2024
by CRC Press
2385 Executive Center Drive, Suite 320, Boca Raton, FL 33431

and by CRC Press
4 Park Square, Milton Park, Abingdon, Oxon, OX14 4RN

CRC Press is an imprint of Taylor & Francis Group, LLC

© 2024 Luis Adrian Zuñiga-Aviles and Giorgio Mackenzie Cruz-Martinez

ISBN: 978-1-032-20047-7 (hbk)
ISBN: 978-1-032-20049-1 (pbk)
ISBN: 978-1-003-26199-5 (ebk)
ISBN: 978-1-032-37784-1 (eBook+)

DOI: 10.1201/9781003261995

Typeset in Times
by Apex CoVantage, LLC

To my wife Sonia, my sons Irving and Kevin, and my daughter Katia—their support and love are my life-balance to continue this fantastic road, collaborating, learning, sharing, and dreaming together to achieve new goals, new ideas, and new books.

Dr. Luis Adrián Zúñiga-Avilés

To my father and mother, without whose partnership and comprehension this book would not have been possible. It is our collective achievement! I love you.

Dr. Giorgio Mackenzie Cruz-Martínez

Contents

Preface

The idea and motivation to write this book emanated from the taste and research interest in the design of exoskeletons the authors share. The authors reflected that currently, the books and courses cover the design of exoskeletons from biomedical, medical robotics, or control points of view, not one that covers all three aspects as a whole and includes materials, manufacturing processes, and usability studies. Considering that both authors are researchers with master's and doctoral degrees, the content of this book on exoskeleton design reflects their experience in developing medical devices in both industrial and academic research.

The book is aimed at designers, research and development workers, engineering, medical bioengineering, design students, and people interested in physical therapy with exoskeletons. The intention is to give the reader knowledge about the development of exoskeletons using modern design tools, which involve design methodologies such as product lifecycle management, quality function deployment, axiomatic design, design for assembly, and platform products. Also, the technology readiness level (TRL), manufacturing readiness level (MRL), and investment readiness level (IRL) are considered. In addition, CAD/CAE/CAM software, rapid prototyping, test benches, materials, heat and surface treatments, and manufacturing processes are covered in the book. Several case studies are presented to provide detailed considerations on the development of specific topics.

An introductory chapter provides a review of the history of exoskeletons, describing how mechanisms formed machines, how the robots were created, and how these robots began to be used in medical applications, progressing to exoskeletons that include control systems, mechanical assemblies, artificial intelligence, and modern motors. This chapter describes the evolution of exoskeletons, manufacturing processes, and design tools used to develop exoskeletons throughout history.

The book continues with the design of the exoskeleton using various design methodologies, beginning with the voice of the customer (VOC) and functional requirements. Subsequently, it delves into collaborative design and solver capabilities through modern software (CAD and CAE simulation) and CAM evaluation until an experimental physical model and test bench are reached.

The book advances to the description of current and emerging materials used in the production of exoskeletons to improve the properties of their components. A review of the main standards that exoskeletons must meet, the intellectual property of the most representative exoskeletons, test benches, energy systems, and usability analysis is carried out.

The topic of exoskeleton design is multidisciplinary, so the various issues of the book are presented in the most accessible way possible, and individual chapters can be consulted as they meet the reader's needs. This book is expected to foster interest and learning in the development of exoskeletons using modern design tools, materials, and emerging manufacturing processes.

Acknowledgments

Dr. Adrian Zuñiga thanks the Faculty of Medicine and the Faculty of Engineering from the Autonomous University of Mexico State, the Military School for Engineers, and the Researchers Program for Mexico (IxM) from the National Council of Humanities, Science and Technology (CONAHCYT). Also, special thanks to Dra. Mariel Davila Vilchis, Dr. Joel Zagoya López, Msc. Jose Luis Medina Valdes, Msc. Nancy Yañes Martinez, and bioengineering student Luis Valdes Aguirre for your collaboration with resources for this book.

Dr. Giorgio Cruz thanks the Faculty of Engineering from the Autonomous University of Mexico State (UAEMex) and the National Council of Humanities, Science and Technology (CONAHCYT).

Both authors thank the CRC Press Taylor & Francis Group team for trusting them and accepting the proposal of this book. A special acknowledgment goes out to Nicola Sharpe and Nishan Bhagat, who promptly followed up on all administrative tasks concerning this book.

Author Biographies

Dr. Adrian Zuñiga is a professor in the bioengineering bachelor of Faculty of Medicine UAEMex, member of Mexican Researchers National System level II, and retired military engineer with vast experience in the development of medical devices. He holds a PhD and a master's degree in science and technology on mechatronics from the Center for Engineering and Industrial Development (CIDESI). He holds a bachelor's degree in military industrial engineering and mechanical engineering specialty from the Military School of Engineers (EMI), Mexican Army and Air Force University. Dr. Zuñiga has led several designs and development of crane systems for lift patients, exoskeletons, rehabilitation devices, aid devices, and prosthetics. Some products are working in the Mexican Central Military Hospital. His experience has focused on new product development, design process, design methodologies, design of mechanisms and machines, test benches, finite element method (FEM) analysis, kinematics, modeling and simulation, manufacturing technologies, and rapid prototypes. He has authored over 200 works, including conference presentations, proceedings, book chapters, patents, articles, projects, and industrial reports. Nowadays, Dr. Zuñiga is a member of the Dynamics and Control Systems in the Faculty of Engineering at the Autonomous University of Mexico State.

Dr. Giorgio Mackenzie Cruz Martínez is an electronic engineer who graduated from the Autonomous University of Mexico State. He also received his master's and PhD studies from this university; in addition, he participates in a military project with the Applied Research Center and Technology Development for the Mexican Military Industry (CIADTIM). He has broad experience in designing and manufacturing rehabilitation robots and exoskeletons. He did a postdoctoral research stay at the informatic, robotic, and microelectronic laboratory of Montpellier in France, working on the development of a robot surgery device. His experience has focused on new product development, design process, design methodologies, medical mechanisms, instrument design, kinematics modeling and simulation, and rapid prototypes. Dr. Giorgio is a member of the research group on Dynamics and Control Systems in the Faculty of Engineering at the Autonomous University of Mexico State and is part of the National Research System.

Abbreviations

1D	One-Dimensional
2D	Two-Dimensional
3D	Three-Dimensional
4D	Four-Dimensional
A2LA	American Association for Laboratory Accreditation
AAMI	Advancement of Medical Instrumentation
ABI	Allied Business Intelligence
ABS	Acrylonitrile Butadiene Styrene
AC	Alternating Current
AD	Año Domini
AEP	Allied Engineering Publication
AQAP	Allied Quality Assurance Publications
AR	Augmented Reality
ASA	Acrylic Styrene Acrylonitrile
ASIMO	Advanced Step in Innovative Mobility
ASME	American Society of Mechanical Engineers
BC	Before Christ
BC	Boundary Conditions
BCL	Binary Cutter Language
BI	Business Intelligence
BLDC	Brushless DC
BOM	Bill of Materials
CAD	Computer-Aided Design
CAE	Computer-Aided Engineering
CAGR	Compound Annual Growth Rate
CAM	Computer-Aided Manufacturing
CDP	Critical Design Parameter
CEN	Committee for Standardization
CE	Conformité Européenne
CFD	Computational Fluid Dynamic
CI	Communality Index
CJM	Customer Journey Mapping
CMM	Coordinate Measuring Machine
CNC	Computer Numerical Control
COBOL	Common Business Oriented Language
COFEPRIS	Federal Commission for the Protection Against Sanitary Risk
CP	Cerebral Palsy
CRM	Customer Relationship Management
CSET	Center for Security and Emerging Technology
CT	Computed Tomography
CX	Customer Experience
D	Difficulty

DAC	Data Acquisition Cards
DC	Direct Current
DFA	Design for Assembly
DFT	Design for Testability
DFX	Design for Excellence
DGI	Dynamic Gait Index
DMD	Duchenne Muscular Dystrophy
DMLS	Direct Metal Laser Sintering
DOD	Department of Defense
DOF	Degrees of Freedom
DP	Design Parameters
DSM	Design Structure Matrix
DT	Digital Twin
EAWS	Ergonomic Assessment Work-Sheet System
EDM	Electrical Discharge Machining
EEG	Electroencephalography
EFTA	European Free Trade Association
EIA	Electronic Industries Alliance
EMG	Electromyography
EOD	Explosive Device Disposal
EPCE	Exoskeleton Performance Case Studies
EPM	Experimental Physical Model
ERP	Enterprise Resource Planning
ESD	Electrostatic Discharge
FDA	Food and Drug Administration
FDM	Fused Deposition Modeling
FEA	Fluid Elastomer Actuators
FGA	Functional Gait Assessment
FHE	Flexible Hybrid Electronics
FISA	Fabric Inflatable Soft Actuators
FMEA	Failure Modes and Effects Analysis
FR	Functional Requirements
FT	Force Torque
GE	General Electric
GOST	Governmental Standard
Gtols	Geometric Tolerances
GUI	Graphical User Interface
HD	Huntington's Disease
HMI	Human-Machine Interface
HOQ	House of Quality
HOQ1	First House of Quality
HOQ2	Second House of Quality
HOQ3	House of Quality 3
HOQ4	House of Quality 4
HOQ4	House of Quality 4
HOQ5	House of Quality 5

HOQ6	House of Quality 6
HOSDB	Home Office Scientific Development Branch
HPC	High-Performance Computing
HTG	Homogeneous Transformation Graphic
IBM	International Business Machines Corporation
IEC	International Electrotechnical Commission
IEDD	Improvised Explosive Device Disposal
IEEE	Institute of Electrical and Electronics Engineers
IFR	International Federation of Robotics
IIoT	Industrial Internet of Things
IMU	Inertial Measurement Unit
IoT	Internet of Things
IPC	International Patent Classification
IRL	Investment Readiness Level
ISO	International Organization for Standardization
ISS	International Space Station
IW	Internet Wave
JIS	Japanese Industrial Standards Committee
JIT	Just in Time
JSA	Japanese Standards Association
JTBD	Jobs io Be Done
LBP	Lower Back Pain
LDPE	Low-Density Polyethylene
LED	Light Emitting Diode
LFP	Lithium Iron Phosphate
LiDAR	Light Detection and Ranging of Laser Imaging Detection and Ranging
LISiN	Laboratory for Engineering of Neuromuscular System
MAP	Manufacturing Automation Protocol
MATE	Muscular Aiding Tech Exoskeleton
MAUDE	Manufacturer and User Facility Device Experience
MBD	Multibody Dynamics
MC	Machining Center
MCM	Monte Carlo Method
MEMS	Micro-Electromechanical System
MER	Mars Exploration Rover
MHLW	Ministry of Health, Labour, and Welfare
MIT	Massachusetts Institute of Technology
MM	Multi-Operation Machines
MRI	Magnetic Resonance Imaging
MRL	Manufacturing Readiness Level
MSD	Musculoskeletal Disorders
NASA	National Aeronautics and Space Administration
NC	Numerical Control
NCAGE	NATO Commercial and Government Entity
NCL	Nice Classification

NDT	Non-Destructive Testing
NIJ	National Institute of Justice
NIOSH	National Institute for Occupational Safety and Health
NIST	National Institute of Standards and Technology
NOM	Official Mexican Standard
NP	New Priority
NPD	New Product Development
NSCISC	National Spinal Cord Injury Statistical Center
NSRDEC	Natick Soldier Research, Development, and Engineering Center
NURBS	Non-Uniform Rational B-Spline
NVH	Noise, Vibration, and Harshness
NVLAP	National Voluntary Laboratory Accreditation Program
OAC	Open Architecture Control
OMPI	World Intellectual Organization of Intellectual Property
PAAD	Performance Augmentation and Amplification Devices
PAM	Pneumatic Artificial Muscles
PCB	Printed Circuit Board
PCT	Patent Cooperation Treaty
PDE	Partial Differential Equations
PDM	Product Data Management
PET	Positron Emission Tomography
PETG	Polyethylene Terephthalate Glycol
pH	Potential of Hydrogen
PLA	Polylactic Acid
PLC	Programmable Logic Controller
PLM	Product Lifecycle Management
PMDA	Pharmaceuticals and Medical Devices Agency
PPE	Personal Protective Equipment
PRM	Performance-Related Measurement
PTP	Point io Point
PV	Process Variable
PVC	Polymerizing Vinyl Chloride
QFD	Quality Function Deployment
ROM	Range of Movement
RP	Rapid Prototype
RT	Rapid Tooling
SAIL	Stanford Artificial Intelligence Laboratory
SAM	Serviceable Available Market
SCI	Spinal Cord Injuries
SCM	Supply Chain Management
SDK	Software Development Kit
SE	Substantially Equivalent
SemiS	Semi-Structured
SLA	Stereolithography
SLS	Selective Laser Sintering
SPA	Soft Pneumatic Actuators

SRI	Stanford Research Institute
SRL	Supernumerary Robotics Limbs
TAM	Total Available Market
TBF	Test Bench Feature
TC	Technical Committee
TDT	Toyota Design Techniques
TIPS	Theory of Inventive Problem Solving
TIR	Technical Importance Rating
TP	Thermoplastic
TPS	Toyota Production System
TPU	Thermoplastic Polyurethane
TRI-HFT	Toronto Rehabilitation Institute Hand Function Test
TRL	Technology Readiness Level
TS	Thermosetting
UCD	User-Centered Design
UI	User Interface
UL	Underwriters Laboratories
UMUX	Usability Metrics for User Experience
UNECE	United Nations Economic Commission for Europe
UnS	Unstructured
UPS	Uninterruptible Power Supply
USA	United States of America
UX	User Experience
VMP	Valuable Minimum Product
VOC	Voice of the Customer
VR	Virtual Reality
VTOL	Vertical Takeoff and Landing
WI	Work Item
WIPO	World Intellectual Property Organization
WWII	World War II

1 History of the Exoskeletons

1.1 INTRODUCTION

To outline the history of exoskeletons, we could start with the meaning of the word exoskeleton, coined in 1841 by the British biologist Richard Owen for his anatomical observations in animals, referring to any rigid external structure, sometimes articulated in some parts, that covers, supports, and protects any animal's internal or soft tissues. This applies especially to invertebrates, in the case of arthropods (insects, arachnids, mites, myriapods, and crustaceans).

In the world of robotics, a mechanical exoskeleton, power exoskeleton, power armor, exoframe, or exosuit is a mobile machine consisting of a soft or rigid external frame worn by a person and including a power system of motors or hydraulics that provides at least part of the energy for the movement of the members. It helps its wearer to move and carry out certain activities, such as carrying weight, mobilizing limbs, training, reducing reaction times, or reducing the energy consumption of geriatric or disabled users. The duration of rehabilitation activities depends on the current consumption of the actuators and the capacity of the energy supply of the batteries. This activity duration is called the autonomy of the exoskeletons.

Now that the word exoskeleton is defined, we will explain its history, starting from the development of mechanisms that gave rise to increasingly complex machines that progressively gave rise to robots. The conception of robots to assist human beings led to various medical applications, among which exoskeletons emerged in the 1960s.

1.2 FROM MECHANISMS TO MACHINES

Several mechanisms have been designed since antiquity, so it would be impossible to mention them all; however, here we highlight the most representative ones for the emergence of robotics as a discipline.

Some authors suggest that the first automatons arose when the statues of some gods and kings gave off fire from their eyes, like the statue of Osiris. Others had mechanical arms operated by the priests of the temple, and others, like that of Memon of Ethiopia, made sounds when the sun's rays illuminated them and thus instilled fear and respect in those who contemplated them. This religious purpose of the automata continued until classical Greece, where statues moved with hydraulic power.

Asian culture, especially China and Japan, has had a great tradition of automata that has been maintained since ancient times. In the year 2000 BC, Chinese legends are told about robots, such as one made of wood and so similar to the man that it confused all who saw it.

DOI: 10.1201/9781003261995-1

In 400 BC, the mathematician Archita designed and built a steam pigeon. In 200 BC, the Greek inventor and physicist Ctesibus of Alexandria designed water clocks with moving figures. Polybius (200–118 BC) invented a contraption in the shape of a woman with nails in her chest and arms, which mortally embraced everyone who defaulted on her payments. Heron of Alexandria (10–70 AD) invented the world's first steam engine and its incorporation of self-regulating feedback control system types as well as a book on the figure of automata robots. The creation of mechanisms is explained, many based on the principles of Archimedes, made mainly for entertainment and imitating movements, such as birds that chirped, flew, and drank; statues that served wine; or automatic doors, all produced by the movement of water, gravity, or lever systems. Also noteworthy is his "The Automaton Theatre", about his mechanical puppet theatre that represented the Trojan War.

The *Book of Ingenious Mechanisms* was written in the year 805 by the Banu Musa brothers (Ahmad, Muhammad, and Hasan bin Musa ibn Shakir), describing a hundred mechanisms and automata and how to use them.

Alberto Magno, born in 1206 in Bavaria, made many works of a magical nature and created artificial beings, two in particular—one of the so-called talking heads and an iron automaton that served him as a butler and on which he worked for 30 years, capable of walking, opening the door, and greeting visitors.

Al-Jazari (1260) invented the crankshaft and the first mechanical clocks that moved by weights and water, among many other automatic control inventions; he was also very interested in the figure of the automaton, creating a work that deals with the history of technology. Within this aspect, his complex elephant clock and a human-shaped robot serving different drinks are worth mentioning.

Leonardo da Vinci (1452–1519) designed an automaton dressed in medieval armor and a mechanical lion. Inventors in medieval times often built machines to amuse royalty.

The entry into the 18th century and the consequent advances in watchmaking were considered to be the time when the most perfect automatons in history were made. Their development, dominated by a scientific nature, highlighted the obsession with reproducing the movements and behavior of living beings.

Born on February 24, 1709, J. Vaucanson wanted to demonstrate the realization of basic biological principles, such as circulation, digestion, or respiration, through his automatons. He wrote about this last function in his first creation, The Flute Player, a life-size figure in the shape of a shepherd who played the drum and the flute with a varied musical repertoire. Vaucanson presented it at the French Academy of Sciences, reaping great success. Later, in 1738, he created his second automaton, The Drummer, as an improved version of the first. The third and most famous was the Duck with Digestive Device, transparent and made up of more than 400 moving parts. It flapped its wings, ate, and thoroughly digested, mimicking the natural behavior of the bird to the smallest detail. Although the duck was a deception because what it ate was not the same as what it defecated; inside the duck, there was a compartment in which the grain it ate was deposited and something similar to excrement came out. Over the years, Vaucanson, tired of his work, sold the figures in 1743.

Another inventor of the 18th century, Friedrich von Knauss (1724–1789), was the creator of one of the first writing automata. This complex creation was formed by a sphere supported by two bronze eagles. In it, the figure of a goddess serves as a muse to the automaton, who, with her long arm, writes on a blank sheet of paper what she has been ordered to do. The operating system could make the robot dip the pen into the inkwell to be able to write and had a method to turn the page after it had been written on. Pierre Jaquet-Droz, a Swiss born in 1721, was responsible for the three most complex and famous automata of the 18th century.

The fame of the Von Knauss and Jaquet-Droz automata led many illusionists and conjurers to incorporate automation tricks into their shows. In 1759 two robots were added to the bell tower built in 1572 on the candle tower. In 18th- and 19th-century Japan, automata achieved high importance and complexity. They were called karakuri, which could be translated as mechanical devices to produce a surprise in a person. In 1738, Jacques de Vaucanson began building automata in Grenoble, France. As mentioned, his duck moved, quacked, flapped its wings, and even ate and digested food [1].

In 1801, a silk weaver, Joseph Marie Jacquard, invented an improved textile loom. The Jacquard loom was the first machine to use punch cards. In 1822, Charles Babbage was an English mathematician, philosopher, inventor, and mechanical engineer who originated the concept of the programmable computer. In 1822 he demonstrated a prototype of his "Difference Engine" to the Royal Astronomical Society. In 1985, the London Science Museum launched a project to build a complete Babbage engine using original designs to explore the practical feasibility of Babbage's schemes. In 1847, as the inventor of Boolean algebra, the basis of Boolean logic, and thus of modern digital computer logic, George Boole was regarded in retrospect as a founder of the field of computer science.

In 1898, Nikola Tesla invented and tested the world's first remote-controlled weapon. Tesla designed and built a couple of radio-controlled boats. The ships were constructed of iron, powered by an electric battery of his design, and equipped with a receiver that accepted commands from a wireless transmitter. The ships were also equipped with a large whip antenna, a modular space that could carry a load, diving rudders, a stanchion, and electric running lights that could be controlled remotely.

In the 20th and 21st centuries modern Japanese robots were designed, with the creation of highly complex anthropomorphic robots such as ASIMO, QRIO, or Repliee Q1, or robotic pets such as Aibo, a direct descendant of the animal automatons of past centuries.

1.3 FROM MACHINES TO MEDICAL APPLICATIONS

1.3.1 IMAGING

The discovery of X-rays by Wilhelm Conrad Röntgen on November 8, 1895, ushered in a new era of medicine. The new technology shone an unprecedented light on the human body, making numerous diseases easier to diagnose. Two predecessor companies of Siemens Healthineers first recognized the massive potential of X-rays—Siemens & Halske and Reiniger, Gebbert & Schall—which soon began producing commercial X-ray equipment. In the early stages, an X-ray image took several minutes to capture, and the patient had to remain motionless. With such long exposure times, organs like the heart would only appear as a blurred shadow on the final image. The decisive breakthrough came with the invention of the "Blitzapparat"—an X-ray device enabling physicians to capture X-ray images in the space of a few milliseconds, on which even the heart was clearly visible [2].

Siemens established the Siemens-Reiniger-Werke AG (SRW) in 1932, bringing together its medical technology business. The following year, SRW created the Pantix rotating anode tube, which served as a precursor to modern X-ray tubes. One year later, Siemens introduced the X-ray Sphere to the market. This device was contained in a spherical casing that was resistant to radiation and high voltages, making it portable, easy to operate, and affordable. It was a popular product, with nearly 30,000 units sold worldwide until the 1970s. In 1950, Siemens introduced the angiograph, which allowed the observation of the catheter on its journey through the blood vessels to the heart on a fluorescent screen. In 1972, Siemens developed the Mammomat, the first mammography unit designed explicitly for examining the female breast. The urograph followed a year later, which combined all urological X-ray exams and instrumental procedures into one dedicated workstation. Other notable innovations included the echocardiography in 1953; the gamma camera in 1958; the Vidoson in 1967, which was the first ultrasound device capable of real-time observations of movements inside the body; and SIRETOM in 1975, a device for cranial computed tomography (CT). In 1983, Siemens introduced Magnetom, the first commercial magnetic resonance imaging (MRI) system, and in 2001, the Biograph, which integrated positron emission tomography (PET) and CT into a single device.

1.3.2 LABORATORY DIAGNOSTICS

During the 1940s, the Clinitest was created, which was a tablet that could quickly test for diabetes in urine by combining all the necessary reagents. The first Clinistix test strips were introduced in 1956, which allowed for the application of the reagents to paper strips. Later versions, like Multistix in 1984, added further test pads to measure other parameters. The AutoAnalyzer was developed in 1957, and the Corning Model 12 in the 1960s. The Corning Model 165, introduced in 1971, was the first device to determine pH, pO_2, and pCO_2 from a single blood sample. In 1976, the Clinitek Analyzer was invented. The development of Clinistix led to the creation of many other urine and blood analysis test strips. The evolution of modern laboratory diagnostics has been influenced by numerous researchers and developers at the predecessor companies of the diagnostics division of Siemens Healthineers. Compared to traditional laboratory conveyor belts, the magnetic sample transport technology is much faster, up to ten times as fast. The Atellica Solution immunoassay system is capable of analyzing over 400 samples per hour. The scheduling software is intelligent and ensures that each sample is registered and prioritized based on its urgency, with urgent samples given priority over routine exams [3].

1.3.3 ADVANCED THERAPIES

For 175 years, Siemens equipment has supported medical therapy in applications ranging from electrical therapy for cardiovascular problems to mitigation of hearing damage or effective treatment of tumors. The history of Siemens medical technology dates back to 1844, when Werner von Siemens first used one of his inventions for medical purposes, treating his brother Friedrich's toothache with the Volta inductor. A few years later, Siemens & Halske presented an improved version of the apparatus: the slide inductor, customized to meet the needs of electrotherapy with built-in voltage and current controls. The device was one of the first-ever pieces of electromedical equipment and enjoyed great commercial success worldwide for decades [4].

The development of the Pantostat universal connection device in 1910 marked a significant achievement in the history of electromedicine, providing a broad range of therapeutic treatments that included the four-cell galvanic bath and vibration massage. Additionally, the Pantostat was adaptable for diagnostic purposes, such as serving as an electricity source for headlamps and endoscopes. This multi-functionality was the key factor behind Pantostat's commercial success, which continued until the 1970s.

Medical professionals started exploring the therapeutic possibilities of X-rays shortly after their discovery in 1896 and conducted initial trials of radiation therapy. By 1910, the first X-ray machines designed specifically for therapeutic use became available. Two areas of therapy emerged from this, namely superficial and deep therapy. To irradiate deep-seated tumors, researchers initially focused on finding ways for X-rays to penetrate deep inside the body, which required high voltages. The Stabilivolt, created by Siemens & Halske in 1922, met many of the requirements for deep therapy and proved successful for several years. The Esha-Phonophor, Siemens's first hearing aid in 1913, was based on telephone technology. Hearing aid technology was revolutionized in the 1940s with the invention of subminiature tubes and crystal microphones. Siemens recognized the significance of these advances and introduced the Fortiphon and Phonophor Alpha pocket hearing aids to replace earlier models that used carbon microphone technology.

The Auriculette 326 was the first behind-the-ear hearing aid system developed by Siemens in 1959, marking a significant transition from earlier models that were carried in a vest pocket. Despite being composed of the same components, the new hearing aids were small and light enough to fit comfortably in a shell directly behind the ear. Another breakthrough was achieved by Siemens in 1966 with the introduction of the Siretta, the first in-the-ear system to be commercially available. The Betatron electron accelerator was also a critical breakthrough in deep radiotherapy, introduced in 1950, which used a magnetic field to accelerate electrons in a circular path to near the speed of light, enabling deep-seated tumors to be effectively treated. This technology paved the way for modern radiotherapy, with circular accelerators eventually being replaced by linear accelerators that accelerate electrons along a straight path. Siemens provided a complete line of linear accelerators, the Megatron series, from 1974 to the 1990s.

Siemens released the Artiste linear accelerator in 2004, which is an all-in-one radio-oncology system that combines imaging and radiation settings. In 1958, the first fully implantable cardiac pacemaker was created by Swedish engineer Rune using miniature batteries and energy-saving transistors. The first pacemakers were large and cumbersome, but as they became smaller, they were still directly connected to the heart through a cable that passed through the skin, which posed a high risk of infection. Modern pacemakers are small and implanted in the patient's chest wall, about the size of a two-euro coin. The development of advanced therapies since 2000 has been supported by modern imaging technology and software applications that assist in the entire therapeutic process, from initial diagnosis and treatment planning to surgery and aftercare. In 2003, Siemens pioneered magnetic navigation in interventional cardiology in collaboration with Stereotaxis, enabling physicians to use remote control guided by precise imaging to navigate a catheter through the heart and coronary vessels to reach previously unattainable locations in the body.

In 2006, the software program syngo InSpace EP enabled the first-ever three-dimensional visualization of the left atrium using real-time X-ray images, which supported the diagnosis and treatment of cardiac arrhythmia. This breakthrough allowed image-guided catheter ablation, which is an effective treatment for atrial fibrillation in the left atrium and reduces the risk of stroke associated with the condition. Siemens released the CLEARstent Live software in 2012, which is available on all its angiography systems. This software helps position stents quickly and accurately by virtually freezing heart movements during a coronary intervention. During complex operations, such as those required to treat heart muscle diseases or valves, cardiologists require information about soft tissue and blood flow from ultrasound diagnostics and detailed vascular imaging from angiography. In 2017, the software application syngo True Fusion merged ultrasound data and live fluoroscopy images to provide all the necessary information in a single image.

1.4 DEVELOPMENT OF ROBOTICS

A science fiction play titled *Rossum's Universal Robots (R.U.R.)* was released in 1921 and is notable for introducing the term "robot". The play begins in a factory that makes artificial people called "robots." Unlike the modern usage of the word, these creatures are closer to the contemporary idea of androids, or even clones, as they can be mistaken for humans and can think for themselves. They seem happy to work for the humans, though changes and a rebellion by hostile robots lead to the extinction of humans. The word robot comes from the word robota, which means serf labor or hard labor in Czech, Slovak, and Polish. While Karel is often thought to have originated the word, he wrote a short letter about an article in the Oxford English Dictionary etymology in which he named his brother, the painter and writer Josef Čapek, as its actual inventor.

In 1926, Fritz Lang's film *Metropolis* was released, where "Maria", the female robot in the film, is the first robot to be projected on to the big screen [5]. In 1936, Alan Mathison Turing was an English mathematician, logician, cryptanalyst, and computer scientist. He was highly influential in the development of computing, providing a formalization of the concept of the algorithm and computing with the Turing machine, which played an essential role in the creation of the modern computer. Turing machines, first described by him in 1936, are simple abstract computational devices intended to help investigate the scope and limitations of what can be computed. Before the invention of the modern digital computer, Turing was interested in the question of what it means to be computable. A task is computable if a sequence of instructions can be specified that, when followed, will result in the completion of the task. Such a set of instructions is called an effective procedure, or algorithm, for the task.

In 1940, Isaac Asimov produced a series of short stories about robots beginning with "A Strange Playfellow" for *Super Science Stories* magazine. The story is about a robot and his affection for a child that he is obliged to protect. Over the next ten years, Asimov produced more robot stories that were finally recompiled in the *I, Robot* volume in 1950.

Asimov is generally credited with popularizing the term "robotics", which was first mentioned in his story "Runaround" in 1942. Issac Asimov's most significant contribution to robot history is the creation of his Three Laws of Robotics [6]:

- A robot may not injure a human or, through inaction, allow a human to come to harm.
- A robot must obey the orders given to it by humans, except where such orders conflict with the First Law.
- A robot must protect its own existence if such protection does not conflict with the First or Second Law.

In 1950, Alan Turing published "Computing Machinery and Intelligence", which proposed a test to determine whether a machine has gained the power to think for itself. It is known as the "Turing Test". The Turing test tests a machine's ability to exhibit intelligent behavior. A human judge engages in a natural language conversation with a human and a machine, each trying to appear human. All participants are separated from each other. If the judge cannot reliably distinguish the machine from the human, the machine is said to have passed the test.

In 1960 the first industrial arm robot was introduced, the Unimate, designed to complete repetitive or dangerous tasks on a General Motors assembly line. It began work in New Jersey in 1961. George Devol created it in the 1950s. Devol and Joseph Engelberger started Unimation, the world's first robot manufacturing company. The machine took on the job of transporting die-cast parts from an assembly line and welding these parts onto car bodies, a dangerous task for the workers, who could be poisoned by exhaust fumes or lose a limb if they weren't careful.

In 1966, The Stanford Research Institute (later to be known as SRI Technology) created Shakey, the first mobile robot that knows and reacts to its own actions. While other robots would have to be instructed on each step to complete a larger task, Shakey could parse the command and break it down into basic chunks. Due to its nature, the project combined research in robotics, computer vision, and natural language processing. Because of this, it was the first project that merged logical reasoning and physical action. In 1969, Victor Scheinman, a mechanical engineering student working at the Stanford Artificial Intelligence Laboratory (SAIL), created the Stanford Arm. The arm design has become a standard and is still influencing robotic arm design today. In 1977, *Star Wars* premiered. George Lucas's film about a universe ruled by The Force introduces viewers to R2-D2 and C-3PO. The film created the most potent image of a human future with robots since the 1960s and inspired a generation of researchers. In 1986, Honda began a robot research program with the premise that the robot "must coexist and cooperate with human beings, doing what a person cannot do and cultivating a new dimension in mobility to benefit in ultimately to society".

In 1989, a walking robot named Genghis was introduced by the Mobile Robots Group at MIT. He becomes known for how he walked, popularly known as the "Genghis gait". Genghis was built at MIT to demonstrate the effectiveness of using numerous small, lightweight mobile robots to explore the Martian surface. In 1996, Honda debuted the P3, the fruit of its decade-long effort to build a humanoid robot. The P series is a chronological progression of humanoid robot prototypes developed by Honda. The research conducted led to the eventual creation of the ASIMO robot.

In 1997, NASA's *Pathfinder* mission landed on Mars. *Sojourner*'s robotic rover rolled down a ramp and onto Martian soil in early July. It transmitted data from the Martian surface through September. After a few days on the Martian surface, NASA controllers turned on *Sojourner*'s hazard prevention system and asked her to make some of her own decisions. This hazard avoidance system distinguished the rover from all other machines that have explored space. *Sojourner* made trips between designated points without the benefit of detailed information to warn her of obstacles along the way.

In 1998, Tiger Electronics introduced the Furby to the Christmas toy market, and it quickly became "the toy" to get for the season. Using a variety of sensors, this "animatronic pet" could react to its environment and communicate using over 800 English phrases and its own language, "Furbish". In 1998, LEGO released its first Robotics Invention System 1.0 and named the product line MINDSTORMS after Seymour Papert's seminal work *Mindstorms: Children, Computers, and Powerful Ideas* published in 1980. In this book, Papert advocates constructionism, or learning by doing.

In 2000, Honda debuted the 12th version of its humanoid robot first introduced in 1986—ASIMO. The name is an acronym for "Advanced Step in Innovative Mobility". The robot has seven DOF in each arm: three DOF in the joints, shoulder, and wrist, giving "six degrees of freedom", and one DOF in the elbow; six DOF on each leg: three DOF on the crotch, two DOF on the ankle and one DOF on the knee; and three DOF in the neck joint. The hands have two DOF: one DOF on each thumb and one on each finger. This gives a total of 34 DOF in all joints. In August 2001, the Food and Drug Administration (FDA) cleared CyberKnife to treat tumors anywhere in the body. The CyberKnife system delivers radiation therapy intended to target treatment more precisely than standard radiation therapy. More than 150 centers, with various generations of equipment, offer treatment worldwide.

On January 4, 2004, NASA's robot rover *Spirit* landed on Mars. On January 23, the second rover, Opportunity, landed safely at Meridiani Planum on Mars. NASA's Mars Exploration Rover (MER) mission is an ongoing robotic space mission involving two rovers. The mission's scientific objective was to search for and characterize a wide range of rocks and soils that contain clues to past water activity on Mars.

Since 2006, Japan's Ministry of Economy, Trade, and Industry has been awarded the Robot of the Year award. The 2007 winner was Fanuc Ltd.'s workhorse industrial robot called the M-430iA. This multi-axis sanitary robot is part of a food and pharmaceutical product handling system. This robot can work non-stop, 24 hours a day, accurately picking 120 items per minute as they roll down a conveyor belt.

It uses rapidly developing machine vision technology to pick items regardless of their position on the conveyor. In 2008, the winner of the award was Takara Tomy's Omnibot 17μ i-SOBOT. The i-SOBOT is the world's smallest humanoid that is aimed at a mass market. The Japanese government praised its low price and advanced technology. In 2009, the winner was the Omni Zero 1000 transforming robot. The Omni Zero 1000 can walk, become a car, and roll on the floor. Initially made for Robot One, a robot competition held twice a year, the robot can also transform into various other forms. When in walking mode, the robot can open its head section to reveal a seat and carry either a human occupant or, more often, its creator Takeshi Maeda.

In 2021, the CRX Collaborative Robot, LOVOT Family Type Robot, MINERVA-II Minor Planetary Exploration Robot, and HUG T1-02 Transfer Support Robot were awarded the award. The general trend for computers is to have faster processing speeds and larger memory capacities. The robots of the future are moving closer and closer to the decision-making capacity of humans and are becoming more independent. Current trends for complete automation and flexible manufacturing are based on computer numerical control (CNC) machines connected to a central computer with program storage and programming functions that are managed by the Internet of Things (IoT).

1.5 MEDICAL ROBOTICS

In medicine, the robotics has the potential to help surgeons and doctors carry out their functions. Robots applied to the medical sector are increasingly common and offer numerous advantages. However, the use is not without certain risks. Next, we delve into medical robotics and its present and future use.

Robotics is the set of sciences aimed at designing, producing, and using robots for tasks intended for humans. In this sense, robotics in medicine consists of the implementation of automated machines for the development of medical functions such as surgery, healthcare, or rehabilitation therapies [7]. The objective of robotics in medicine is to facilitate the work of surgeons and professionals in the hospital sector in general, maximizing the precision of processes such as operations or surgeries and minimizing the limitations and deficiencies of the human being.

The origin of robotics in medicine dates to 1985, when the PUMA 560 robotic arm was first used to perform neurosurgery successfully. This same robot was used in successive years to perform minimally invasive surgeries, and in 1987 it performed a transurethral resection. In 1990, the AESOP system became the first FDA-approved robot. One of the significant advances in robotics in medicine occurred in the year 2000, when the Da Vinci robot came to light—the first FDA-approved system for performing medium-complexity surgeries. This robot, with regular updates, is still in use today. Since then, robotics applied to medicine has not stopped evolving; today, it is used in different medical fields.

The evolution of robots in medicine has made their use in surgical operations possible. Thanks to them, less invasive surgical techniques have been implemented. In this way, surgeries can be performed in less time, and the patient's recovery time is also shorter. Robots in surgery can work with greater precision, avoiding errors and limitations of the human being. These machines have sensors that allow them to analyze or diagnose processes and carry out interventions based on exact parameters.

Robots in medicine are also used in rehabilitation processes. Initially, they were mainly intended to help people with motor disabilities. Over time, these systems have become more effective and have a greater range of action. One of the most widespread uses in medical robotics is the storage and transport of medicines. Currently, there are robots capable of efficiently managing the dispensing and dosing of medicines. In addition, the most advanced robots have artificial intelligence that allows them to move independently and find the most efficient route between two points. The advantages of using this type of robot became apparent during the coronavirus COVID-19 epidemic.

The use of robot assistants in medicine is also becoming more frequent, for example, to provide service in contaminated areas or with a high presence of viruses or bacteria. They can even serve as a companion and distraction for children and patients of all ages. Currently, almost all kinds of prostheses can be used as substitutes for lost limbs. However, robotics in medicine wants to go a little further and is committed to robotic exoskeletons. These are instruments capable of imitating the normal movements of a limb by collecting neural impulses from the brain.

The advancement of these electronic prostheses allows the replaced limb to be moved or even to feel through the said prosthesis. Thanks to robotics in medicine, it is now possible to recover senses that were thought to be lost. For example, in 2014, a woman named Joanne Milne underwent a cochlea transplant that allowed her to hear for the first time at the age of 40, and in 2015, Alle Zderad was able to regain her sight thanks to the implantation of a bionic eye. Robotics in medicine is also allied with artificial intelligence in the search for vaccines and new treatments. Thanks to the union of these two technologies, a much more considerable amount of data can be processed and laboratory tests carried out with the highest precision.

The main advantages of robotics in medicine are the following: greater precision, avoiding human tremors, less invasive procedures, faster and more effective interventions, patient recovery in less time, less risk of tissue damage, and the ability to access delicate areas or complex areas. In addition, medical robotics has applications in many tasks: rehabilitation, assistance, and transportation; development of new techniques for study, diagnosis, and treatment; equipment capable of working under challenging conditions, such as environments with high radiation or contamination; other instruments can be added, such as video cameras for subsequent visualization of operations; possibility of performing or directing surgical procedures from anywhere in the world; and allows professionals in the health sector to free themselves from doing more mechanical or repetitive tasks.

However, it must be considered that robotics in medicine also has a series of aspects to improve, such as:

- Developing technology. There is still a lot to improve, and many of these systems are still experimental.
- High costs. Not all health facilities may have access to instruments of this type, and their use is limited to hospitals or private health research centers.

- These are systems whose programming and management are complex, and specialized and trained personnel are needed in both cases.
- They are not exempt from failures, especially in operations with a certain degree of complexity. There are cases of patients who have reported burns or damage to adjacent organs.
- Lack of regulations. A controversial issue surrounding implementing these new technologies is the responsibility for an error if a surgical robot makes a mistake that has negative consequences for the patient.

The union between robotics and medicine has already given rise to the appearance of numerous devices whose objective is to facilitate the task of medical professionals. At this point are mentioned seven robots for robotic surgery and medicine that have achieved great success in hospitals.

The Da Vinci surgical robot. The Da Vinci robot is best known in the medical and surgical fields. The first version came out in 1990, and since then, it has become a significant help for surgeons worldwide. This robot comprises a display console, a displacement cart, four robotic arms, and all the necessary instruments to perform a surgical operation (which are fixed at the end of the robotic arms). It is a system capable of receiving orders in real time and accurately reproducing the movements made by the surgeon. The professional uses a series of master controls and visualizes the entire operation through a display screen that offers images of the whole process in 3D.

The Tug is one of those medical robots that transports or stores medication. In addition, Tug can perform many other tasks with a high degree of efficiency, such as transporting samples to laboratories, taking food to patients on the floor, or even performing additional cleaning tasks. All of this makes it possible to help non-health personnel exercise their functions and to minimize the errors that humans can make.

Riba is a Japanese robot used to help in hospitals or health centers for the elderly. Among other things, this robot can help the elderly to carry out daily tasks that, due to their delicate state of health, can be complicated, as well as something as practical such as assisting them to get out of bed and get into their wheelchair. And it can not only be used with older people—the main objective is to offer greater independence to any patient with mobility problems. The robot was initially designed for domestic assistance, although its use has been limited almost exclusively to hospitals.

The ViRob is an exploration robot that is designed to reach places inside the human body that would not be accessible with the usual medical instruments. It is a medical robot with a minimal size, only 14 mm, and that can move inside the body at a speed of 9 mm/s. Among its many functions is the ability to treat diseases by taking drugs to delicate or difficult-to-reach areas or to perform incisions and minor internal surgeries. Due to its small size, it can move through veins, arteries, and other interior cavities, which is why it is also used to uncover blood clots. In addition, no operation is necessary since it can be introduced with a simple injection or even swallowed.

The Jibo robot was also created as a home assistant, but its use was eventually limited almost exclusively to hospitals. It is a robot whose objective is to contribute to the well-being of hospitalized little ones. Jibo can perform many functions, all of them aimed at entertaining children. This robot can sing, dance, tell stories, and offer different games so that the stay in the hospital is as bearable as possible.

IntellIFill IV is an intelligent robot used for drug administration. Its objective is to eliminate errors, mainly when administering drugs intravenously. This robot reads the barcode of the order and fills the syringes that are later used on the patients based on their barcode, thus avoiding human errors and medical negligence. In addition, it is much faster than a human—filling and sterilizing up to 600 syringes per hour.

Relay Robot is another robot that effectively transports medicines, supplies, and samples in the hospital. The most exciting thing is that the robot does not need to be oriented with markers or sensors. Instead, this robot is guided by an electronic map and uses laser detection to ensure safe and efficient movement, always taking the fastest route. It even has a voice message alert to report the user's presence.

All these robots have led to significant advances in the field of medicine. However, it is a very young technology, and it is still in development, so it is to be expected that much more advanced and efficient systems will be developed in the future. On the other hand, one of the most significant challenges of robotics in medicine and health is that these systems are applied without risk.

1.6 TECHNOLOGY INTEGRATED INTO ROBOTS

1.6.1 SENSORS

Humans can experience sensations such as heat, cold, hard or soft, solid or unpleasant, heavy or light. Similarly, in a robot, a sensor is any device with a property sensitive to a magnitude of the medium capable of varying a property in the face of physical or chemical magnitudes, called instrumentation variables, and transforming them with a transducer into electrical variables. The instrumentation variables can be light intensity, temperature, distance, acceleration, inclination, pressure, displacement, force, torque, humidity, movement, or PH [8]. The first proximity sensor was the one that Pepperl Fush introduced to the world for the first time in 1958. Honeywell developed the first intelligent sensor in 1969. It was devised as a solution to the problem of temperature compensation in sensors. Willard Boyle invented the first sensor used in digital still cameras in the year 1969. Sensors are everywhere in the refrigerator and heating systems and are distributed in an electrical system's fuses. And some are distributed in various thermostats and mobile devices such as phones or smartwatches.

The first connected sensor in history dates to 1874, involving French scientists, a 4,695-meter-high mountain, and a new type of shortwave technology. The old mercury thermometers were a perfect example of a sensor and an indicator. In addition to recording the temperature from the expansion of mercury in a tube, they showed it with lines placed at different heights to indicate the degrees. Nowadays, a sensor can be accessed through Bluetooth or Wi-Fi networks.

The first temperature-controlled sensor in history is attributed to Daniel Gabriel Fahrenheit and was very similar in shape to the one that has been used until recently. After testing various materials, he decided in 1714 to use a glass thermometer with mercury inside. For more than a century, various French scientists improved thermometers. Most history books list 1873 as the year Maxwell formulated the theory of electromagnetic waves, 1887 as the year that Hertz discovered radio waves, and 1894 as the year that Tesla publicly demonstrated that radio transmissions were viable. But in 1874—decades before the Eiffel Tower became a gigantic antenna wired from top to bottom—a French team decided that Parisians would enjoy getting to know the temperature on top of Mont Blanc as well as the speed of the wind, its direction, and the height of the snow surface, for which the weather station became the first connected sensor in 1874. The word "wireless" has caught on nowadays, probably because in the 19th and 20th centuries we aimed to fill the world with cables. In 1926, long after the Mont Blanc experiment, Tesla said in an interview that radio was the future.

The first safety sensors for robots are those with 2D vision; they have a video camera that can perform different activities such as detection of robot and peripheral movements, location, and detection of parts in the complete robotic system, including transporters and coordination of positions of the pieces. It helps the robot to later adapt its actions and movements to the information it receives, even for emergency stops. Another of the safety sensors for robots contemplates 3D vision, a three-dimensional vision system that must have two cameras at different angles or, in any case, use laser scanners in addition to detecting the third dimension of objects and parts. They are used in specific applications, such as those where it is required to re-create the part in 3D to analyze and select it.

On the other hand, entering safety sensors for specific robots, the so-called FT sensor is described as force and torque for the robot's wrist. To know and detect the force, the robotic arm is applying controlled movements and can perform applications such as assembly, manual guidance, teaching, and force limitation. Most of the time, the FT sensor will be between the robot and the tool to monitor all the forces applied to them. Another of the safety sensors for robots will be one specialized in collision detection, which occurs mainly through tactile recognition that sends signals to the robot to limit or stop its movements, direct integration into the robot, accelerometers and similar feedback, and detection of abnormal forces. Its primary function is to provide a safe working environment through emergency stops.

Safety sensors for robots require the robot to pick up parts, providing it with information about the position of its gripper or another similar tool, automatic error detection, and repetition of the operation to ensure that the part is well grasped. Many other sensors can be installed in a robotic cell that is very application specific, for example, in seams or tactile types, where the position and grip force of the end effector can be monitored and even detect variations of heat. Early accelerometers were analog electronic devices that evolved into microprocessor-based electronic and digital designs. Airbag controls in the hybrid automobile industry use micro-electromechanical systems (MEMS). Brüel & Kjær has led the industry since its inception: from developing the first charge accelerometer in 1943 to innovative solutions for 21st-century satellites.

In 1942 Per V. Brüel and Viggo Kjær founded their company and received a license to market their products. In 1949 they developed the 2301 Level Recorder. In 1958 the company began its international expansion. In this year the first condenser microphones were manufactured, which became a benchmark within the industry. In 1960, the 2203 was launched, the world's first solid-state portable sound level meter. Over the years, new features and functions were added, selling more than 32,000 units. Brüel & Kjær Airways was founded in 1962. This small fleet of in-house-managed aircraft was used to deliver orders and visit customers worldwide, even as far away as Thailand, the United States, or Egypt. In 1966 the first airport noise monitoring system was installed in the French town of Toulouse. In 1977 the 2131 was released, the world's first digital filter analyzer, designed to measure and represent octave and one-third octave spectra in real time. In 1980 Brüel & Kjær became the first Western electronics company to open a service center in the People's Republic of China [9].

In 1981, the first commercial sound intensity analysis system appeared, capable of measuring the flow direction and magnitude of sound energy. In 1986, the first commercial acoustic holography system was launched, which made it possible to build complete sound field models. In 1996 Brüel & Kjær developed the PULSE system for Windows. This program introduced a revolutionary concept: multi-analysis, allowing engineers to conduct all their analyses simultaneously and see the results in real time on one screen. Since then, the PULSE platform has not stopped evolving. Today, it is a complete and flexible software and hardware package (including the LAN-XI modular acquisition system and PULSE Reflex software).

Another of the most-used sensors in robotics is a rotary encoder, also called an axis encoder or pulse generator. It is usually an electromechanical device used to convert the angular position of an axis to a digital code, which makes it a kind of transducer. These devices are used in robotics, state-of-the-art photographic lenses, computer input devices (such as the mouse and trackball), and rotating radar platforms. There are two main types: absolute and incremental (relative) [10].

The absolute type generates an exclusive digital code for each angle of the axis. To achieve this, a complicated design is cut out of sheet metal and positioned on an insulating disk fastened to the shaft. A row of sliding contacts is also located along the radius of the disk. The sheet metal is linked to an electrical current source, and each contact is associated with a distinct electrical sensor. The sheet metal design is created in such a way that every position of the shaft generates a unique binary code in which some contacts are joined to the current source.

The relative rotary encoder is used when the absolute encoding methods are impractical due to the disk's size. It utilizes an optical switch like a photodiode to produce an electric pulse each time a line passes through its field of view. An electronic circuit counts these pulses to determine the angle of the shaft. However, the system can only determine the change in angle relative to some arbitrary data when the power is switched on, and it cannot measure the absolute shaft angle. This limitation does not affect computer input devices, such as mice and trackballs. To determine the absolute shaft position, a second sensor can be added to detect the zero position; to detect the direction of rotation, two sensors placed at different angles around the axis can be utilized. This type of encoder is known as a quadrature encoder. The TR Electronic brand, a pioneering German company in positioning systems, produces various encoders, including rotary and linear encoders, for industrial applications.

Position encoders directly offer a digital signal from an analog input. They are used to carry out measurements generally of linear or angular positions and can be incremental or absolute. The incremental rotation encoder is made up of a disk with radial slots typically located close together around its entire circumference or alternating light and dark lines, which rotate in front of a photosensor, generating a pulse for each slot or changing color. A typical example of this type of encoder can be seen inside computer mice: small disks with spaces on each axis of movement. A circuit keeps track of the pulses, through which it is possible to know both the advanced angle and the rotation speed.

Absolute encoders provide an encoded output indicating the position of the movable element concerning a reference. The mobile segment has zones that allow distinguishing and assigning them values of one or zero. The main difference with incremental encoders is that it has several tracks with differentiated and grouped zones so that the reading system obtains the coded number that gives its position at each point of the mobile element. Each track represents one bit of the output, with the innermost track corresponding to the highest resolution bit.

In this case, the most widely used sensors are optical, with opaque and transparent areas, and to a lesser extent, contact sensors, with conductive and insulating regions. Position encoders are related to the measurement and control of linear and angular positions with high resolution. Therefore, they are used in robotics, cranes, hydraulic valves, plotters, machine tools, and positioning of reading heads on magnetic disks and sources of radiation in radiotherapy, radar, and orientation of telescopes.

1.6.2 Motors

Linear actuators are a type of actuator that converts the rotary motion of motors into linear or straight push/pull motions. Linear actuators are ideal for all kinds of applications in which it is necessary to use a tilt, lift, pull, or push kilos of force. Electric linear actuators are the perfect solution for applications requiring easy, safe, clean motion with smooth motion control and exact precision. LINAK created the first electric linear actuator in 1979 and has been a leader in the linear motion industry ever since.

1.6.3 Virtual Reality

In 1956, John McCarthy, Marvin Minsky, and Claude Shannon invented the term artificial intelligence at the Dartmouth Conference. Ivan Sutherland's 1965 postdoctoral work laid the foundations for a computer-based multisensory system, which he called "The Ultimate Display". The term virtual reality was coined in 1987 by Jaron Lanier, who, together with Tom Zimmerman, would be one of the main actors who developed the "data glove", which was a significant step in the field of haptic virtual reality. The first technological implementation based on augmented reality came in 1957 by Morton Heiling. The first time the concept of augmented reality was used was in 1901 by the writer Frank Baum, who first imagined electronic glasses to display additional information about the people in front of him.

In 1973, computer artist Myron W. Krueger created the first augmented reality installation that mixed video cameras with a projection system to create an interactive environment that responded to user movements through shadows and movement. During the 1990s, applications that used the concept of augmented reality began to be implemented to solve problems in fields such as industry or design. It is worth noting that Tom Caudell coined the term "augmented reality" in 1992 while developing the Boeing 747 aircraft to describe an application designed to support the assembly of complex electrical wiring. Although this concept was invented many years ago, augmented reality is still an emerging technology today, and it has taken many technological advances in computing and visualization to reach maturity. This is how augmented reality companies arise, which, in the heat of the evolution of these technologies, take advantage of the enormous potential that augmented reality has in a multitude of sectors [10].

1.6.4 PROGRAMMING

The first finding of something related to programming was discovered in 1801 by Joseph Marie Jacquard and his programmable loom. The first programming language was an algorithm created by Ada Lovelace in 1883. Ada Lovelace created this algorithm for Charles Babbage's analytical engine to calculate the Bernoulli numbers [11].

In 1936, for the first time, computer codes were studied by Alonzo Church and Alan Turing. In 1952 Autocode was developed by Alick Glennie, the first compiled language that was directly converted to machine code using a compiler. FORTRAN was the first popular programming language developed in 1954 by a team at IBM, including John W. Backus. Its purpose was to clarify and facilitate understanding, bringing it closer to a typical mathematical notation. COBOL was the first high-level programming language that could run on any type or brand of computer. It was developed in 1959 and stood for Common Business Oriented Language. It was used in credit card processing, ATMs, and even in the *Terminator* movie for the visual display of the Terminator. Later, in 1964, BASIC was born, a family of programming languages that emerged as a support tool focused on teaching but ended up acquiring surprising relevance. Pascal was created in 1970, which, like BASIC, was born as a teaching tool that was soon used for application development. Even though its influence has been reduced over time, Pascal is still primarily used in programming schools. In 1972 the C language arrived, and the rest is history. Dennis Ritchie created C as a basic programming language, which would soon acquire vital relevance, eventually becoming one of the most widely used languages today. In 1979 another historical milestone for programming took place: the C++ language was created with the idea of adding mechanisms to manipulate objects to the C language. C was the first systems programming language, and Prolog was the first logic programming language.

In 1973, the first programming language for computer-type robots for research under the name WAVE was developed at SRI, and the AL language followed it in 1974. The two languages were later developed into the commercial VAL language for Unimation by Victor Scheinman and Bruce Shimano.

One of the merging of programming languages was C++. C++ was developed by Bjarne Stroustrup in 1983. It is an extension of C with an important feature: object-oriented programming. Today, C++ is one of the most used programming languages. It is widely used in game engines and web development. Popular software like Adobe Photoshop also uses C++. Another significant trend added during this time was the use of modules, or simply coding organizational units on a large scale. Modules became an essential part of the world of programming at that point. Also, object-oriented features like polymorphism originated in the 1980s.

Numerous new programming languages emerged in the 1990s and the Internet decade. Many of them achieved great popularity and are still widely used today. Among them, we highlight some such as HTML, Python, Visual Basic, Java, JavaScript, and PHP, which are present in almost all web pages and applications today. Java was an important high-level programming language that came out in the 1990s. In the modern world, anyone who is even slightly involved in programming knows about Java. But initially, it was developed for cable boxes and handheld devices. Without a doubt, Java is the most popular programming language today.

In 1991, Guido Van Rossum created a very easy-to-use programming language. He named it Python because he loved the British comedy group Monty Python very much. Python became a prevalent language in the following years. Today, along with Java and JavaScript, Python is among the most popular languages. Other notable languages created during this period were Haskell in 1991, Visual Basic in 1991, Lua in 1993, R in 1993, Ruby in 1995, Ada 95 in 1995, PHP in 1995, and Rebol in 1997. R became popular for its use in parsing, while PHP and Ruby are widely used in web development.

Other more recent languages are C#, created in 2001, and Scratch, a programming language created in 2006 with a reduced complexity to facilitate more visual learning for children, adolescents, and adults. Go from Google in 2009; Kotlin in 2012, today dubbed one of the best languages for programming on Android; and Swift in 2013, created by Apple to program on iOS are more recent languages.

1.6.5 Relays

A relay works like a switch controlled by an electrical circuit in which, by means of a coil and an electromagnet, a set of one or more contacts is activated, allowing other independent electrical circuits to be opened or closed. It was invented by Joseph Henry in 1835 [12].

1.6.6 The Programmable Logic Control (PLC)

The history of the PLC began when the purpose of eliminating the enormous cost of replacing a control system based on relays appeared in the late 1960s. The company Bedford Associates (Bedford, MA) proposed a system called Modular Digital Controller (MODICON) to a car manufacturing company in the United States. The MODICON 084 was the first commercially produced PLC. The new PLCs had to be easily programmable, have a long useful life, and resist harsh environments. This was accomplished using familiar programming techniques and by replacing the relays with solid-state elements. In the mid-1970s, AMD 2901 and 2903 were very popular with MODICON PLCs. In those days, microprocessors were not that fast and could only be compared to small PLCs. With the advancement in the development of microprocessors, more and more large PLCs were based on them. The ability to communicate between them appeared around 1973. The first system to do so was MODICON's Modbus.

In the 1980s, an attempt was made to standardize communication between PLCs with the General Motors manufacturing automation protocol (MAP). In those times, the size of the PLC was reduced, and its programming was carried out through personal computers (PCs) instead of terminals dedicated only to that purpose. In the 1990s, new protocols were introduced, and some previous ones were improved. The latest standard (IEC 1131-3) has attempted to combine PLC programming languages into a single international standard. Some PLCs are programmed based on block diagrams, instruction lists, and C languages [13].

PLCs today constitute the brain of all control logic—in their micro, medium, and maxi PLC versions up to the integrated PLC+HMI. They will be the first alternative for general control for domestic uses such as in smart washing machines or coffee makers, or for industrial uses such as in oil refineries and the nuclear industry, or for commercial uses, such as in intelligent buildings, within their specific regulations.

1.6.7 BATTERIES

The battery was invented in Italy 200 years ago by Alessandro Volta. In recent years, batteries have come a long way and can drastically change power management. The basis of its development is lithium, hydrogen, and lead. Alessandro Volta dedicated his life to finding practical applications for electricity, and the unit of electrical voltage was named volt in his honor. Despite the revolution with the voltaic battery, the device could not supply electricity for an extended period. John F. Daniell, a friend of Michael Faraday (the chemist who discovered the laws of electromagnetic induction), decided to improve it. The British devised the Daniell battery in 1836 using zinc and copper electrodes. It was the first to acquire practical use in homes.

In 1887 the German Carl Gassner patented the zinc-carbon battery, a "low-cost" battery that is still used in low-power devices. The inventor Samuel Ruben from the USA created mercury batteries, which withstood extreme temperatures, which is why they were widely used during World War II. Later Ruben would improve alkaline manganese batteries, which were more resistant and longer lasting than zinc-carbon batteries until the Duracell was introduced in 1964.

In 1859, Gaston Plante invented the lead-acid battery, the first rechargeable battery in history that is regenerated by passing a current in reverse. Another scientist, Camilo Faure, managed to increase its capacity in 1881, allowing its production on a large scale. In 1900, the Swedish Waldemar Jungner developed the nickel-cadmium battery that was used to power an electric vehicle in Stockholm. Nickel-cadmium batteries have continued to be used, but in 2013 the European Parliament banned the use of toxic metals such as mercury and cadmium in batteries, cells, and accumulators.

Jungner decided to replace cadmium with iron so that the battery would be cheaper, but he was not the only one with this idea; Thomas Alba Edison also began to work on nickel-iron batteries. The inventor and entrepreneur got the first manufacturers of electric vehicles to buy them. Edison investigated new designs, but internal combustion engine vehicles began to take over, and nickel-iron batteries were reduced to applications in wind and photovoltaic installations.

During the 1950s and 1960s, there were several significant innovations in car batteries. The so-called gel cells were developed, batteries that were protected with a spill-proof gel. The batteries were getting smaller and capable of offering a higher voltage, which reduced the size of the batteries and increased their autonomy and power. In the 1970s, one of the most outstanding improvements in the field of lead acid batteries was introduced, with the appearance of the so-called AGM batteries, absorbent batteries with fiberglass mesh. They are like gel batteries but offer even more durability and power.

American physicist John B. Goodenough was obsessed with finding a scientific answer to the 1973 oil crisis, so he investigated the possibilities of lithium. His research opened up a new world of options for rechargeable batteries versus lead-acid batteries, which are too heavy for small devices. In 1985, the Japanese Akira Yoshino perfected this system and developed the prototype of lithium-ion batteries with carbonaceous material.

The nickel-hydrogen battery entered the market as an energy storage subsystem for commercial communications satellites. The first consumer-grade nickel-metal hydride (NiMH) batteries for smaller applications appeared on the market in 1989 as a variation on the nickel-hydrogen battery of the 1970s. NiMH batteries tend to have a longer life than NiCd batteries (and their lifespan continues to increase as manufacturers experiment with new alloys), and since cadmium is toxic, NiMH batteries are less harmful to the environment.

In 1991, Sony and Asahi Kasei (the company Yoshino worked for) began marketing the first rechargeable lithium-ion battery, a milestone in battery history. Lithium batteries continue to improve their design to make them more energy efficient and cheaper, especially to give the final push to electric cars. In 1997, Sony and Asahi Kasei launched the lithium-polymer battery. These batteries keep their electrolyte in a solid polymer compound instead of a liquid solvent, and the electrodes and separators are laminated together. The latter difference allows the battery to be wrapped in a flexible wrap instead of a rigid metal casing, which means such batteries can be specifically shaped to fit a particular device. This advantage has favored lithium-polymer batteries in the design of portable electronic devices, such as mobile phones, personal digital assistants, and radio-controlled aircraft, as these batteries allow for a more flexible and compact design. They generally have a lower energy density than typical lithium-ion batteries [14]. In 1999 the creators of the Li-ion battery returned with a new version called the Li-ion polymer battery. Due to its composition with lithium salt contained in a type of gel, this device is more responsive to spills, with greater flexibility, which allows it to adapt to curved structures, making it less susceptible to deformation. In 2019, John B. Goodenough, M. Stanley Whittingham, and Akira Yoshino received the Nobel Prize in Chemistry for developing lithium-ion batteries [15].

The batteries meet design criteria such as the memory effect, an undesired effect that alters batteries. The voltage or capacity is limited at each recharge (due to a long time, high temperature, or a high current). The consequence is a reduction of its ability to store energy. Another criterion is the initial charge, where lead sulfate loses electrons or is reduced to lead metal at the negative pole (cathode), while lead oxide is formed at the anode. Therefore, it is a dismutation process. No hydrogen is released, since the reduction of protons to elemental hydrogen is kinetically prevented on the lead surface, a favorable characteristic reinforced by incorporating small amounts of silver into the electrodes. The release of hydrogen would cause the slow degradation of the electrode, helping parts of it to crumble mechanically, leading to irreversible alterations that would shorten the duration of the accumulator. During download, the charging processes are reversed. Lead oxide, which now functions as the cathode, is reduced to lead sulfate, while elemental lead is oxidized at the anode to lead sulfate as well. An external circuit uses the exchanged electrons in the form of an electric current. It is therefore a commutation. The lifecycle is a function of the charge and discharge capacity since this process cannot be repeated indefinitely. When the lead sulfate forms crystals, it no longer responds well to the indicated methods, thus losing the essential reversibility feature. It is then said that the battery has leaked, and it is necessary to replace it with a new one. Batteries of this type that are currently sold use a paste electrolyte, which does not evaporate and makes its use much safer and more comfortable.

Lithium-polymer (LiPo) batteries are different from lithium-ion (Li-ion) batteries. Their characteristics are very similar, but allow for a higher energy density and discharge rate. These batteries have a smaller size compared to other components. Compared with other lithium and lead-acid batteries, LiFePO4 batteries have a longer lifespan, are highly safe and maintenance-free, have higher charging efficiency, and have better discharge.

The lithium-iron-phosphate battery (LiFePO4) is a lithium-ion battery that uses LiFePO4 as the cathode material and a graphitic carbon electrode with a metal backing as the anode. The energy density of LiFePO4 is lower than that of lithium cobalt oxide, and it also has a lower operating voltage [16]. The main drawback of LiFePO4 is its low electrical conductivity due to its low cost, low toxicity, well-defined performance, and long-term stability. LiFePO4 is finding several roles in vehicle use, utility-scale stationary applications, and backup power. LFP batteries do not contain cobalt [17].

The LiFePO4 battery uses chemistry derived from lithium ions and shares many advantages and disadvantages with other lithium-ion battery chemistries. However, there are significant differences. LFPs do not contain nickel or cobalt, which are expensive and in limited supply. Human rights concerns have been raised regarding using mined cobalt in batteries for distributed power, home storage, and electric vehicles. LFP chemistry offers a longer cycle life than other lithium-ion approaches. Like nickel rechargeable batteries and other lithium-ion batteries, LiFePO4 batteries have a constant discharge voltage. The voltage remains near 3.2V during the discharge until the cell is depleted. This allows the cell to deliver virtually its full power until discharged and can significantly simplify or even eliminate the need for voltage regulation circuitry. Due to the 3.2V nominal output, four cells can be placed in series for a nominal voltage of 12.8V. This is close to the nominal voltage of six-cell lead-acid batteries. Together with the excellent safety features of LFP batteries, this makes LFP a suitable potential replacement for lead-acid batteries in applications such as automotive and solar applications, provided the charging systems are adapted so as not to damage the cells. LFP from excessive charging voltages (beyond 3.6V DC per cell while under charge), temperature-based voltage compensation, equalization attempts, or continuous trickle charging. LFP cells must be at least initially balanced before the package is assembled, and a protection system must also be implemented to ensure that no cell can be discharged below a voltage of 2.5V, or severe damage will occur in most cases.

The use of phosphates avoids the cost of cobalt and environmental concerns, particularly concerns about cobalt entering the environment through improper disposal. LiFePO4 has higher current or peak power ratings than lithium-cobalt-oxide. The energy density (energy/volume) of a new LFP battery is approximately 14% lower than that of a new LiCoO battery [18]. Also, many brands of LFPs and cells from a certain brand of LFP batteries have a lower discharge rate than lead-acid or LiCoO2. Since the discharge rate is a percentage of the battery's capacity, a higher rate can be achieved by using a larger battery (more amp hours) if low-current batteries must be used. Better still, a high-current LFP cell will have a higher discharge rate than a lead acid or LiCoO2 battery of the same capacity. LiFePO4 cells experience a slower rate of capacity loss (also known as a longer lifespan) than lithium-ion battery chemistries such as LiCoO2 cobalt or LiMn2O4 manganese spinel lithium-ion polymer batteries (LiPo battery) or lithium-ion batteries. After one year on the shelf, a LiFePO4 cell typically has about the same energy density as a LiCoO2 lithium-ion cell due to the slower decay in energy density of LFP.

LiFePO4 has uses such as energy storage in the home; the characteristics of these cells make them ideal for this purpose. Thanks to their size, safety, and high power and storage capacities, multiple possible configurations are easily adaptable to each type of home. Transportation, the higher discharge rates needed for acceleration, lower weight, and longer life make this battery ideal for forklifts, bicycles, and electric cars. 12V LiFePO4 batteries are also gaining popularity as a second (household) battery for a caravan, motorhome, or boat; LFP cells are now used in some solar-powered landscape lighting instead of 1.2V NiCd/NiMH. The higher working voltage of the LFP (3.2V) allows a single cell to drive an LED without circuitry to boost the voltage. Its higher tolerance to modest overcharge (compared to other Li cell types) means that LiFePO4 can be connected to PV cells without circuitry to stop the recharge cycle. The ability to drive an LED from a single LFP cell also avoids battery holders and the corrosion, condensation, and fouling problems associated with products that use multiple removable rechargeable batteries. In 2013, better solar-charged passive infrared security lamps emerged. The AA-size LFP cells have a capacity of only 600 mAh (whereas the bright LED in the lamp can draw 60 mA), and the unit glows for 10 hours. However, if tripping is only occasional, these units can be satisfactory even charging in low sunlight, as the lamp electronics ensure quiescent currents of less than 1 mA.

Many domestic electric vehicle conversions use the wide-format versions as the car's drive package. With good power-to-weight ratios, high safety features, and chemical resistance to thermal runaways, there are few barriers to use by homebuilders. Motorhomes often convert to lithium-iron-phosphate due to increased consumption, and some electronic cigarettes use these types of batteries. Other applications include flashlights, radio-controlled models, portable powered equipment, amateur radio equipment, industrial sensor systems, and emergency lighting [19]. After starting Tesla's construction to produce 500,000 lithium-ion batteries per year for its vehicles, Elon Musk has launched his famous Powerwall batteries capable of storing energy from solar or wind generation and reducing our dependence on the conventional electrical grid.

1.6.8 BATTERY RECYCLING

Most batteries contain heavy metals and chemical compounds, many of which are harmful to the environment. In most countries, throwing them away is not allowed, and taking them to a recycling center is mandatory. Also, most dealers and specialty stores take care of spent batteries. It is essential to comply with these preventive measures. The rupture of some batteries can release mercury vapor, increasing the risk of mercury poisoning. The release of mercury in batteries has occurred due to the use of three types of batteries: mercury oxide, C-Zn, and alkaline. In the first type, the content of the said metal is 33%, and they were used both in the button model and in other sizes starting in 1955. Theoretically, production stopped in 1995, although there are sources of information that indicate the process continues in Asia and they are distributed on the international market. For the second and third types of batteries, it is known that, for several decades, before 1990, mercury was added (between 0.5% and 1.2%) to optimize their operation, with alkaline being the ones with the highest content; also, the carbon they contain is sometimes naturally contaminated with this metal.

In 1999, the INE of Mexico requested an analysis of samples of three brands of AA-type batteries of typical consumption in that country, of which two were of Asian origin (of C-Zn) and one alkaline of European origin. The results were as follows: For those of Asian origin, the values obtained were 0.18 mg/kg and 6.42 mg/kg. As for the one of European origin, the result was 0.66 mg/kg. These quantities, equivalent to parts per million, do not exceed the limits of 0.025% established in the Protocol on Heavy Metals adopted in 1998 in Aarhus, Denmark, by the member countries of the United Nations Economic Commission for Europe (UNECE). In Mexico, other sources of mercury are the chlorine/soda industry, which uses it as a cathode in the electrolytic process and in products such as thermometers, various types of switches, and fluorescent lamps. According to official information, mercury is no longer extracted in Mexico. Mercury is a local and global pollutant par excellence. Regarding the adverse effects caused to human health by this substance, various studies suggest serious neurological effects from oral exposure to manganese.

1.7 ROBOTS THAT HAVE SET RECORDS

Since our existence on this planet, *Homo sapiens* have developed a technology that will adapt to their needs and facilitate their day-to-day living. Over the years, these innovations have become more sophisticated and intelligent. Since man saw the opportunity to use machines instead of labor, a revolutionary development began. Today various robots have been given awards in different categories in competitions as popular as the Guinness World Records.

The Japanese humanoid robot Kirobo set two Guinness records at the same time: on the one hand, it became the first companion robot in space by boarding the International Space Station (ISS) on August 9, 2013, and on the other hand, the robot had a conversation (with the Japanese astronaut Koichi Wakata) at the highest altitude in history, 414.2 km above sea level, on December 7, 2013. Kirobo spent 18 months on the ISS.

Although many robots have tried to come up with the fastest resolution of this scientific toy (among the human competitors, Collin Burns is the fastest with only 5.25 seconds), it was CubeStormer 3 that managed to win the coveted Guinness record. He solved the Rubik's Cube in just 3,253 seconds in March 2014.

Developed by Liquid Robotics, the Wave Glider Robot is an autonomous aquatic robot that is hybrid in nature (it uses solar energy and wave energy to power its sensors and move) and also uses Linux as its operating system. This robot covered 14,703 kilometers across the Pacific Ocean.

The Partner type Personal Robot (PaPeRo), developed by NEC, was designed for maximum interaction with human beings and especially to take care of children since the robot can sing, dance, and spin. It has a vocabulary of 3,000 words and reacts to touch through nine sensors. In 2013, Papero became the first babysitter robot with its friendly look.

In 2015, Xingzhe N°1, or Walker One, developed by the Chongqing University of Posts and Telecommunications (China), broke the distance record for a robot without assistance or battery recharge. He managed to cover 134.04 kilometers in 54 hours on a running track. He had time to do 1,405 laps between October 24 and 27, 2015, until his energy ran out. Walker One has outdone the previous record set at 65 kilometers by the Ranger robot from Cornell University (USA).

Robot Kitchen, a restaurant opened in July 2006 in Hong Kong, China, comprises several robots capable of taking orders from customers and delivering their meals. A third robot performs simple culinary tasks such as preparing tortillas or cooking hamburgers.

The Fanuc M-2000iA/1200 is a robot with an impressive load capacity of 1,200 kilograms. According to Guinness World Records, this robot is currently the strongest in the world (the previous record was set at 1,000 kg).

In 1937 Elektro was born, considered the first human-like robot in history. Its structure was very robust, as it was 2 meters tall and weighed approximately 120 kg. Elektro could walk on command through voice recognition and recognized about 700 words. His success was such that he came to appear in movies like *Sex Kittens Go to College* and *Beauty and the Robot*. Currently, it is owned by the Mansfield Memorial Museum (England).

The Chinese company WL Intelligent Tech set a world dance record with the most significant number of robots dancing simultaneously. One thousand and seven robots completed this record in 60 seconds of the dance in the middle of the Qingdao Beer Festival in Shandong. This mark surpassed that of the Chinese company UBTECH Robotics Corp., which had the previous record with 540 robots.

Sophia is the name of what is currently considered the most advanced robot in the world. It was created and activated in 2015 by the Hanson Robotics company. Its primary function is to learn and adapt to human behavior and work with humans. It is a computer platform, and its programmers have given it a compassionate and caring personality. Sophia has over 40 individual motors and over 62 facial expressions. In addition to having the record for the most advanced technology, it achieved one more merit in 2017. In this case, it became the first robot to obtain citizenship, specifically that of Saudi Arabia. The robot publicly thanked the distinction that it had been awarded and assured it was a historic moment.

A robot designed by another Japanese company, in this case, Omron, achieved the Guinness Record as the first robotic ping-pong teacher in the world. The award winner, dubbed FORPHEUS, assesses a human player's abilities to adjust his gameplay and advises his opponent to improve his technique.

In July 2017, the first intelligent sex robot in history was presented to the public. Harmony is capable of interpreting feelings in the eyes of those observing it, learning the desires of its owner, and improving relationships with them.

One hundred and six jumps in less than a minute was enough to establish the new Guinness Record for jumping rope by a robot. Jumpen is the brainchild of the Nara College National Institute of Technology in Chiba, Japan, and he presented his skills at the Robocon tech event in Tokyo.

Octobot, the first "soft" robot without batteries or cables that propels itself through fluids, was designed to save lives. Octobot is shaped like an octopus, moves autonomously, and is flexible. Scientists and engineers have spent years looking at soft, lightweight materials that allow machines to fit into spaces more efficiently and flexibly than metals like steel. Materials such as plastic or steel had to be replaced by others that were more malleable and where movement could be achieved without external help through a chemical reaction. When its small legs were filled with gas, movement was produced.

1.8 FAMOUS BRANDS IN ROBOTICS

1.8.1 General Electric

General Electric (GE) was born in 1892 thanks to the merger of two American companies: Edison Electric Light Company, later called Edison General Electric, owned by Thomas Alva Edison, and Thomson-Houston, called Electric of Massachusetts. The architect of this merger was J. P. Morgan, a businessman who skillfully handled corporate finance; he decided to buy the shares of the Edison company. After this, he created some modifications; for example, he changed the drive from direct current to alternating current, which was developed by Nikola Tesla. In short, he imprinted an innovative spirit: he developed electric locomotives, fans, transformers, kitchen stoves, and toasters; increased the life of light bulbs; and produced some of the first plastics and X-ray equipment [20].

The company decided to follow the line of the companies that gave it life; General Electric focused on energy and lighting. Still, it broadened its scope over the years, buying companies in various strategic areas. Starting in the 1950s (GE created the Hardiman exoskeleton between 1965 and 1971), the company increased its income and popularity considerably because its laboratories began to produce Lexan, or polycarbonate, one of the most used plastics to manufacture optical lenses, kitchen utensils, artificial diamonds for industrial use, and the solid-state laser, among others.

1.8.2 HONEYWELL

Honeywell grew out of Albert Butz's invention of the thermostat in 1885 and with the subsequent innovations in electric motors and control processes by the Minneapolis Heat Regulator Company, which had been tracked since 1886. In 1906, Mark C. Honeywell founded Honeywell Heating Specialty Co., Inc., in Wabash, Indiana. Honeywell's company merged with the Minneapolis Heat Regulator Company in 1927. After that, it was called the Minneapolis-Honeywell Regulator Company. Honeywell was its first president, and William R. Sweatt was its head of the board of directors [21].

James H. Binger (1916–2004) grew up on Summit Avenue in St. Paul, Minnesota. He attended the Blake School, where he met his wife, Virginia, who graduated in economics from Yale University and in law from the University of Minnesota. In 1943 James joined Honeywell and became its president in 1961 and its chairman in 1965. Following this, he renewed the company's sales focus, emphasizing profits over production volume. In addition, he furthered the company's international expansion—it had six plants producing 12% of the other companies' revenues. He also changed the company's corporate name from the Minneapolis-Honeywell Regulator Co. to Honeywell. From the 1950s to the mid-1970s, Honeywell was the U.S. importer of Pentax cameras and photographic supplies. These products were labeled in the United States as Honeywell Pentax.

Under Binger's administration from 1961 to 1978, he expanded the company into fields such as the arms industry, the aerospace industry, computers, and cameras. Honeywell originally got into the computer business with a venture with Raytheon, better known as Datamatic Corp., but soon bought out a piece of Raytheon, making it a division of Honeywell. In addition, he purchased a small computer control corporation, renaming it Honeywell's Computer Control Division. In 1970, Honeywell bought General Electric's computer division. The company was reorganized into two operating units: Honeywell Information Systems and another dedicated to the arms industry. Honeywell entered the arms industry in World War II, producing aviation elements for the first time. During and after the Vietnam War, Honeywell's defense division made many products, including cluster bombs, missile guidance systems, napalm, and land mines. In 1990, Honeywell's defense division became Alliant Techsystems, headquartered in Edina, a suburb of Minneapolis. Honeywell continued to build aerospace products, including jet engines. In 1996, Honeywell acquired Duracraft and began selling home comfort products. Today, Kaz, Inc., owns home comfort lines (Duracraft and Honeywell).

Honeywell's specialty materials heritage began with a small sulfuric acid company owned by chemist William H. Nichols in 1870. Toward the end of the 19th century, Nichols created several companies and became recognized in the growing American chemical industry. Nichols's vision of a bigger and better company began when he teamed up with researcher Eugene Meyer in 1920. Nichols and Meyer combined five small chemical companies to create the Allied Chemical & Dye Company, which later became Allied Chemical Corp. and was usually part of AlliedSignal, the forerunner of Honeywell's specialty materials business.

General Electric tried to acquire Honeywell in 2002 when Honeywell was valued at more than $21 billion. The merger was allowed by the American authorities but was blocked by Mario Monti, a European Commission commissioner. In 2007, General Electric acquired Smiths Aerospace, which has a similar product portfolio.

The American firm that would give rise to the turbo era in the new continent was founded by John C. Garrett in Los Angeles, California, in 1936 under Garrett AiResearch. Initially, it specialized in the manufacture of turbochargers and turbines for engines in the aerospace industry. The previous AiResearch Industrial Division, established in Phoenix, Arizona, was renamed Garrett Automotive, and in 1955 the T15 turbo that assembled the first vehicle came out of its facilities based on the industry equipped with this technology in America: The Caterpillar D9 crawler tractor. Since 1999, Garrett has been part of Honeywell International, and almost all SUV manufacturers have opted for its products to equip their models. We owe this company the appearance of the variable nozzle turbine (VNT) variable blade technology. Honeywell International is the product of a merger between AlliedSignal and Honeywell, Inc.

Honeywell International is known for its implementation and daily practice of Six Sigma and Lean manufacturing techniques, commonly called Six Sigma Plus. Six Sigma Plus focuses on reducing errors/failures, improving cycle time, and reducing costs. Recently, Honeywell announced the implementation of a corporate philosophy known as the Honeywell Operating System (HOS), which incorporated methods from the Toyota Production System. Honeywell Technology Solutions (HTS) is a research laboratory within Honeywell that is dedicated to investigating new products. HTS has development centers in Hyderabad, Madurai, Shanghai, Borneo, and Mexico City. Most of the flight control systems are created and tested in these laboratories. HTS provides R&D and technology services to various business units of Honeywell International.

1.8.3   ABB

ABB and its predecessor companies have a history of excellence in innovation dating back more than 130 years. In 1990, ABB presented Azipod, a family of electric propulsion systems that are fixed to the exterior of ships, giving them thrust and guidance capacity. They improve maneuverability, efficiency, and the space available on board. In 1998, ABB introduced the FlexPicker, a three-arm robot (delta robot) designed specifically for the pick and pack industry. In 2000, ABB supplied the first commercial ship power system from shore, reducing greenhouse gas emissions from ships docked in the Swedish port of Gothenburg. In 2002, ABB linked South Australia and Victoria's alternating current (AC) grids with the world's longest underground line, a 177-km high voltage direct current (HVDC) light cable with a capacity of 220 megawatts (MW). ABB also linked Connecticut and Long Island with the world's first extruded HVDC submarine cable, a 40-km HVDC light cable with a power rating of 330 MW [22].

In 2004, ABB presented its Extended Automation System 800xA, which has since been installed in thousands of medium and large process plants in the oil, pulp, and gas industries. In 2005, ABB supplied electricity to a gas extraction platform in the

North Sea 70 km from the coast through a direct current line, thereby avoiding the annual emission of 230,000 tons of CO2 and 230 tons of NOX. In 2010, ABB linked the Xiangjiaba hydropower plant in southeast China with Shanghai, located some 2,000 kilometers away, with an ultra-high voltage direct current (UHVDC) connection, at ±800 kilovolts (kV) and with a power of 7,200 MW.

In 2012, ABB successfully designed and developed a hybrid DC switch suitable for creating large inter-regional DC networks. This discovery represented the solution to a technical problem that has taken more than a hundred years to solve and has been perhaps one of the most important in the "war of the currents". In 2015, ABB introduced the world's first genuinely collaborative robot: YuMi. This human-friendly double-arm robot with innovative functionality unlocked the industry's vast global additional automation potential. In 2017, ABB launched ABB Ability, its industry-leading digital solutions offering, connecting customers to the power of the Industrial Internet of Things (IIoT). ABB Ability turns data insights into direct action that "closes the loop" and creates value for the customer. In 2018, ABB joined the FIA Formula E Championship as the series' lead partner to form the newly named ABB FIA Formula E Championship. In 2019, ABB revolutionized low-voltage control substations: bus board technology combined with ABB Ability platform connectivity marks the next leap in innovation, making ABB NeoGear the safest choice for operators, maximizing efficiency and reducing costs for digitized industries. In 2020, ABB Ability Genix Industrial Analytics and AI Suite combined the power of data management, domain knowledge, technology capabilities, and implementation expertise. The suite helps make timely, accurate, and insight-based decisions to achieve a high degree of optimization and control.

1.8.4 KUKA

Johann Josef Keller and Jakob Knappich founded an acetylene gas plant in Augsburg in 1898, which enabled the profitable operation of public and domestic lighting. In 1939, KUKA built the first electric spot welding system in Germany. The product range extends beyond welding systems and large containers to the compact "Princess" typewriter with excellent precision mechanics and to the "Selecta" machine that enables fast and flexible manufacturing in the textile industry. In 1956 KUKA launched the first automatic welding equipment for refrigerators and washing machines on the market; in addition, KUKA delivered the first multi-spot weld transfer line to Volkswagen [23].

In 1971, KUKA launched the robots on the market, and built Europe's first robot-operated weld transfer line for Daimler-Benz. In 1973, Famulus, the robot pioneer of robotics, was the world's first industrial robot, with six axes driven by an electric motor. In 1996, KUKA was the first robot manufacturer to risk a paradigm shift toward the PC-based robot controller. In 1998, it was one of the first global companies to export robots to China, specifically to the Audi factory. In 2001, they were using the world's first robot-controlled "Cyberknife" radiosurgery system. The system allows the treatment of inoperable and surgically complex tumors. In 2006, commissioned by the Chrysler Group, KUKA Toledo Production Operations was created for the integrated production of the Jeep Wrangler body in North America.

In 2007, the payload capacity exceeded the magic mark of 1,000 kg. The KUKA KR 1000 TITAN is listed in the Guinness Book of Records as the world's most robust six-axis industrial robot. In 2010, the KUKA KR QUANTEC quickly became the best-selling robot series in the world. In 2013, the LBR iiwa was the world's first mass-produced sensitive robot approved for human-robot collaboration (HRC). The cobot success story continues with the LBR iisy, which can be used in both serial industrial production and dynamic and unstructured workstations. In 2014 KUKA AG merged with Swisslog Holding AG and gained access to attractive growth markets in the logistics and healthcare sectors. As of 2018, it is one of the world's leading providers of intelligent automation solutions for Industry 4.0.

1.8.5 HONDA

The company was founded in 1948. Honda's primary purpose since its founding has been to develop technologies that make people's lives easier and happier. In this sense, all the years of research dedicated to making the Advanced Step in Innovative Mobility (ASIMO) turned into applications grouped under the Honda Robotics brand and at the service of society [24].

ASIMO was born in 1986 when the first Honda robots were legs that tried to simulate the walk of a human to develop assistance systems for dependent people or replace humans in dangerous tasks. For the first time, a bipedal robot with human dimensions and shapes could maintain its balance when walking perfectly and even go up and down stairs. This incredible breakthrough perfectly and artificially simulated the human balance system, making it the world's first humanoid robot capable of autonomous interaction in a human environment.

The latest version of the friendly robot, the sum of Honda's advances in robotic technologies since 1986, was presented in Europe in 2014. With a height of 1.3 m and a weight of 50 kg, it runs at 9 km/h and can walk on even slopes and climb stairs without problems. Thanks to the levels reached in terms of mobility, speed, and stability and its advanced level of artificial intelligence, the latest ASIMO has a greater awareness of its surroundings and the ability to react. Not only does it walk and run, but it can also jump, kick a ball, walk on one leg, pour coffee, and even dance. And that is only on a physical level! Thanks to advances in artificial intelligence, ASIMO can recognize sounds and voices, faces and gestures, and receive simple commands.

1.8.6 MITSUBISHI

The company was founded in 1870 by Yataro Iwasaki. Mitsubishi creates collaborative robots. The concept of collaborative robots, or cobots, is not new. Still, it has taken a couple of decades for cobots to be light and agile enough to be attractive to a company like Hella Electronics Corporation. Located in Flora, Illinois, Hella designs and manufactures lighting and electronics products for the rapidly evolving automotive industry. The ASSISTA collaborative robot was designed to change the perception of what a robot can be. Light, agile, and low maintenance, the ASSISTA requires fewer safety protections than a traditional industrial robot. Human employees can not only work in their environment safely, but there is less hardware that needs to move along with the robotic arm. ASSISTA also offers direct education by moving the robotic arm by hand; each memorized position is fixed, which allows preparation and commissioning times to be reduced to a minimum [25].

1.8.7 Fanuc

The company was founded in 1956 by Dr. Seiuemon Inaba, who introduced his pioneering numerical control (NC) concept; Fanuc has been at the forefront of a true global revolution in manufacturing processes. Dr. Inaba began this transformative breakthrough when he invented the first electric pulse motor, programmed a numerical control, and included it in a machine tool. The evolution has continued over the following decades to automating entire production lines. In 1972 Fanuc's first CNC machining center was called ROBODRILL. In 1975, Fanuc's first ROBOCUT was introduced. In 1958, the shipment of Fanuc's first commercial NC started exporting industrial robots. In 1984 the first Fanuc ROBOSHOT was installed in Japan. In 2018 Fanuc introduced the new SCARA robot series in Europe [26].

1.8.8 Siemens

Another company that has contributed to multiple sectors is Siemens, a technology company formed in 1847, among which its components for medical devices, automation, and robotics stand out. An essential element in any robot is the electric cable; some think it was created by Alessandro Volta in 1870 when he invented the electric battery and required conductive metals to conduct electric energy; however, in 1835, Samuel Morse invented the first model of the electric telegraph, which was in the form of an electrical switch. Likewise, Siemens in 1890 had a cable plant in Woolwich, England. Later in 1866, Siemens invented the dynamo machine. From 1880 to 1945, the company transitioned to an electrical conglomerate. In 1953, Siemens introduced the first infrared-heated oven onto the market. In 1957, Siemens pooled the development, production, and sale of its entire line of home appliance products—together with radios and television sets—at its Munich subsidiary Siemens-Electrogeräte AG. Finally, in 1967, the joint venture Bosch Siemens-Hausgeräte GmbH brought a breakthrough to rationalized, modernized mass production. In 1958, Siemens began a worldwide triumph with the SIMATIC system, supplemented in 1960 with the SINUMERIK machine tool controller. The two systems stood out for their novel control elements. Constantly improving, enhanced versions of these remain in use today wherever there is a need to automate industrial systems effectively and reliably. In the mid-1960s, it had become the only producer of medium-size and large computer systems. In response to the broad need for medical care among large population segments, the Allies had already given Siemens-Reiniger-Werke in Erlangen permission to resume production in 1945. The internationally respected specialists in electromedical technology were ready to go into action; by 1948, they were already producing "technology for health" again under normal conditions. In 2008, Siemens began making selective acquisitions to build up a digital portfolio of software and services. By 2022, it will have invested 13.6 billion euros in companies such as UGS, Mentor Graphics, LMS, and Mendix.

These acquisitions laid the foundation for the creation of today's leading industrial software business [27].

With its digital factories business, Siemens was the first to place its hopes in systematic industry digitalization. Siemens became the frontrunner in Industry 4.0 as it emerged. In 2022, Siemens welcomed a leader in cloud-based asset management software with the acquisition of Brightly—a perfect complement to Siemens' digital offerings for buildings.

In terms of medical technology, in 2001, Siemens brought the Biograph onto the market—a hybrid system that combined computed tomography and nuclear medicine. The device can precisely image body functions, metabolic processes, and anatomical details of organs, which means it can play a key role in the early detection and treatment of diseases. And with SOMATOM Definition, which uses two X-ray tubes and detectors, Siemens greatly enhanced the performance of computed tomography while at the same time reducing radiation exposure. Beginning in 2006, the company entered laboratory diagnostics through various acquisitions, and today, it is a pillar of Siemens Healthineers. One crucial element is the Atellica diagnostics platform, a flexible solution for clinical chemistry and immunodiagnostics.

In 2016, Siemens rebranded its healthcare business as Siemens Healthineers. In 2021, Siemens Healthineers acquired U.S. cancer therapy specialist Varian. It brought the company the potential to fight cancer even better in the future—with a whole portfolio of products for imaging, laboratory diagnostics, artificial intelligence, and therapy innovators.

In 2022 Siemens Xcelerator was introduced: an open, digital business platform intended to make digital transformation simpler, faster, and scalable for customers of every size and in every sector. The company offers many core technologies defining the industrial metaverse, including 5G, artificial intelligence, edge computing, and the industry's most comprehensive, physics-based digital twin. The Siemens Xcelerator will relate to NVIDIA's Omniverse as a first step in this arrangement, and this 3D design platform will be a shared base for developing immersive digital twins.

1.8.9 Boston Dynamics

Boston Dynamics is an American engineering and robotics company specializing in building robots. The company was founded in 1992 by engineer Marc Raibert, a former Massachusetts Institute of Technology professor. In June 2021, Hyundai Motor Group acquired a majority interest in Boston Dynamics and now holds an 80% stake in the company. SoftBank, through one of its affiliates, has the remaining 20%. Boston Dynamics operates as an independent business within the more extensive Hyundai portfolio. In 2005 Boston Dynamics created the quadrupedal robot BigDog. In 2016, Boston Dynamics released the Atlas, The Next Generation, showing a new humanoid robot approximately 5' 9" tall. In 2017, a range of new abilities for Atlas was presented, including jumps, 180-degree jumps, and reverse jumps.

In 2016, Boston Dynamics revealed the four-legged, canine-inspired SpotMini9, which weighs just 55 pounds and is lighter than its other products [28].

1.8.10 TOYOTA

Toyota has been developing multitasking robots for elderly care, manufacturing, and entertainment. The Frontier Research Center in Japan is the epicenter of Toyota's advanced technology and robotics research. Its sophisticated robots include humanoid technologies, medical rehabilitation aids, emotion management, and even enormous accuracy for shooting, such as the CUE4, a robot that plays basketball. T-HR3 is a humanoid robot capable of moving flexibly, mimicking the movements of its human operator, who can be located 100 km away. The robot operator uses the main maneuvering center that shows the vision of the robot and its environment in real time. Also, T-HR3 was designed to move in environments designed for humans and not for machines [29].

The Toyota robot called Welwalk WW-200 is already marketed for medical assistance in the recovery of mobility for patients affected by paralysis of the lower limbs due to cerebrovascular accidents, trauma, or other causes. Patients use a robotic leg and a treadmill. The patient's stride is reflected on a screen, where they can track their recovery progress in real time. In addition, it has a game function to motivate the patient to reach his or her goal and speed up recovery.

Kiboro comes from combining the Japanese words "robot" and "hope". This Toyota robot rose to fame after spending 18 months orbiting the earth. Its function is to be operational in zero gravity, with voice functions, video recording, and facial recognition. Kiboro gave rise to Kiboro Mini, a robot that fits in the palm of your hand and aims to keep people company, recognizing their emotions and expressing support and encouragement. In Japan, it is already marketed together with its specific mobile application.

Toyota has developed a range of humanoid robots known as the Toyota Partner Robots. These robots made their first public appearance at the 2005 World Expo in Aichi, Japan, where they played music on drums and trumpets. There are five robots in the series, each with a unique movement system: Version 1 is bipedal, Versions 2 and 3 have Segway-like wheels, Version 4 uses a unique wire system, and the i-Foot can be mounted on two legs. In 2009, Toyota shared a video demonstrating the running and standing abilities of their partner robot, which can reach a speed of 7 km/ hour but is only able to walk and run on flat surfaces.

1.8.11 YASKAWA

In 1915 Yaskawa Electric was founded by Daigorou Yasukawa in collaboration with his older brothers. In 1917 they introduced their first custom product: the 20-hp three-phase induction motor. In 1927 synchronous motors with 4,000 hp and 250 rpm were introduced. In 1937 a transportation system was adapted for small electronics and switches and ready for industrial production. In 1950, a revolutionary and easy-to-use motor with variable speed and remote control was developed. In 1958 its new Minertia engine multiplied the response speed by a hundred. It is the prototypical figure of current servomotors. In 1969 "Mechatronics" was born, and the term was invented by the engineer Tetsuro Mori. In 1977, the company's legendary Motoman L10 robot, the basis of today's industrial robots, came onto the market. It became the cornerstone of today's motion control business. In 2003 the company created Mecha-trolink—suitable for motion control, and they founded the Mechatrolink Members Club. In 2020 the company sold 30 million variable frequency drives [30].

1.8.12 BALLUF

It started in 1921 with a repair shop for bicycles, motorcycles, and sewing machines. Today Balluff is a leading provider of sensor and automation solutions. The repair shop founded by Gebhard Balluff in 1921 grew into a craft business, initially man-ufacturing turned and milled parts. In 1960, inductive proximity switches emerged, marking the transition from mechanical to electrical products. Over the years, there were more and more products and developments; milestones followed inductive proximity switches in product development, such as the first RFID systems in the 1980s and magnetostrictive transducers and magnet-encoded position sensors. The introduction of IO-Link as the first standardized digital interface at the sensor/actu-ator level marked the company's entry into Industry 4.0 in 2006. In 2016, intelligent camera systems expanded the inspection task. Since 2017 the company has been pushing more digitization solutions based on software development [31].

1.9 EVOLUTION OF EXOSKELETONS

1.9.1 EXOSKELETONS

Passive mobilization consists of the movement of a joint in all possible directions without muscle contraction by the patient. In bedridden patients, it serves to maintain joint range of motion in addition to preventing adhesions and retractions.

An exoskeleton is an external structure that supports and protects a subject's body. Powered exoskeletons are wearable robots or portable devices attached to a subject's limbs, using principles of electro-simulation first to detect a subject's movements and then replace or enhance them. These are typically used after an accident, disease, or periodic/permanent paralysis across hospitals and rehabilitation centers that address the needs of elderly and disabled persons or even those afflicted with spinal cord injury and stroke [32]. The goal is to facilitate walking by providing additional force to swing the legs with each step.

The ancient Greeks and the Chinese were the first to combine chairs and wheels to provide medical solutions. King Philip II of Spain, who reigned from 1527 to 1595, used a custom-built wheelchair with arm rests and footrests. However, he had to be pushed and couldn't propel himself. Canadian George Klein and his team are considered to have invented the first motorized wheelchair, and he developed it in the 1950s to help World War II veterans. In Germany in 1665, Stephen Farfler, a paraple-gic watchmaker, built a wheelchair with three wheels and a hand crank on the front wheels, meaning that users could move without assistance.

For decades, engineers and sci-fi buffs have dreamed of an exoskeleton that could boost human strength, turning an average person into a real-world Iron Man. In the 1960s, GE set out to build its human exoskeleton. Dubbed Hardiman, the suit was funded by the U.S. military and designed to mimic the user's natural movements, capable of lifting 1,500 lb. The suit weighed 1,500 lb and included 28 joints and two grasping arms connected by a complex hydraulic and electronic network. The Hardiman survives today in the form of the Man-Mate industrial manipulator. Western Space and Marine, founded by a GE engineer who worked on the Man-Mate line in the 1970s, continued to develop and improve it, using force feedback to allow the operator to lift loads up to 10,000 lbs. It is today primarily used in the forging and foundry industries.

In 2017 Toyota launched a rental service for the Welwalk WW-1000 robot. The Welwalk WW-1000 was designed to aid in the rehabilitation of individuals with lower limb paralysis as a result of stroke and other causes. The Welwalk WW-1000 comes with a range of rehabilitation support functions based on motor learning theory, including adjusting the difficulty level to suit the patient and providing feedback about the patient's gait characteristics. The robot's simple construction and functions, such as easy fitting and central touch panel operation, ensure ease of use in clinical settings [33].

Toyota is developing partner robot technologies related to senior life support, medical support, personal life support, and welfare support. The development will help to assist the elderly by enabling them to live more independent lives and provide support for their caregivers. Development of rehabilitation robots in the field of medical support began at the end of 2007 with the collaboration with Fujita Health University Hospital in Toyoake, Aichi Prefecture. Since 2011, pilot testing has been conducted at the hospital's medical facilities. Between 2014 and the end of March 2017, walk training assist robots were installed in 23 medical facilities throughout Japan for clinical research [34].

The Honda walking assist device (Stride Manager) builds on the company's experience with walking robots like ASIMO. The walking assist device has been in research since 1999. This exoskeleton is based on the inverted pendulum model, a theory of bipedal walking, and designed as a device to be used in the training of walking. The onboard controller activates motors based on data obtained from hip angle sensors. The main goal is to improve the symmetry of the timing of each leg lifting from the ground and extending forward. It also promotes a longer stride for easier walking. In 2015, the Honda walking assist device went on lease to businesses in Japan. The Honda wearable robot weighs 2.7 kg. It is built using proprietary motors and a control system. It is a minimalistic design attached to the body with simple straps. The device is made to be highly adaptable to various body sizes [35]. As mentioned, the control computer activates motors based on data obtained from hip angle sensors during walking to improve the symmetry of the timing of each leg.

Three training modes are available. In following mode, the walking assist device influences the user's walking motions based on their walking pattern. Symmetric mode is based on the walking patterns of the user—the walking assist device influences the user to achieve bilaterally symmetric motions such as bending and extending both legs. In step mode, the walking assist device influence the user's steps repeatedly to recover the rocker functions (rocker functions are leg motions which enable smooth shifting of weight from heel to sole and sole to toe), which allows the smooth shifting of weight. Key specifications include the following: overall width approximately 430 mm to 495 mm; weight approximately 2.7 kg (including the battery); operating time by charge approximately 60 minutes; lithium-ion battery, 22.2V to 1 Ah; motor output, maximum torque: 4Nm; and use environment, indoor or outdoor (except when raining) on flat floor or ground [36].

In Japan, Cyberdyne developed (1997–2012) another wearable robotic suit called HAL that is already on the market. The battery-powered suit was designed to help the disabled and people in rehabilitation therapy. It is being tested in hospitals, with nurses wearing it to lift heavy patients.

At the beginning of the 21st century, the first exoskeleton products made their way to the market and were accessible to an increasing number of users. One of the first applications was gait rehabilitation in stroke and spinal cord–injured patients.

An early example is the gait rehabilitation exoskeleton Lokomat, released in 2001 and used in hospitals and rehabilitation centers worldwide. In 2013, Hocoma-AG announced the shipment of the 500th device.

Development continued in the first decade of the 21st century at an increasing number of research labs and companies. Toward the end of the decade, several prototypes of military exoskeletons that aim to augment their user's strength and endurance were presented. Raytheon XOS is a full-body exoskeleton, and Lockheed Martin's "Human Universal Load Carrier" (HULC) supports its users in carrying a heavy backpack [37].

Starting in 2010, various exoskeletons for gait assistance and restoration have been introduced to the market. The majority of these devices are created to provide support for paraplegic individuals, allowing them to stand and walk upright without the need for a wheelchair. Examples include the ReWalk device produced by ReWalk Robotics and the Indego exoskeleton by Parker Hannifin, which originated from a Vanderbilt University research system. Many of these exoskeletons are now being certified for clinical use and outside medical facilities, such as receiving the Conformité Européenne (CE) certification in Europe or the Food and Drug Administration (FDA) in the United States, which is a crucial step toward their release in the home market. In September 2016, ReWalk announced that they had delivered their 100th exoskeleton designed for home use.

In addition to medical and military purposes, exoskeletons have been created by various companies for industrial use. The first systems for this use were introduced around 2014–2015. Passive systems, which do not require actuators to alleviate the payload or body weight of the user, are gaining popularity for this purpose. For certain applications, a single articulated exoskeleton can offer sufficient support, resulting in devices that are less heavy and less expensive than their actuated counterparts.

In addition to all the development efforts, exoskeleton producers started to promote their systems to a broader audience to demonstrate their capability and increase awareness. In 2012, Claire Lomas, who has paraplegia, used a ReWalk to participate in the London marathon and crossed the finish line after 16 days. In 2016, she participated in a half-marathon and finished after 5 days.

In 2014, a paralyzed person used an EEG-controlled exoskeleton to kick off the World Cup in Brazil. The exoskeleton was developed as part of the Walk Again project. In October 2016, ETH Zürich in Switzerland held the first Cybathlon, a sporting competition for people with disabilities using robotic assistive aids. One of the disciplines was an exoskeleton race on an obstacle course for paraplegic users.

The users had to complete tasks such as sitting on a couch and standing up again, walking on slopes and stones, and climbing stairs. None of the pilots were able to complete all obstacles, and the fastest teams took more than 8 minutes to finish the 50-meter course.

To address the size, weight, and rigidity constraints of exoskeletons, the concept of exosuits emerged in 2016. Exosuits are soft, robotic devices made mostly of textiles that can be worn like clothing. They provide support through actuated cables integrated into the textiles or soft and lightweight actuators located at the joints. SuitX has developed the MAX, a passive, unpowered workplace exoskeleton that redirects loads to the attachment points on the body, transferring the strain to the hips and then down to the ground, using a lightweight metal frame. The MAX is part of Kazerooni's "design simplification" approach.

Although limited power supply is still a considerable constraint, today's batteries may be enough as exosuit tech morphs into new forms. Many new exoskeletons have gone soft (soft exosuits), eschewing metal frames altogether for flexible fabric and artificial muscles. This kind of exoskeleton seeks to prevent damage to injury-prone areas of the body and minimize fatigue. The XOS 2 suit is arguably an advanced exoskeleton. Recently unveiled by Raytheon and funded by the U.S. Defense Advanced Research Projects Agency, XOS 2 allows its wearer to "do the work of two to three soldiers", according to its creators—including the function of lifting hundreds of pounds for long periods [38].

The Wyss Institute conducted pioneering work at Harvard University that developed exosuits to support walking. Today, several research labs around the world are developing exosuits. In 2017, ReWalk Robotics licensed an exosuit technology from Harvard; later, Rewalk released the first exosuit for stroke patients in 2018. ReWalk Robotics is a medical device company that designs, develops, and commercializes powered solutions that provide gait training and mobility for individuals with lower limb disabilities. They currently offer solutions for stroke rehabilitation and spinal cord injury: ReStore Exo-Suit for Stroke Rehabilitation. ReStore is a powered, lightweight, wearable soft exosuit for rehabilitation of individuals with lower limb disabilities due to stroke. ReStore is a versatile and efficient gait training solution that provides dorsiflexion and plantarflexion assistance. The ReStore Exo-Suit received CE marking and FDA clearance in 2019. ReWalk users can operate the systems independently. ReWalk received FDA clearance to market in 2014. It was the first exoskeleton in the United States to earn this clearance. CE and additional regulatory approvals exist in select geographies [39]. Some of the recent exoskeletons are the 2016 Levitation 2 knee brace, 2016 Dephy exo-boot, 2017 Indego, 2017 fortis K-SRD, 2017 Airframe, 2018 Ekso Vest, 2018 Ekso NR, and 2020 Guardian XO Alpha.

All ASTM F48 technical subcommittees will be addressing the safety, quality, efficiency, and performance of exoskeletons and exosuits. The objectives will focus on all applications, including industrial, medical, military, and consumer use. To support the development and maintenance of F48 international consensus standards, the committee will host workshops and coordinate with various related stakeholder organizations. Therefore, the companies develop their testing protocols for evaluating the benefits and limitations in five focus areas with separate subcommittees: design and manufacturing; human factors and ergonomics; task performance and environmental considerations; maintenance and disposal; and security and information technology. Technical considerations include passive and active systems; enhancing and decreasing effects; and physical and cognitive factors. The lifecycle approach includes aspects such as before the device is on a person; putting on the product; on the user and in use; and software [40].

In November 2018, Kentucky was the first plant of Toyota to require exoskeletons as PPE, and the Indiana plant followed suit, and this was implemented across all plants by the end of 2019. In performing overhead work, company surveys showed that those who wore the exoskeletons reported a lower Rating of Perceived Discomfort (RPE). An electromyography (EMG) study noted a statistically significant reduction of shoulder and back muscle maximum voluntary contraction (MVC), which translates to less muscle fatigue. So, in November 2018, Toyota plant in Ontario, Canada, became the first that required exoskeletons for specific jobs. Even though relatively few exosuits exist, the list of potential users is growing long. Beyond the many disabled and older adults who could use the technology, so too could their nurses and caregivers, with health insurance covering the bill [38].

1.9.2   EQUIPMENT USED IN THE EXOSKELETON DESIGN

Exoskeletons commonly use miniature brushless DC motors with additional products such as gearboxes for high torque and encoders for positional feedback. Typical application requirements include high torque, long battery life, and the ability to work under load. Flat brushless DC and DC servo motors are designed for long battery operating times with a lightweight package, making them ideal for powering exoskeleton applications. The benefits are high torque with compact size; extended battery operating time; long lifetime, high efficiency with low power consumption, weight, and volume; and ability to work under load (sitting position, walking on a staircase) [32]. Robots depend on miniature motors for their motion, so evolution within robotics relies on technological advances in motor design. The use of robots proliferates in applications that span from surgical suites to the battlefield. While robots become more specialized, a commonality is the corresponding development of miniature motors on which robots depend for their motion. Therefore, advances in the development of robots must be matched by advances in the motors that drive them, so let's look at the key trends in miniature motor technology [41].

The design of robots, especially collaborative robots, must prioritize compactness and mobility. To achieve human-like dexterity, the motors powering them need to be small and lightweight while still providing high power density. Brushless DC (BLDC) motors have an advantage over conventional DC motors because they offer a higher power density in a smaller and lighter package. By using slotless BLDC motors and efficient planetary gearboxes, this combination can be achieved, and these components can be integrated into standard robot designs that require a small footprint.

For robots in manufacturing automation and similar tasks, speed and precision are critical factors. When it comes to pick-and-place applications, coreless DC motors and disk magnet stepper motors are suitable due to their low inertia, which enables rapid acceleration and deceleration. For applications that require dynamic but smooth control, such as camera systems, slotless BLDC motors are the preferred choice due to their lack of cogging or detent torque. In many robotic applications, battery power is crucial, and thus energy efficiency is an essential factor, Ironless brushless DC motors can achieve up to 90% efficiency, making them the motor of choice when extended robotic running time is required. It's also crucial to ensure that the gearbox is efficient and matched to the motor for high torque/low speed applications.

Protection against extremes of temperature and pressure is required for robotic applications such as surgical robots undergoing autoclave sterilization. The robot's motor depends on a high degree of resilience; setting components within a thermoset epoxy maximizes robustness and extends the lifecycle. When it comes to robots, safety and productivity are inextricably linked. Inaccurate control can cause physical harm, whether in a surgical setting or on the factory floor. At the same time, machine stoppage resulting from a safety breach can damage the product and cause downtime. Robots will therefore continue to rely on high-accuracy feedback devices to ensure their protection and that of the environment around them. High-resolution encoders enable accurate and fast motor control in applications that demand control and high-speed combinations. In a robotic welding system, high-resolution feedback achieved within a robust package is crucial to ensure precise robotic motion.

Autonomy and machine learning are crucial in robotic development, and this is evident in autonomous vehicles and surveillance robots. LiDAR technology is used to capture 3D imagery of the environment, which aids in self-guided navigation and scanning at high refresh rates. LiDAR-based mirror systems now use brushless, slotless mini motors because they are more efficient and have lower heat dissipation. Multiple-axis control is required for some complex robotic applications, such as surgical robots, and sensors equipped with serial interface communication can provide position information with high accuracy. To minimize the footprint in multi-axis applications, miniature motors are combined with communication protocols to reduce wiring. Customization of tiny motors is a growing trend in robotic control, and motor manufacturers are tasked with developing highly compact, lightweight motors that balance torque and speed to meet specific application needs.

In the 1960s, Yaskawa developed a succession of innovative DC servo motors, and in 1983, an AC servo motor was launched, creating a new wave in the motor industry. And now, almost 100% of factory automation (FA) uses AC servo motors. While a general motor is designed to continuously rotate the load, a servomotor is designed to rotate the load and respond accurately and quickly to the target. In the late 1980s, the all-digital AC servo motor was commercialized. In the 1990s, the use of ASICS, 16-bit microcomputers, and serial communications to increase the speed of detector position data dramatically improved control performance. In parallel with these amplifier and control performance improvements, using powerful neodymium, iron, and boron magnets for the motor's permanent magnets has resulted in dramatic miniaturization and responsiveness. In the 1990s and 2000s, the semiconductor and liquid crystal industries became active, and a large amount of AC servo motors were mounted on this manufacturing equipment.

In 2017, Japanese companies' global production of servo motors increased to approximately 7.9 million units, according to a survey by Fuji Keizai. The need for cleaner and more accurate servomotors has increased, and new types of motors, such as linear motors and direct drive motors, were developed [42]. Harmonic Drive strain wave gear and actuator products are customizable. Most of the products sold by Harmonic Drive LLC are made at a manufacturing facility in Massachusetts in the United States. Harmonic Drive Group Companies in Japan (Harmonic Drive Systems, Inc.) and Germany (Harmonic Drive SE) provide additional products. With over 60 years of experience, its motors have high precision and zero backlashes. Harmonic Drive strain wave gears and Harmonic Planetary gears have, and continue to play, critical roles in robotics, spaceflight applications, semiconductor manufacturing equipment, factory automation equipment, medical diagnostics, and surgical robotics. The mechanism was the brainchild of C. Walton Musser [43].

1.10 KINESITHERAPY

The historical antecedents of physical exercise go back to the oldest times, in which it was included under the name of gymnastics, which is defined as the practice that pursues the physical development of man and whose essential purpose was hygienic, aesthetic, and sports. Ancient civilizations, such as the Egyptians, Assyrians, and Hindus, empirically practiced exercise together with massage. The Greeks and Romans also attached great importance to physical exercise. Physical education evolved in the following centuries toward its modernization. In the last half of the 19th century, therapeutic exercise's purposes, biological actions, and indications were defined and systematized.

Dr. Pehr Henrik Ling is owed the greatest push given in his time to developing kinesitherapy. Ling removed it from the empiricism in which he found himself and gave it a true scientific height by establishing his fundamental principles on the laws of mechanics and the principles of anatomy and physiology.

Exercise produces local effects on the corresponding muscles and joints and general repercussion effects. Exercise improves circulation since the movement of muscles and joints exerts a mechanical pump action that contributes to venous and lymphatic return. It also produces an increase in muscle volume due to hypertrophy of the fibers and/or an increase in the capillary network. Muscle contractions cause the burning of glycogen and increased blood flow to the muscle (hyperemia), which gives it greater functional range and increased contractility. Active movements strengthen the muscles and their resistance and favor muscular power; passive movements can stretch fibrous structures that may be shortened or retracted. The joints are also favored by exercises since the stretching of capsules and ligaments, together with a stimulation of the synovial secretion, makes it easier to carry out the movements. The peripheral nerves are also favored by the mobilizations, since their stretching stimulates their functioning and the transmission of the nerve impulse to the motor plate, which translates into an improvement in balance and coordination of movements.

Thus, exercise has favorable psychic effects and leads to a satisfactory physical state, an important factor due to its repercussions on the desire for the recovery of patients. In addition, we must bear in mind that immobility in elderly or bedridden patients causes a decrease in muscle and bone mass, upsets the balance, alters the integrity of the skin, facilitates the appearance of pressure ulcers, and favors the presentation of various cardiovascular and respiratory and digestive complications. These complications/consequences of immobility or bedrest can be intervened or prevented in different ways, such as postural changes, hygiene, massage, padding, and general hydration. Kinesitherapy can be classified into passive and active kinesitherapy.

1.10.1 Passive Kinesitherapy

Passive kinesitherapy is where the patient does not actively participate in the mobilization: mobilization, postures, joint tractions, musculotendinous stretches, and manipulations are examples of this. Passive motion therapy includes relaxed passive motion therapy and forced passive motion therapy. In relaxed passive kinesitherapy, it is carried out in cases where the joints are free, and no cause prevents them from moving. There are no adhesions, no retractions, no spastic contractures, and no pain that opposes mobilization. In forced passive kinesitherapy, it is used in the opposite cases—in situations where the joints are not accessible due to adhesions or retractions that totally or partially prevent their mobilization, spasms, or contractures that oppose the movement. This type of mobilization can be carried out momentarily or maintained.

The best-known form of momentary passive mobilization is manipulation, consisting of high-speed maneuvers carried out energetically and without danger if carried out with sufficient knowledge and experience. Sustained passive mobilization involves continuous action on the joint using external forces, which may be the therapist's hands, the action of gravity, or mechanical means such as pulleys or mechanical splints.

With passive assisted mobilization, both auto-passive and instrumental passive, the patient's muscles and joints are set in motion with these techniques. The mobilization is produced exclusively as a force external to the patient. According to the external force applied, we distinguish between assisted passive mobilization when performed by the therapist manually or by mechanical means; self-passive mobilization, when it is the patient himself who performs it manually or using pulleys; instrumental passive mobilization, when executed by electromechanical devices or machines; and assisted passive mobilizations, which can be analytical or global. In the first case, the mobilization tends to be directed to a single joint, while global mobilization is required to manipulate different joints.

The passive mobilization we use in each case will depend on our intended purpose—careful maneuvers with continuous and sustained movements without causing pain. Applying gentle moist heat to the joints can further stretch and reduce pain. We must explain what is going to happen. Before starting the mobilizations, explain to the person what will be done, how, and how many repetitions (10–15), and tell them that they will be smooth movements without forcing any joint and having to present any pain. The positions that the therapist adopts for each movement will be significant to be able to make a complete tour of the joint and protect himself or herself from possible back injuries when performing the mobilization.

1.10.2 ACTIVE KINESITHERAPY

Active kinesitherapy is where the patient actively participates in mobilization, such as assisted or antigravity active kinesitherapy, free or gravitational active kinesitherapy, and resisted active kinesitherapy. Active kinesitherapy includes a set of analytical or global exercises performed by the same patient with their strength, voluntarily or self-reflexively, and controlled, corrected, or helped by the physiotherapist.

Muscle contraction is a key point in the execution of the movement. Remember that the muscles are composed of contractile fibers gathered in fascicles, which serve to move. The muscles are elastic and contractile, and even in a state of rest, they have a permanent partial contraction or muscle tone that contributes to the static balance of organs and limbs.

The complete loss of the contractile process of a muscle is known as paralysis, and the partial loss is called paresis. An excited muscle can shorten if one of its limbs is fixed and the other is free, or it can change tension without changing its length if both limbs are fixed. In isometric contraction, there is an increase in muscle tension without changes in its length. Types of active kinesitherapy depend on whether the patient voluntarily initiates muscular activity helped by an external force, freely or overcoming opposition. Active kinesitherapy is divided into assisted active kinesitherapy, free active kinesitherapy, and resisted active kinesitherapy. Assisted active kinesitherapy is applied when the patient cannot perform the exercise that causes movement against gravity (muscle balance less than 3), which means they need help. The intensity of the external force that constitutes the aid will complete the action of the muscle but will not replace it. Free active kinesitherapy is also called gravitational kinesitherapy. The patient executes the movements of the affected muscles exclusively, without requiring any help, and voluntarily performs contraction of synergists and relaxation of antagonists without external assistance or resistance except gravity; in these cases, the muscle assessment should be 3. In actively resisted kinesitherapy, the movements are made to overcome the resistance that the therapist opposes with the hands or by instrumental means. Therefore, muscle contraction takes place against external opposition.

Resisted active kinesitherapy is the best method to increase muscle power, volume, and resistance, factors on which muscle function depends, along with the speed of contraction and coordination. The muscular balance must have at least a value of 4. Ultimately, the goal is neuromuscular strengthening: strength, speed, resistance, and coordination.

George and Liedreichk published "General Fundamentals of Gymnastics". In 1845 George suggested the word kinesitherapy should be used. Ling (who was Swedish) promoted mobilization and subtracted the physiotherapeutic methods from the dominant empiricism, taking it to a more scientific place and laying the foundations and fundamental principles of the laws of anatomy and physiology. The main merit of it was to introduce a new element in teaching: the use of systematized exercises capable of locating the effort in specific points, producing changes in habitual attitudes. Ling's disciples—George (from Paris) and Zander (who was Swedish)—invented devices for mobilization, spread their use, and contributed to greater and more complete knowledge. For Ling, gymnastics had three purposes: educational, hygienic, and therapeutic.

The current theory of resistance exercises is based on the contribution of Adolfo Eugenio Fick (1829–1901); he studied the mechanics of muscular movement using the terms isometric and isotonic. Jules Amar, in 1920, worked extensively in the field of kinesiology on the efficiency of muscular work and its mechanics. The improvement of devices and instrumental kinesitherapy have contributed to the evolution of exoskeleton design concerning new physical therapy techniques.

1.11 EVOLUTION OF MATERIALS

The materials employed for the manufacturing of components have progressed over the years. The materials range from stone, wood, and bone, through different metals, to modern materials such as polymers, composites, and ceramics. Native copper was the first metal used by humans. However, this metal in its pure form is soft. Arsenical bronze, an accidental alloy made of copper (Cu) and arsenic (As), was used to obtain valuable forms. Considering the Cu-As phase diagram and depending on the content, the melting point of arsenical bronzes was above 600 °C. Nowadays, bronze is an alloy of copper and other elements, including tin, aluminum, silicon, and nickel [44]. Considering bronze is made of copper (Cu) and tin (Sn), according to the Cu-Sn phase diagram, the melting point of bronze may vary from 830 to 1020 °C.

When humans acquired knowledge to obtain and process iron, it gradually replaced bronze. Ferrous alloys are a combination of iron (Fe) as the prime constituent, and they are classified as steels and cast irons, depending on the carbon (C) content [44]. Cast irons may contain between 2.14 and 6.70 wt% C and are today classified into gray, ductile, white, malleable, and compacted graphite irons. However, in ancient times they were generally known as cast irons. Another kind of iron was wrought iron, which contained a deficient carbon (<0.25 wt%) content compared with cast iron. Wrought iron fell into disuse, but its modern equivalents are low-carbon steels [44]. According to the Fe-C phase diagram, the compositions of most cast irons are around the eutectic point. Their melting point ranges from 1150 to 1300 °C, which man could reach in those times. China produced cast iron as early as 200 BC.

Steels are the other types of ferrous alloys, which are iron-carbon alloys (0.008–2.14 wt% C) containing appreciable concentrations of alloying elements, usually added to improve mechanical and corrosion-resistance properties [44]. The melting point of most steels is about 300 °C higher than for cast irons. The earliest proof of steel production dates back to 300 BC when humans discovered that iron became harder, stronger, and more durable if it was combined with charcoal. There is evidence that the first high-carbon steel productions were carried out in India with the steel known as wootz, which had 1.0–2.0 wt% C. The modern age of steel began with Sir Henry Bessemer in 1856, who invented a pneumatic process for steel production to improve gun construction and reduce costs [45].

Aluminum is the most abundant metal in the earth's crust. Among other properties, aluminum and its alloys have a relatively low density (2.7 g/cm^3 compared to 7.9 g/cm^3 for ferrous alloys) and good resistance to atmospheric corrosion [44]. Thanks to these properties, aluminum alloys are essential materials in manufacturing exoskeleton components.

Polymers are classified depending on their thermomechanical properties [46]. One of these classes is thermoplastics, commonly known as plastics. Plastics can be molded into numerous shapes through various manufacturing processes, such as injection molding and extrusion. Plastics have very low densities compared to steel and aluminum, which saves weight. For instance, the density of the polyamide 66 (Nylon 66), which is used in the manufacture of exoskeleton components, is around 1.17 g/cm^3 (versus 2.7 g/cm^3 for aluminum alloys and 7.9 g/cm^3 for steels) [47]. It is worth mentioning that plastics are often blended with fillers, additives, and modifiers to improve their properties. Another class of polymers is elastomers, which are rubbery materials that can be stretched many times their original dimensions and that recover their initial dimensions when the applied stress is released [46]. The fabrication of polymer components for exoskeletons is usually cheaper and faster than metallic elements. Further, they offer excellent corrosion and recoil impact resistances, are thermal insulators, and their color can be customized, among other advantages. Different exoskeleton components are produced from polymers: frames, handguards, mechanisms, and covers, among others.

A composite is a material produced from two or more materials to obtain a combination of properties that differ from the original materials. Composites may be selected to achieve unusual combinations of stiffness, strength, weight, high-temperature performance, corrosion resistance, hardness, or conductivity [48]. According to the nature of the matrix, the composites are classified into metal-matrix, polymer-matrix, and ceramic-matrix composites. The reinforcing phase may be particulates, fibers, or laminates, and they are typically stiffer, stronger, and harder than the matrix.

About polymer-matrix composites, the plastics used for manufacturing exoskeleton components are habitually reinforced with particles or fibers. In addition, there are investigations where hybrid materials (ceramic-matrix reinforced with fibers + metal matrix-material reinforced with fibers) are used.

A ceramic is an inorganic compound made of metallic and non-metallic elements whose crystal structure is generally more complex than metals [48]. Compared to metals, ceramics possess high hardness and stiffness, superior wear and heat resistance, high-temperature capability, and relatively low density. For example, the density of alumina (Al_2O_3) is around 3.8 g/cm^3 [49]. The main drawback of ceramic materials is their disposition to catastrophic brittle fracture; thus, their processing of finished products is typically slow, laborious, and costly. Due to these disadvantages, they are somewhat limited in applicability [44].

1.12 EVOLUTION OF MANUFACTURING PROCESSES

The history of manufacturing can be divided into two periods. First, the discovery and invention by humans of materials and processes to make things. Second, the development of production systems [50]. Processes such as forging, casting, machining, and stamping have been used since ancient times, with the difference that before, they were done manually, while today, they are done with the help of machinery.

Nowadays, the production of robot components requires tight dimensional tolerances; hence, selecting suitable technology and manufacturing processes is necessary. There are multiple methods for producing such parts. For metals, casting (sand, die injection molding, investment, lost foam), powder metallurgy, machining, welding, forging, stamping, rolling, and additive manufacturing processes, among others, are used; they may be complemented by heat and surface treatments. For polymers, injection molding, extrusion, and additive manufacturing processes are used.

1.13   EVOLUTION OF DESIGN TOOLS

The evolution of design tools concerning the production systems, starting with World War II (WWII) as a reference point, can be divided into the following three periods: The first period comprises the use of sequential design. The project performs the production of systems. The production in mass was gradually growing with the production of the automobile. One technique was Fordism, a manufacturing technology that served as the basis of modern economic and social systems in industrialized, standardized mass production and mass consumption [51]. The second period arises after WWII with the new design techniques. Overall, the design techniques that are highlighted are the Toyota Design Techniques (TDT) as Toyota Production System (TPS), kaizen (change for better—continuously improve). Ishikawa diagram (also called fishbone diagrams, herringbone diagrams, cause-and-effect diagrams, or Fishikawa), just in time (JIT), poka-joke (mistake-proofing), and waterfall Toyota. Other design techniques also arose, such as the theory of inventive problem solving (TIPS in English or TRIZ in Russian) in 1946; failure modes and effects analysis (FMEA) in 1949; design for test or design for testing or design for testability (DFT) in 1950; supplier development in 1951; bill of materials (BOM) in the early 1960s; design structure matrix (DSM) in 1960; and quality function deployment (QFD) developed in Japan in the late 1960s. The third period arose with computer-aided design (CAD) in 1959. Unisurf software was a pioneering surface CAD and computer-aided manufacturing (CAM) system designed to assist with car body design and tooling; it was developed in 1968 [52]. Later, the Sketchpad system was developed in 1963 [53]. As computers became more affordable, the application of CAD gradually expanded into exoskeleton development. Table 1.1 summarizes the evolution of CAD software.

The design techniques were consolidated and new techniques arose, such as technology readiness level (TRL), during the 1970s; user-centered design (UCD) in 1977; design thinking in 1978; product lifecycle management (PLM) in 1985; Six Sigma in 1986; Lean manufacturing in 1988; platforms (products families, modular architecture, commonality index) in 1990; enterprise resource planning (ERP) systems in 1990; axiomatic design in 1998; product data management (PDM) in 2001; design for inspection in 2014; and several design techniques developed in 1996, including the design for X, or design for excellence [49], as seen in Table 1.2.

Thanks to the aforementioned design techniques, skills for design, and CAD software, the behavior of exoskeletons was improved.

Evaluation activity. Please answer the next quiz.

https://forms.office.com/r/xbU9kueMaw

1. According to Richard Owen, what is an exoskeleton?
   A. Any rigid external structure, sometimes articulated in parts, that covers, supports, and protects any animal's internal or soft tissues

TABLE 1.1

Evolution of CAD Software

1963: Sketchpad	1986: SLA format	2007: NX
1968: Unisurf	1987: Pro-engineer	2011: LibreCAD
1970: Mouse device	1989: FDM format	2012: Autodesk 360
1971: Adam	1994: Step format	2013: 3D CAD apps
1977: Catia	1995: Solidworks	2014: Selective laser sintering
1978: Unigraphics	1995: Solidedge	2015: Onshape
1980: Iges format	1996: Catia conferencing	2017: Virtual reality in CAD
1981: Geomod	groupware	2019 Extended reality in
1982: Autodesk AutoCAD	1999: Autodesk inventor	Solidworks
(DXF and DWG file formats)	2002: FreeCAD	

TABLE 1.2

Design for X

Design for Six Sigma (DFSS)	Design to cost	Design for ergonomics
Design for reliability	Design for logistics	Design for aesthetics
Design for minimum risk	Design for user-friendliness	Design for serviceability
Design for environment	Design for repair-reuse-recyclability	Design for maintainability

    B. Any rigid internal structure, sometimes articulated in parts, that covers, supports, and protects any animal's internal or soft tissues

    C. Any rigid external structure, sometimes articulated in parts, that covers, supports, and protects any human's internal or soft tissues

    D. Mobile machine consisting of a soft or rigid external frame worn by a person and a power system of motors

2. What is the purpose of a mechanical exoskeleton in robotics?
   A. To assist in carrying weight
   B. To mobilize limbs
   C. To reduce reaction times
   D. All of the above

3. Who invented the crankshaft and the first mechanical clocks moved by weights and water?
   A. Archimedes
   B. Al-Jazari
   C. Jacques de Vaucanson
   D. Leonardo da Vinci

4. According to the text, what was the purpose of early automatons?
   A. Entertainment
   B. Religious
   C. Scientific
   D. Both A and B

5. Where was the first industrial robot, the Unimate, implemented?
   A. On a Unimation assembly line
   B. On a General Motors assembly line
   C. NASA's exploration missions
   D. In a pharmaceutical product handling system

6. What was the first robotic arm used to perform neurosurgery successfully?
   A. PUMA 560
   B. AESOP
   C. Da Vinci
   D. ViRob

7. The main advantages of robotics in medicine are the following: greater precision, avoiding human tremors, less invasive procedures, faster and more effective interventions, patient recovery in less time, less risk of tissue damage, and the ability to access delicate areas or complex
   A. True
   B. False

8. A sensor is any device that has a property that is sensitive to a magnitude of the medium capable of varying a property in the face of physical or chemical magnitudes, called instrumentation variables, and transforming them with a transducer into electrical variables.
   A. True
   B. False

9. What was the main purpose of the development of PLCs?
   A. To reduce the cost of replacing control systems based on relays
   B. To improve communication between systems
   C. To standardize programming languages
   D. To reduce the size of control systems

10. Who invented the battery?
    A. John F. Daniell
    B. Michael Faraday
    C. Alessandro Volta
    D. Samuel Ruben

11. What is an exoskeleton?
    A. An external structure that supports and protects a subject's body
    B. A device that contracts muscles
    C. A machine used to prevent adhesions and retractions
    D. A tool to enhance muscle strength

12. What's the first human exoskeleton invented?
    A. Welwalk WW-1000
    B. Hardiman
    C. Aichi
    D. None of the above

13. What are the typical application requirements for exoskeletons?
    A. High torque and long battery life
    B. High speed and precision
    C. Autonomy and machine learning
    D. All of the above

14. Nowadays, the production of robot components requires tight dimensional tolerances; hence, the selection of suitable technology and manufacturing process is necessary.
    A. True
    B. False

15. What is the advantage of polymer components over metallic elements for exoskeletons?
    A. Cheaper and faster fabrication
    B. Excellent corrosion and recoil impact resistances
    C. Thermal insulators
    D. All of the above

Chapter 2 describes the types and applications of exoskeletons.

REFERENCES

1. Di Liberto, A., Robotic Surgery: Practical Examples in Gynecology. Walter de Gruyter, 2013.
2. Siemens, Imaging; Available from: www.siemens.com/global/en/company/about/history/technology/medical-technology/imaging.html.
3. Siemens, Laboratory diagnostics; Available from: www.siemens.com/global/en/company/about/history/technology/medical-technology/laboratory-diagnostics.html.
4. Siemens, Advanced therapies; Available from: www.siemens.com/global/en/company/about/history/technology/medical-technology/advanced-therapies.html.
5. Constancia, P., The art & science of ROBOTICS (1) – A brief history. April 19, 2022, 2012. Available from: https://wp.me/p4Gxxr-FC.
6. Mitchell-Evans, W.O., et al., Why Do Humans Imagine Robots? Worcester Polytechnic Institute, 2010.
7. Taylor, R.H., et al., Medical Robotics and Computer-Integrated Surgery. Springer Handbook of Robotics, 2016: p. 1657–1684.
8. Input devices, 2021; Available from: http://fabacademy.org/2021/labs/zoi/students/jeffery-naranjo/input.html.
9. Brüel & Kjær History—Sound and Vibration | Brüel & Kjær; Available from: www.bksv.com/en/about/history.
10. Sreenivasulu, M.C., M.A.G. Kumar, and G.M. Rao, Position control for digital DC drives and PLC. International Journal of Engineering Research and Development, 2013.6(7): p. 61–68.

11. The History of Programming Languages—A Complete Guide, in Web Solutions Blog.
12. Hernandez, L. and M. Ospina, Scheme and creation of a prototype for the supervision of lights and electronic devices with a PBX, using a WLAN solution based on IoT. In 2019 IEEE Colombian Conference on Communications and Computing (COLCOM), 2019, Barranquilla, Colombia. p. 1–6.
13. Hristu-Varsakelis, D. and W.S. Levine, Handbook of Networked and Embedded Control Systems. Springer, 2005.
14. History of the battery, in Wikipedia.
15. Ankit, V., Sustainable Processes for Critical Metal Recovery Using Oxalate Chemistry. University of Kansas, 2021.
16. Lithium Iron Phosphate vs Lithium Cobalt Oxide | Battery Monday, 2020; Available from: www.grepow.com/blog/lithium-iron-phosphate-vs-lithium-cobalt-oxide-battery-monday.html.
17. Lithium metal battery. Wikipedia.
18. ABOUT LIFEPO4 2021; Available from: https://leadinglithium.co.za/about-lifepo4/.
19. Mongird, K., et al., 2020 Grid Energy Storage Technology Cost and Performance Assessment. U.S. Department of Energy, 2020: p. 6–15.
20. GE History; Available from: www.ge.com/about-us/history#/.
21. Honeywell, The history of Honeywell; Available from: www.honeywell.com/us/en/company/our-history.
22. ABB, ABB Group. Leading Digital Technologies for Industry. ABB, 2023; Available from: https://global.abb/group/en.
23. Kuka, Kuka robotics; Available from: www.kuka.com/.
24. Honda, American Honda Motor Co., Inc.—Official Site; Available from: www.honda.com/.
25. Mitsubishi, Global Website | MITSUBISHI MOTORS; Available from: www.mitsubishi-motors.com/en/index.html.
26. FANUC, FANUC America | Automation Solutions that Redefine Productivity; Available from: www.fanucamerica.com.
27. Siemens, Siemens USA; Available from: www.siemens.com/us/en.html.
28. Dynamics, B., Boston dynamics | Changing your idea of what robots can do; Available from: www.bostondynamics.com/.
29. Toyota, Toyota motor corporation official global website; Available from: https://global.toyota/en/index.html.
30. Yaskawa, Yaskawa America Inc. Home; Available from: www.yaskawa.com/.
31. Balluff, Balluff; Available from: www.balluff.com/en-mx.
32. Siviy, C., et al., Opportunities and challenges in the development of exoskeletons for locomotor assistance. Nature Biomedical Engineering, 2022: p. 1–17.
33. Clifford, J., Toyota launches loan service for Welwalk rehabilitation robot, 2017; Available from: https://mag.toyota.co.uk/toyota-launches-loan-service-for-welwalk-rehabilitation-robot/.
34. Asgharian, P., A.M. Panchea, and F. Ferland, A review on the use of mobile service robots in elderly care. Robotics, 2022.11(6): p. 127.
35. Walking Assist, 2016: Exoskeleton Report.
36. Honda, Honda Global | Walking Assist; Available from: https://global.honda/innovation/robotics/WalkingAssist.html.
37. The history of robotic exoskeleton development; Available from: www.eduexo.com/resources/articles/exoskeleton-history/.
38. Robotic exoskeletons are changing lives in surprising ways, 2017; Available from: www.nbcnews.com/mach/innovation/robotic-exoskeletons-are-changing-lives-surprising-ways-n722676.
39. ReWalk, About ReWalk robotics; Available from: https://rewalk.com/about-us/.

40. Schram, R. Introducing exoskeletons into the Toyota manufacturing environment. In 2018 Ergo-X Symposium Exoskeletons in the Workplace—Assessing Safety, Usability, and Productivity. National Institute for Occupational Safety and Health, 2018.

41. Top motor trends in the continuing evolution of robots, 2020; Available from: www.controlengeurope.com/article/182488/Top-motor-trends-in-the-continuing-evolution-of-robots.aspx.

42. Yaskawa, History of Servomotors | Yaskawa global site; Available from: www.yaskawa-global.com/product/servomotor/history.

43. Harmonic Drive® gears—Over 50 years of experience | Harmonic Drive | Harmonic Drive; Available from: www.harmonicdrive.net/about-us.

44. Callister, W.D. and D.G. Rethwisch, Materials Science and Engineering: An Introduction, Vol. 7. John Wiley & Sons, 2007.

45. Birat, J.-P., The relevance of Sir Henry Bessemer's ideas to the steel industry in the twenty-first century. Ironmaking & Steelmaking, 2004.31(3): p. 183–189.

46. Ramirez, J.H. and L.Z. Aviles, Designing Small Weapons. CRC Press, 2022.

47. Hamley, I.W., Introduction to Soft Matter: Synthetic and Biological Self-Assembling Materials. John Wiley & Sons, 2013.

48. Askeland, D.R., The Science and Engineering of Materials: Solutions Manual. 1st ed. Springer Dordrecht, 1991: p. 268.

49. Eastman, C.M., Design for X: Concurrent Engineering Imperatives. S.S.B. Media, 2012.

50. Groover, M.P., Fundamentals of Modern Manufacturing: Materials, Processes, and Systems. John Wiley & Sons, 2020.

51. Thompson, F., Fordism, Post-Fordism and the Flexible System of Production. Center for Digital Discourse and Culture, 2003.

52. Gannon, M., Reverberating Across the Divide: Bridging Virtual and Physical Contexts in Digital Design and Fabrication. ACADIA, 2014.

53. Bhoosan, S., Collaborative design: Combining computer-aided geometry design and building information modelling. Architectural Design, 2017.87(3): p. 82–89.

2 Types and Applications of Exoskeletons

2.1 INTRODUCTION

Robotics is guided by important bodies such as the International Organization for Standardization (ISO), the Institute of Electrical and Electronics Engineers (IEEE), the American Society of Mechanical Engineers (ASME), and the International Federation of Robotics (IFR). In addition, the World Intellectual Organization of Intellectual Property (OMPI) and the associations of the countries that support the technological development of robotics, such as China, the USA, Japan, and Germany have guidelines. A robot is classified as follows: industrial robot, service robot, and military robot. The IFR's use of the term "industrial robot" is based on the definition of the ISO: an "automatically controlled, reprogrammable multipurpose manipulator programmable in three or more axes". The International Organization for Standardization defines a "service robot" as a robot "that performs useful tasks for humans or equipment excluding industrial automation applications" [1]. Military robots are autonomous or remote-controlled mobile robots designed for military applications, from transportation to search and rescue, and attack [2]. An exoskeleton can be part of the three classifications according to its application. There are various exoskeletons for industrial, medical, and military applications.

Specifying the classification, we will say that an exoskeleton is part of wearables, part of service robots that can be used in service, industrial, and military applications. Broadening the panorama, the IFR does not consider military robots due to their ethical implications; however, we will describe some of their military applications in this chapter.

2.2 GENERAL CLASSIFICATION

In general, an exoskeleton is wearable; however, some applications require stationary exoskeletons, so we could say that, in this case, they are portable. However, we maintain the criteria that an exoskeleton is a wearable device, given the large number of applications where most are wearable. The classification in Figure 2.1 shows a subclassification first by mobilization zone divided into full body, upper body, and lower body. Later soft and rigid refer to the subclassification by type of structure. Then active and passive belong to the subclassification by type of action. Thus, conventional and mechatronic refer to a technology subclassification. Another subclassification relates to scope, which includes research, test bench, patent, and

DOI: 10.1201/9781003261995-2

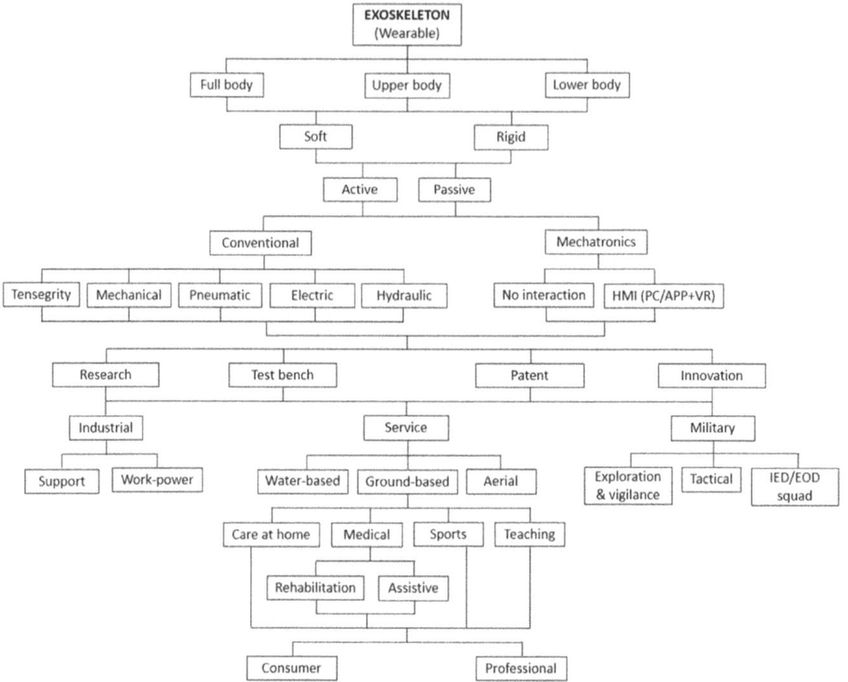

FIGURE 2.1   Exoskeleton classification.

innovation. Finally, industrial, service, and military belong to the subclassification by application.

In the exoskeleton classification, it is possible to observe that an exoskeleton can be, for example, full body, soft, passive, mechanical, research, and industrial application in terms of work power. In contrast, another configuration can be lower body, rigid, active, with a human-machine interface (HMI) using virtual reality and an app for innovation due to intending commercialization, for service application, for knee rehabilitation, and for professional users.

2.3   SUBCLASSIFICATION BY MOBILIZATION ZONE

The subclassification by mobilization zone includes the upper body divided into complete when the range of movement (ROM) is covered by both arms or by segment when any arm or segment of the arm is covered like the wrist, elbow, or shoulder. Full body when is the arms and legs are covered, and lower body includes complete when both legs are covered and by segment when any leg, ankle, knee, heel, or foot is covered. This subclassification is shown in Figure 2.2.

The authors Shuang Qiu, Zhongcai Pei, Chen Wang, and Zhiyong Tang generated the classification of exoskeletons by extremity, as follows: TH Trunk–Hip, HK Hip–Knee, KA Knee–Ankle, THK Trunk–Hip–Knee, HKA Hip–Knee–Ankle, and THKA Trunk–Hip–Knee–Ankle [3].

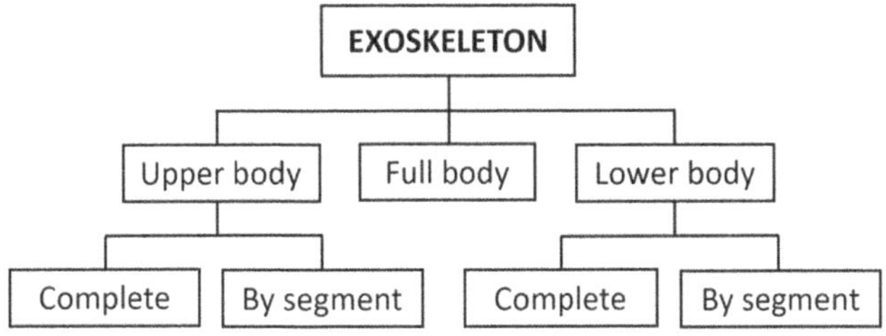

FIGURE 2.2   Exoskeleton subclassification by mobilization zone.

2.4   SUBCLASSIFICATION BY STRUCTURE

The subclassification by structure includes rigid and soft exoskeletons. **Rigid exoskeletons** are the classical exoskeletons; they have a metal frame and usually include sensors such as encoders and potentiometers in robotic joints. However, these sensors are incompatible with the soft exoskeleton; therefore, new sensors suitable for soft exoskeletons need to be created. Due to their application, some rigid exoskeletons include a rigid structure covered by soft material, allowing for flexible structures. However, they are not part of soft robotics; they still belong to rigid robotics. **Soft exoskeletons**, or exosuits, are made of soft materials. Some components, such as battery packs and controllers, have to remain rigid. The power is transmitted by flexible materials only, such as Bowden cables, air muscles, or filaments that shrink due to heat or electrical current. Some features of soft exoskeletons are the following: custom fitting and the use becomes simpler; they are smaller and much lighter and require less energy to use; exosuits are easier to wear: they provide fewer limitations to the user's joints; exosuits can be worn underneath clothing, because current exoskeletons are viewed as ugly and unattractive; soft exoskeletons could be significantly less expensive than rigid exoskeletons. Soft exoskeletons have difficulty transferring power from any area of the body to the ground. Motors and sensors will be more difficult to mount; torque and force generated by actuators will enter the user's body; therefore, the use of exosuits is complicated in elderly and disabled people [4]—Figure 2.3 shows subclassification by structure in a general way.

Soft exoskeletons include exogloves and exosleeves. An **exosleeve** is an exoskeleton mounted on the forearm, while an **exoglove** is mounted over the hand. Hand exoskeletons or exogloves have become a popular technological solution for assisting people suffering from neurological conditions and enhancing healthy individuals' capabilities. Despite the progress in the field, most existing devices do not provide the same dexterity as the healthy human hand [5].

Actuators for exosuits are called soft actuators; some are air muscles that have many ways of operating. Some soft actuators or soft pneumatic actuators (SPAs) are the following: fabric inflatable soft actuators (FISAs), which integrate a set of pneumatic chambers made of 200D TPU-nylon that creates bending-extending motions using a modular assembly that allows FISAs to adapt to any size of limb or easily replace them [6]; pneumatic artificial muscles (PAMs); and fluid elastomer actuators (FEAs) [7].

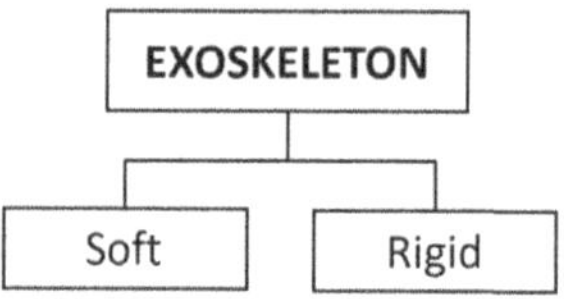

FIGURE 2.3 Exoskeleton subclassification by structure.

In recent years, inflatable soft actuators have increasingly attracted more interest than other SPAs, since they are considered the most straightforward design with high payload capacity and low stiffness [8]. They are composed of a set of lightweight chambers that are flat but become bulky when inflated [9]. Usually, chambers are made of thermoplastic polyurethane (TPU)–coated nylon [10] or electrostatic discharge (ESD) plastic sheets [11]. The chambers have the ability to emulate natural human movements by adapting to different shapes inside pockets with a single air input that can support twice their own structure [12].

In the literature, several designs of inflatable actuators have been proposed for soft robotics applications using different parameters, constraints, materials, electro-pneumatic configurations, and computational or fabrication methods to enhance their performance [13]. Air chambers or bladders are mainly determined by their geometry and dimensions of gap, height, and thickness of the wall or number of chambers, depending on the target trajectory and required pressure to achieve a specific motion on a surface. The higher the number of chambers, the less pressure required; however, voluminous structures are obtained [14]. Moreover, using thin and high walls increases the force output, which means less pressure to reach maximum bending [15].

Inflatable structures have outperformed other SPAs since they do not require high forces during contraction nor sophisticated equipment for their fabrication, nor are they time-consuming compared to FEA development. Usually, chambers are pleated in serial with a single layer [16] or multiple layers with thin films of polymerizing vinyl chloride (PVC) [17] or low-density polyethylene (LDPE) [18] to reduce their weight. However, forces are restricted since they are more likely to explode. Most assemblies are joined in a single piece [19], but chambers cannot be replaced when air leaks occur or designs are oriented to a custom user [20].

2.5 SUBCLASSIFICATION BY ACTION TYPE

According to the type of action, the exoskeletons are active or powered and passive. It should be noted that there is confusion depending on the approach. From the perspective of kinesitherapy, the names active and passive refer to movement with manual or instrumental assistance (exoskeletons). Specifically, it refers to the patient's participation, being passive when the patient does not participate actively in mobilization (mobilizations, postures, joint traction, musculotendinous stretching, and manipulations) and activating when the patient participates in the mobilization.

Passive exoskeletons are not motorized and are often used for ergonomic support, to prevent repetitive stress injuries, or to help hold tools or equipment. In contrast,

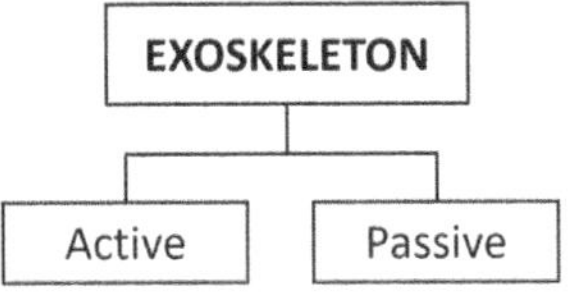

FIGURE 2.4 Exoskeleton subclassification by action type.

active or powered exoskeletons can aid in lifting heavy objects while reducing the potential for musculoskeletal injuries [21]. Figure 2.4 shows the exoskeleton subclassification by action type.

Passive kinesitherapy is divided into relaxed passive kinesitherapy (joints are free, and nothing prevents movement) and forced passive kinesitherapy (can be carried out momentarily or maintained). Passive kinesitherapy includes assisted passive mobilization (when the therapist performs it manually or by mechanical means), auto-passive mobilization (when it is the patient himself who performs it manually or through pulleys), and passive instrumental mobilization (electromechanical devices or machines carry it out).

Active kinesitherapy is divided into assisted or antigravitational active kinesitherapy (applied when the patient is unable to perform the exercise that causes movement against gravity, which means that they need help to perform it, and the intensity of the external force which constitutes the aid will complete the action of the muscle, but will not replace it); free or gravitational active kinesitherapy (the patient executes the movements of the affected muscles exclusively, without the need for help); and resisted active kinesitherapy (the movements are performed trying to overcome the resistance that the therapist opposes with his hands or by instrumental means [the muscular contraction is carried out against external resistance to increase power, volume, motor coordination, and muscle endurance). Table 2.1 describes a summary relationship between exoskeletons with kinesitherapy.

2.6 SUBCLASSIFICATION BY TECHNOLOGY

Exoskeletons are a perfect example of a mechatronic product, not only for their technology but also for their design methodology, which due to its complexity, must be carried out with an engineering concurrent approach, which is a central part of mechatronics design. Exoskeletons in terms of technology can be conventional or mechatronic. Figure 2.5 shows the detail of exoskeleton subclassification by technology.

2.6.1 Conventional Technology

Conventional exoskeletons are divided into tensegrity, mechanical, pneumatic, electric, and hydraulic, as shown in Figure 2.6.

Tensegrity is a design principle that applies when a discontinuous set of compression elements is opposed and balanced by a continuous tensile force, thereby creating an internal prestress that stabilizes the entire structure [22]. Architect Buckminster Fuller is credited with coining the term "tensegrity," which is a combination of the

TABLE 2.1

Relationship Between the Type of Exoskeleton With the Type of Kinesitherapy

Exoskeleton	Passive Kinesitherapy	Active Kinesitherapy
Active (free movement)	Relaxed passive kinesitherapy (assisted or self-assisted)	
Active (position held)	Forced passive kinesitherapy (assisted)	
Active (complementary movement)		Actively assisted kinesitherapy
Passive (postural and corrective)		Free active kinesitherapy
Active (configurable resistive force)		Resisted active kinesitherapy

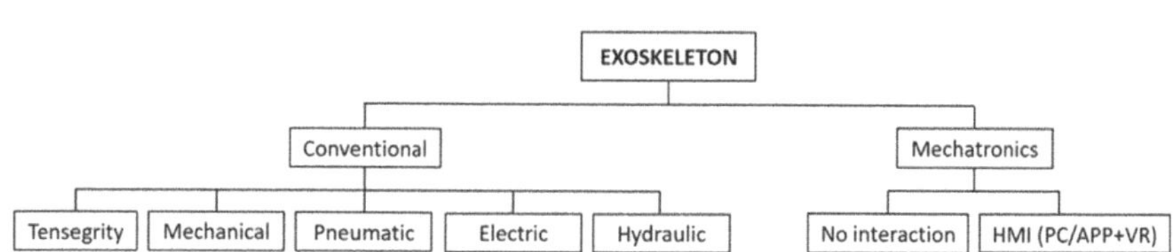

FIGURE 2.5 Exoskeleton subclassification by technology.

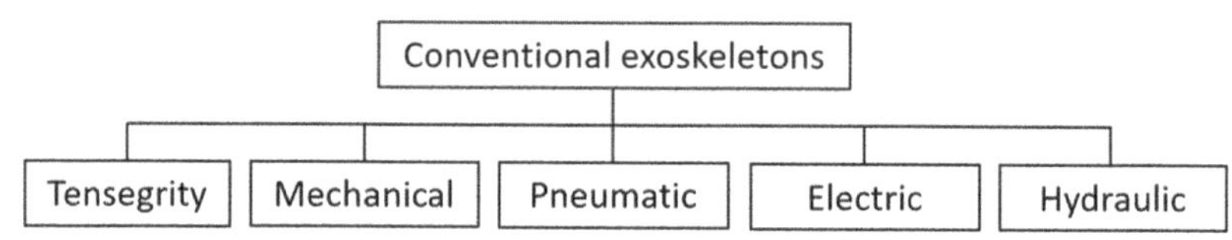

FIGURE 2.6 Exoskeleton subclassification by conventional technology.

words "tensional" and "integrity." These unconventional structures are held together by tensional forces, which provide their stability. In 1949, sculptor Kenneth Snelson created the first structure that was officially recognized as a tensegrity. This structure consisted of two X-shaped wooden struts suspended by a taut nylon cable. Snelson captured the defining features of tensegrity [23]:

- Biotensegrity: mimics the human skeleton: bones for compression, tendons for tension.

- Pervasive tension and separation of rigid elements, a condition Snelson and Fuller called "continuous tension, discontinuous compression".
- Stable. This stability is because the tension and compression components are always in mechanical equilibrium.
- Prestressed. This mechanical equilibrium results from how the compression and tensile components interact to bring out each other's essential nature: the cables pull in on both ends of the struts while the struts push out and stretch the cables, a condition known as "self-stress" or "prestress."
- Resilient. While they are stabilized by prestress, tensegrity structures are also exquisitely responsive to outside perturbation. Their components immediately reorient when the structure is deformed, and they do so reversibly and without breaking.
- Globally integrated. Because the components are so intimately interconnected, all feel what one feels, producing a truly holistic structure.
- Modular. Though complete on its own, a tensegrity structure can combine with other such structures to form a larger tensegrity system. Individual tensegrity units can be disrupted in these systems without compromising overall system integrity.
- Hierarchical. Smaller tensegrity structures may function as compressive or tensile components in a larger tensegrity system.

Tensegrity exoskeletons have joints that use the tensegrity principle; that is, they use systems of tensioners attached to support points. Mechanical exoskeletons provide postural and ergonomic support, movement correction, and force augment using mechanisms. They work with the user to enhance their strength and performance to complete tasks or rehabilitate their bodies. Mechanical exoskeletons take the weight of users' arms off their necks, backs, and shoulders and transfer it to their cores. Workers' energy becomes more evenly distributed, reducing strain and stress on the muscles and joints [24]. Also, there are mechanical exoskeletons based on complaint mechanisms; in mechanical engineering, a compliant mechanism is a flexible mechanism that achieves force and motion transmission through elastic body deformation. It gains some or all of its motion from the relative flexibility of its members rather than from rigid-body joints alone [25].

Pneumatic exoskeletons are manufactured based on pneumatic actuators, either by pneumatic cylinders or soft pneumatic actuators (SPAs). Electric exoskeletons are structures that use motors in their joints, either rotational or linear motors.

Soft exoskeletons used electric actuators such as electroactive polymers. Electroactive polymers change shape or size when stimulated by an electric field and are widely used in robotics as actuators or sensors [26]. Other actuation methods of soft exoskeletons consist of a servomotor, a flexible Bowden cable transmission, and a force feedback loop based on a series elastic actuation (SEA) [27].

The hydraulic exoskeleton is one research hotspot in the field of robotics, which can take a heavy load due to the high-power density of the hydraulic system. However, the traditional hydraulic system is ordinarily centralized, inefficient, and bulky during the application, which limits its development in the exoskeleton [27].

2.6.2 MECHATRONICS TECHNOLOGY

Mechatronics exoskeletons are devices with more recent technology integrated into their operating and user interaction. Mechatronics exoskeletons are divided into non-interactive mechatronics exoskeletons and interactive exoskeletons. Figure 2.7 shows the categorization of mechatronics technology.

Non-interactive mechatronics exoskeletons are systems that include the latest technology in motors, sensors, and control strategy to assist in medical rehabilitation according to pathology requirements, such as stroke, cerebral palsy (CP), hemiplegia, spasticity, Duchenne muscular dystrophy (DMD), and neurological disability, among others. Some examples of exoskeletons are adaptive mechatronic exoskeletons for force-controlled finger rehabilitation; exoskeletons controlled by a neuroelectric signal, specifically electroencephalography (EEG); electromyography (EMG)–controlled exoskeletons; event-triggered sliding mode impulsive control for lower limb rehabilitation exoskeleton robot gait tracking [28]; and real-time supervisory control to exoskeletons, among others.

Interactive exoskeletons illustrate the close integration and interdependence of mechanical design, drive trains, sensors, control strategy, and user interface [29]. In this category, the latest technologies working in a collaborative environment include artificial intelligence, gaming, deep learning, machine learning, virtual reality (VR), augmented reality (AR), Internet of Things (IoT), gait recognition, prediction model by a neural network, robust adaptive-fuzzy-proportional-derivative controller, mixed perception model, EMG-controlled knee exoskeleton to assist home rehabilitation in a game context, and clouding, among others.

Three exoskeletons became slightly more popular in use: ARMin, Bi-Manu Track, and ArmeoSpring [30]. Most gaming exoskeletons aim to exert a reactive force on the user while using a virtual reality headset. It is the exact opposite of exoskeletons for teleoperation, which are only used to extract position and movement data from the user. This is the same direction in which medical and military exoskeletons have gone [31].

AxonVR's goal is to create a fully suspended exoskeleton that can simulate various experiences, such as walking, swimming, and interacting with virtual objects by providing appropriate resistance. This could be achieved using different types of exoskeletons, including gloves, that can resist specific body parts while using virtual objects. Other VR exoskeletons include Dexmo, Manus, AxonSuit, AxonSkeleton, and Hypersuit VR. It is essential to try VR technology personally to understand its level of immersion, which is difficult to describe without experience. Exoskeletons for gaming provide a sense of touch in the VR world and are an intersection between virtual reality and exoskeleton technology.

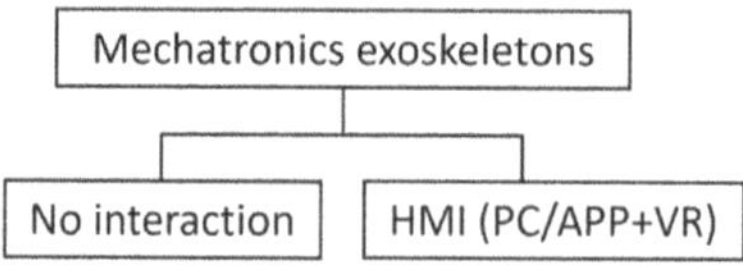

FIGURE 2.7 Exoskeleton subclassification by mechatronics technology.

2.6.3 Haptic Exoskeletons

The ability to wear haptic devices has expanded their potential applications in various areas, including social interaction, healthcare, virtual reality, remote assistance, and robotics. However, the challenge of designing compact and kinesthetic haptic devices that can be comfortably worn for extended periods remains due to the smaller form factor and wearability requirements. Hand exoskeletons have been developed for commercial and research purposes to address this challenge. [32]

Haptic or force-reflecting interfaces are robotic devices that display touch- or force-related sensory information from a virtual or remote environment to the user [33].

CyberGrasp is a commercial haptic exoskeleton developed by CyberGlove Systems LLC. The CyberGrasp device is a lightweight, force-reflecting exoskeleton that fits over a CyberGlove data glove (wired version) and adds resistive force feedback to each finger and the palm. There are five actuators, one for each finger. Grasp forces are produced by a network of tendons routed to the fingertips via the exoskeleton; low friction tendons are used to transmit forces with a peak force of 12N on the fingertip. CyberGrasp has a relatively large weight: 453.6 g. [34].

The RMII-ND glove from Rutgers is a force feedback device that operates using a direct drive actuation system, with actuators on the palm. Unlike the CyberGrasp, this exoskeleton is lighter and can control four separate fingers through four pneumatic actuators, offering force feedback of up to 16N. Unlike other devices, the RMII-ND provides forces on the intermediate phalanx, leaving fingertips free to interact [32].

Many other haptic exoskeletons have been developed, and one of the main characteristics to be improved is lightness; for this purpose, Bowden cables have become popular as remote controllers.

The Wolverine is a mobile, wearable haptic device designed for simulating the grasping of rigid objects in a virtual reality interface. The project focused on creating a low-cost and lightweight device that directly renders a force between the thumb and three fingers to simulate objects held in pad opposition (precision)-type grasps. Integrated sensors are used both for feedback control and user input: time-of-flight sensors provide the position of each finger, and an inertial measurement unit (IMU) offers overall orientation tracking [35].

2.7 SUBCLASSIFICATION BY SCOPE

The scope-based subclassification of exoskeletons refers to the design of an exoskeleton created from scratch for research, testing, patenting, or innovation. A research exoskeleton is a system dedicated to experimental objectives, outlining lines of research, looking for alternative solutions to performance or performance problems, and establishing new operating principles. Tests on the test benches are run according to test protocols to validate the performance of different exoskeletons. Exoskeleton patents are intellectual property ready to be transferred or licensed to healthy companies. Exoskeleton innovations are fabricated to propose commercially, reach a trade position, or lead the market—Figure 2.8 shows the exoskeleton subclassification by scope.

2.8 SUBCLASSIFICATION BY APPLICATION

Exoskeletons subclassified by application are industrial exoskeletons, service exoskeletons, and military exoskeletons, as shown in Figure 2.9.

2.8.1 INDUSTRIAL APPLICATION

Industrial exoskeletons are mechanical devices worn by workers whose construction mirrors the structure of the operator's limbs, joints, and muscles. They work in tandem with them and are utilized as a capabilities amplifier or fatigue and strain reducer. Body weight support, lift assistance, load maintenance, positioning correction, and body stabilization are common capabilities of industrial exoskeletons [36]. Industrial exoskeletons can be divided into support exoskeletons and work-power exoskeletons as shown in Figure 2.10.

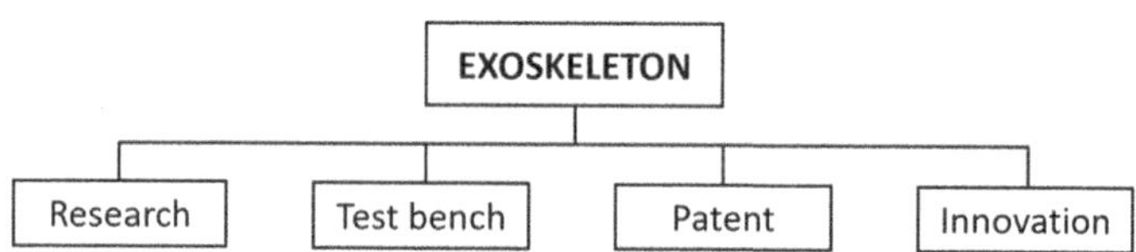

FIGURE 2.8 Exoskeleton subclassification by scope.

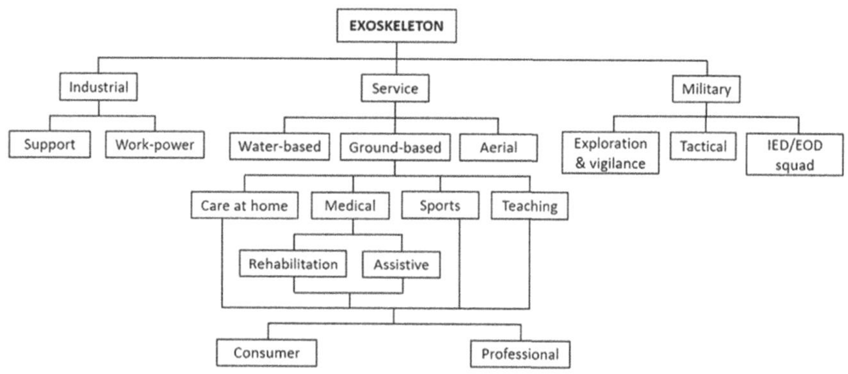

FIGURE 2.9 Exoskeleton subclassification by application.

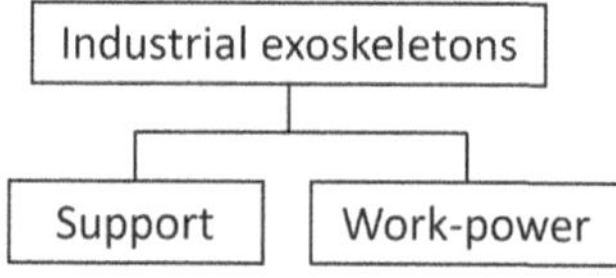

FIGURE 2.10 Exoskeleton subclassification by industrial application.

Exoskeletons have the potential to revolutionize the way people work in labor-intensive industries by reducing physical strain and fatigue, preventing injuries, and increasing productivity. These devices come in various forms, power requirements, and construction materials and can support different parts of the body, such as the arms, upper and lower body, and hands.

In the industrial sector, exoskeletons are commercially available and used by sizable companies, particularly in the automotive, logistics, retail, and construction fields. The acquisition of these devices is not dependent on high insurance, and the ROI is convenient, making them an attractive option for companies looking to improve worker safety and productivity.

However, while standards and regulatory issues related to using exoskeletons in industrial settings are significant, they are not nearly as complex as their medical counterparts. Nevertheless, companies need to ensure that the exoskeletons they acquire meet safety and quality standards and that their workers receive proper training.

Examples of exoskeletons designed to support manual labor tasks in industrial environments include Lockheed Martin's FORTIS and Noonee's Chairless Chair, which attach at the hip and carry weight by the exoskeletons to the floor, acting as a seat when needed. Other devices, such as StrongArm Technologies' FLx ErgoSkeleton, are upper body systems that support the shoulders, arms, and upper back. In contrast, others assist hands in gripping, such as Bioservo Technologies' Ironhand.

Most commercially available exoskeleton solutions, whether powered or unpowered, use batteries to operate the actuators and provide assistance, although some unconventional power sources like compressed air are also used. There are numerous examples of powered exoskeletons, such as ATOUN's Power Assist ARM, Innophys' Muscle Suit, Cyberdyne's HAL for Labor Support, RB3D's HERCULE, Sarcos Robotics' Guardian XO, and Noonee's Chairless Chair. On the other hand, unpowered or "passive" exoskeletons use mechanisms to increase strength and provide stability through a combination of human-guided flexion/extension and locking mechanisms. Examples of unpowered industrial exoskeletons include Ottobock's Paexo, Levitate Technologies' AIRFRAME, suitX's MAX Exoskeleton Suit, StrongArm Technologies' FLx ErgoSkeleton, Laevo's Laevo, and Lockheed Martin's Fortis.

There are many business benefits to using industrial exoskeletons, including increased efficiency and productivity. The primary advantage and reason for adopting industrial exoskeletons are to reduce the number of worker injuries and reduce healthcare and disability costs.

In October 2018, Hyundai Motor Group announced they would begin testing their Hyundai Vest Exoskeleton (H-VEX), exoskeleton technology that reduces pressure on workers' necks and back, at a North American Hyundai-KIA factory. This follows the start of trials at the same plant beginning in August 2017 of the Hyundai Chairless Exoskeleton (H-CEX), a knee joint sustainability device that maintains the sitting position of workers. According to Hyundai the H-CEX is light and straightforward but is endurable enough to bolster a body weight of up to 150 kg. Both the H-CEX and H-VEX systems are designed to reduce injuries and increase worker efficiency [36]. Figure 2.11 shows the Hyundai Chairless Exoskeleton (H-CEX).

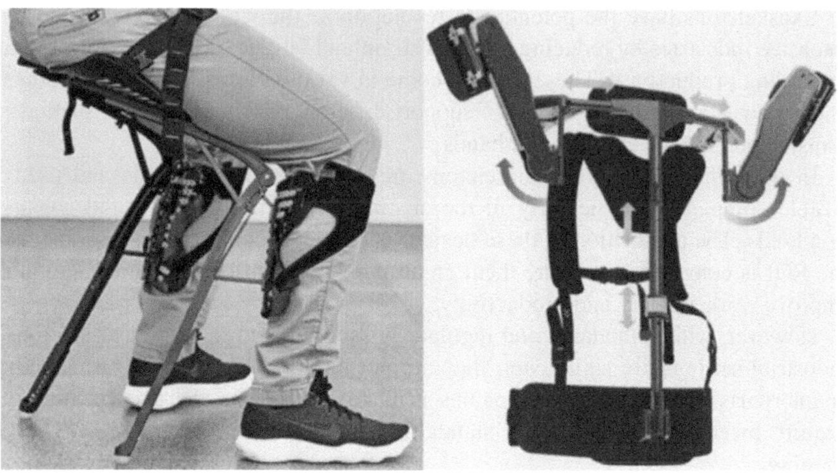

FIGURE 2.11   H-CEX and H-VEX exoskeletons.

(*Credit*: Hyundai)

In August 2018, Ford declared that they would implement 75 upper body exoskeletons from Ekso Bionics at 15 automotive factories worldwide. This move aimed to minimize repetitive motion injuries that result from carrying out overhead tasks. Meanwhile, the BMW assembly plant located in South Carolina is currently utilizing the unpowered AIRFRAME upper body exoskeleton from Levitate Technologies. Furthermore, other BMW plants are also conducting trials of these systems.

Industrial exoskeletons are becoming more affordable and functional thanks to advances in enabling technologies, particularly in actuators, batteries, and advanced materials. As a result, these exoskeletons are being adopted more widely and quickly. Many of these technological breakthroughs are happening in the robotics sector, where medical technology and robotics converge, particularly in robotic rehabilitation and quality-of-life systems. Examples of these advancements include Harmonic Drive's lightweight, brushless FLA Rotary Actuators and igus' polymer bearings, which are used in Levitate Technologies' unpowered exoskeletons. Maxon has also introduced a new product, the Exoskeleton Drive joint actuation unit, which is compact, lightweight, and consists of a brushless DC motor with an optimized rotor and high-resolution encoders.

Industrial exoskeletons can be divided into the following categories [37]:

- Tool-holding exoskeletons: This category includes a type of exoskeleton that uses a spring-loaded arm, like the zero-G mechanical arm, to support a heavy tool on one end. The other end is connected to a lower body exoskeleton and a counterweight. Typically, these exoskeletons are passive, although at least one prototype uses motors in the legs. The weight of the tool is directly transferred to the ground. Some examples of tool-holding exoskeletons are the Ekso Works by Ekso Bionics, Fortis by Lockheed Martin,

Prototype by Falltech, Robo-Mate by the European Union, and O-ArmX by BAE Systems.

- Chairless chairs: Lightweight exoskeletons designed to be worn over work pants can be stiffened and locked in place to reduce fatigue when crouching or standing for extended periods. Examples of such exoskeletons include Honda's Body Weight Support Assist, Wearable Chair's Archelis, and StrongArm Technologies' V-22 Ergoskeleton.
- Back support: Exoskeletons are also available to help maintain proper posture when lifting objects. These exoskeletons can help reduce the back muscles or spine load during bending. Examples of such exoskeletons include StrongArm Technologies' V-22 Ergoskeleton, Laevo by Laevo, SuitX's MAX, Innophys' Hip Auxiliary Muscle Suit, CYBERDYNE's Hal for Labor Support Lumber, and Panasonic's AWN-03.
- Powered gloves: Mechanized gloves designed to assist workers with a weak grip by providing mechanized support to help them hold onto tools more securely. Additionally, some exoskeleton gloves can be used in reverse to help workers who have difficulty opening certain fingers to grasp tools by mechanically opening them. Examples of these exoskeleton gloves include the SEM Glove by Bioservo Technologies and the Pneumatic Power Assist Glove by Daiya Industries.
- Full-body powered suits: In the past, it was thought that large, full-body powered suits would be used for work and industry, but in recent years, most developers have shifted their focus to smaller, specialized exoskeletons. However, there are still a few examples of full-body powered suits being developed, such as the MS-2 by Panasonic, the Prototype Shipyard Exoskeleton by Daewoo, the Body Extender by PERCRO Lab, the HULC by Lockheed Martin and Ekso Bionics, and the XOS 2 by Sarcos/Raytheon.
- Additional/supernumerary robotics: Exoskeletons that provide a second set of hands are considered the most ambitious wearable robotics project for work and industry. These exoskeletons consist of two or more powered arms that the wearer can control to hold tools or materials in place. While tool-holding exoskeletons are also considered to be supernumerary, the arms in those exoskeletons are typically passive, spring-loaded, and cannot be independently controlled. An example of an exoskeleton that provides a second set of hands is the Supernumerary Robotics Limbs (SRL) developed by MIT.

2.8.2 SERVICE APPLICATION

ISO 8373:2012 defines terms used concerning robots and robotic devices operating in both industrial and non-industrial environments. A service robot performs useful tasks for humans or equipment, excluding industrial automation applications. It explicitly states that a robot's mechanical type/kinematics is insufficient to distinguish industrial robots from service robots. Hence, by ISO definition, the application is a sufficient criterion to distinguish industrial from service robots, but the

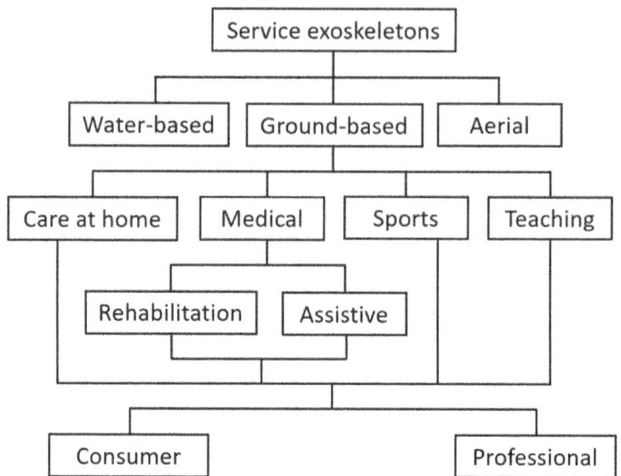

FIGURE 2.12 Exoskeleton subclassification by service application.

kinematics are not [38]. Service exoskeletons are designed to mimic, augment, or enhance the body's natural movements and are deployed in various applications. These exoskeletons provide important support for human motion and can be used for both consumer and professional applications. Figure 2.12 shows the exoskeleton subclassification by service application.

Water exoskeletons are structures to assist users in activities in water. An example is the exoskeletons for underwater swimming. These designs are biologically inspired and based on observations of dolphins, sea turtles, and penguins. Biologically inspired designs have the advantages of stealth, maneuverability, and a natural interface compared to propeller-driven underwater propulsion devices. The dolphin-based concept has the benefits of using the wearer's most powerful muscle groups, being the most natural to swim with, and leaving the user's hands free for other tasks. The sea turtle–based concept has the advantage of novelty and may have appeal as a recreational device. It is expected that with actuation and energy storage components available today, an exoskeleton that produces a cruising speed of over 1 m/s and a top speed of over 1.5 m/s is feasible. It is estimated that cruising at 1 m/s can be achieved with less than 504 watts of power consumption, which translates into 2.4 kg of off-the-shelf silver-zinc batteries per hour of operation [39].

Aerial exoskeletons are structures to assist users in aerial activities. There are three main uses: vertical takeoff and landing (VTOL), astronaut training, and airport exoskeletons. Airport exoskeletons are industrial exoskeletons, only their performance is in airline activities. VTOL exoskeletons have several denominations, such as personal VTOL flight, jet pack, jet suit, turbojet pack, and flight pack. Some famous companies with aerial exoskeletons are Gravity Industries, Daedalus Flight Pack, Trek Aerospace, and JetPack Aviation.

ISO 8373:2012 further distinguishes personal or consumer from professional service robots. A personal service robot is a service robot used for a non-commercial task, usually by laypersons. In contrast, professional service robots are used for commercial tasks, usually operated by a properly trained operator. An operator is a person designated to start, monitor, and stop the intended operation of a robot [38].

Care-at-home exoskeletons are devices that either require capacitation for their use or clearance of the FDA. Some exoskeletons are dedicated to assisting in the bathroom or to help the user up the steps. Teaching exoskeletons are exoskeletons dedicated to teaching dancing and hand guides to acquire skills such as drawing.

Sport exoskeletons are devices to assist athletes during training or in competition. Roam Robotics' Elevate exoskeleton is specifically designed to assist experienced skiers by reducing the pressure on their quads and knees, allowing them to continue enjoying skiing without discomfort. It is the first powered and actively actuated exoskeleton for skiing. It can support up to 30% of the user's body weight using actuators that rapidly inflate and deflate, powered by a small air compressor in a backpack-like pouch. The Elevate's onboard software is a crucial component that adjusts and anticipates the level of support required by the knees and quads. The device does not take over the skiing experience from the user, but rather extends their skiing time while improving their safety.

The RoboGolfPro exoskeleton is the first swing training system and is an end effector that uses seven motors to generate precise replicas of complex golf swings. The golf swings that the machine can execute do not have to be in the same plane, and the swings can be either theoretical or copies of those by successful professional golfers [40]. RoboGolfPro can repeatedly execute the same golf swing hundreds of times with precision. This can be extremely useful for activities like golf, which require high accuracy and repetition. However, the technology can also be utilized for other activities, such as archery and shooting firearms.

The Ski~Mojo is a passive knee exoskeleton for skiing. It works as a spring dampener for the knees. It operates similarly to a shock absorber system found in cars and takes advantage of the fact that skiers wear stiff boots by attaching to them. The Ski~Mojo can be worn on top of or underneath clothing, minimizing the effects of bumps and shocks during skiing. The device is also effective in preventing muscle fatigue and reducing leg pain. The Xnowers exoskeleton for skiing and snowboarding is a passive exoskeleton with an adjustable suspension system. The springs are meant to support the athlete's weight and dampen the impact on their body. The Xnowers' goal is to reduce the impact on the knees and provide more security and control.

Medical exoskeletons are structures where commercial products are more complex than industrial exoskeletons due to FDA rules. So, there are several medical applications, such as exoskeletons in geriatric work. Medical exoskeletons wrap around the user's limbs to support them physically. This offers tremendous assistance to those with disabled limbs, and rehabilitation is where exoskeletons initially made much progress in healthcare.

The Mihajlo Pupin Institute in Belgrade, Serbia, created the first functional medical exoskeleton in 1972. After several years, the development of exoskeletons aimed at helping medical professionals lift and transport patients. However, research efforts shifted to focus more on patients and their needs. Researchers discovered that exoskeletons could mimic movements consistently and accurately, which enables patients to perform exercises more effectively with greater consistency in less time.

In the field of wearable medical devices, as patients improve their strength and confidence, the level of assistance provided by the exoskeleton is gradually reduced. This results in a key distinction between two types of devices: rehabilitation and mobility aids. A rehabilitation device is designed to supplement a physical rehabilitation program and is typically discontinued once the program is completed. On the other hand, a mobility aid is intended to be used permanently, with the user not expected to make a full recovery. In this context, the exoskeleton functions as an assistive device.

Medical exoskeletons and orthotics are a diverse field with two major groups: rehabilitative and augmentative. Rehabilitation exoskeletons are designed for users who will improve after a supervised training regimen and will no longer need the device after rehabilitation. On the other hand, augmentative exoskeletons are intended for users who will rely on the device for the rest of their lives.

Two examples of exoskeletons that illustrate this difference are the Ekso GT and the REX. The Ekso GT by Ekso Bionics is used by individuals who still have some mobility and can shift weight from one leg to the other. It has variable assist software that provides targeted assistance and gradually decreases the assistive force as the patient becomes stronger during rehabilitation. In contrast, the REX by REX Bionics takes complete control of walking, including transferring weight from one leg to the other, and the operator rides the suit, not using their muscles to walk. Individuals can use it with complete paralysis to stand up and walk. Thus, these devices cater to different needs and capabilities.

There are different design challenges for medical orthotics used for rehabilitation versus augmentation. A rehabilitation exoskeleton needs to be adjustable, execute the same motion multiple times accurately, and track information for each patient. It is typically used in 1- to 2-hour sessions per user. On the other hand, an augmentative exoskeleton needs to be fitted for only one user, have a longer battery life (if powered), and be comfortable to wear for an entire day. Comfort over long periods is a significant challenge for mobility-assist exoskeletons. Even though wearables have become smaller and more useful, wearing an exoskeleton for extended periods while performing everyday tasks remains challenging. Medical exoskeletons can also be categorized by their target region, such as the upper or lower body. Lower-body medical exoskeletons aim to improve walking or aid individual joints, while upper-body medical orthotics focus on strengthening or augmenting the arm or hand. Both upper- and lower-body medical wearable robotics can be used for rehabilitation or augmentation.

A third way to classify medical exoskeletons can be according to their size and mobility, with three main categories: stationary, tethered, and mobile. Stationary exoskeletons are fixed to a wall or the ground. In contrast, tethered ones can be suspended on an overhead rail, supported by a metal frame on wheels, or directly attached to a mobile robot. Stationary and tethered exoskeletons are typically heavy and do not distribute their weight to the user. In contrast, mobile medical exoskeletons are designed to be worn by the user and are suitable for use inside and outside the home. They require lighter motors, controllers, and a battery pack that can be fitted into a small space. Another way to categorize medical exoskeletons is by the control strategy they use. The most straightforward strategy is a preprogrammed exoskeleton that follows predetermined movements. More complex exoskeletons wait for specific conditions to be met before initiating a motion. The most advanced exoskeletons read electrical signals from the spine, arms, and legs and can even provide functional electrical stimulation while controlling the exoskeleton.

The following is a list of commercial medical exoskeleton research projects that are close to becoming commercial products and research projects that have had a significant influence on the health field: stationary lower body exoskeletons (Lokomat Pro by Hocoma, RoboGait by Bama Teknoloji, InMotion Ankle by Interactive Motion Technologies, Alex 3 by University of Delaware, and ANKLEBOT by MIT); stationary upper body and arm and wrist exoskeletons for rehabilitation (InMotion Arm by Interactive Motion Technologies, InMotion Wrist by Interactive Motion Technologies, Armeo by Hocoma, ALEx by KineteK Wearable Robotics, Tack-Hold by KineteK Wearable Robotics, Power Jacket REALIVE by Panasonic ActiveLink, and HARMONY by ReNeu Robotics Lab, UT Austin); stationary upper body and hand exoskeletons for rehabilitation (Amadeo by Tyromotion, InMotion Hand by Interactive Motion Technologies, and Hand of Hope by Rehab-Robotics); mobile upper body exoskeletons for rehabilitation and augmentation (MyoPro Motion G by Myomo, CARAPACE by Lorenzo Masia, Robotic Soft Extra Muscle (SEM) Glove by Bioservo, Pneumatic Power Assist Glove by Daiya, Inflatable Soft Exoskeleton by Otherlab Orthotics, Inflatable Soft Robotic Glove—Wyss Institute, and Affordable Tremor Suppression Arm by MedEXO Robotics); and mobile lower body rehabilitation exoskeletons (HANK by Gogoa, ReWalk by ReWalk Robotics, Hal Medical by CYBERDYNE, Ekso GT by Ekso Bionics, Indego by Parker Hannifin, and ExoAtlet by ExoAtlet [41].

With back pain being the cause of one in every four medical leaves in Japan, some of the largest hospitals and manufacturers now use our Archelis suits as a form of personal protective equipment (PPE). Surgeons who have adopted the Archelis have found it comfortable and easy to use [42].

2.8.3 Military Application

Information on military exoskeletons is not disclosed or found in scientific communications. However, some of the data has been found in patents and information from companies that develop military and defense equipment. The exoskeletons for military applications can be divided into exploration and vigilance exoskeletons, tactical exoskeletons, and improvised explosive device disposal (IEDD)/explosive device disposal (EOD) squad. See Figure 2.13.

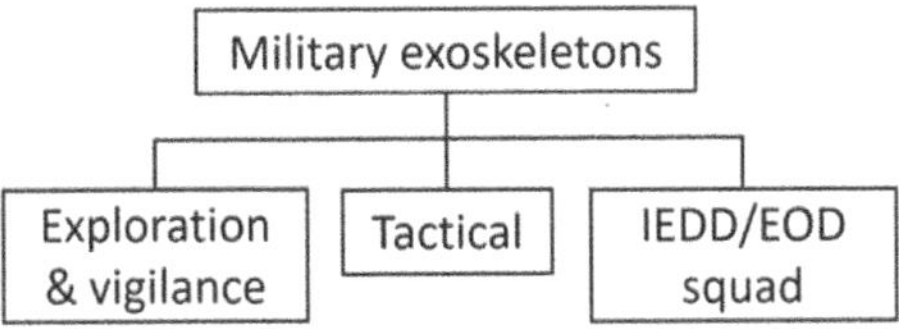

FIGURE 2.13 Military exoskeleton classification.

The exploration and vigilance exoskeletons are external removable structures that support the human musculoskeletal system, usually using full body, energy scavenging, and stationary exoskeletons. The goal is to increase strength and the capability of load vision, X-ray, and LiDAR systems and reduce fatigue. Most military exoskeletons are intended for tactical tasks such as combat, defense, fighting, attack, incursion, carrying and approaching ammunition, and shooting firearms. Tactical exoskeletons usually used are full body, lower-body-powered, and upper-body-powered exoskeletons. The exoskeletons for assisting a bomb squad or IEDD/EOD squad are full-body, passive, and energy-scavenging exoskeletons. The IEDD/EOD squad has a mission to search, detect, disarm, and dispose of explosive devices.

Full-body military exoskeletons are wearable robots that cover both the legs and arms. These full-body suits are typically large and have numerous actuators, making them challenging to power and control. As a result, the current design architecture is modular, so the exoskeletons can be configured based on specific requirements. Some examples of prototypes include the HULC by Lockheed Martin and Ekso Bionics, as well as the XSO and XSO2 by Sarcos/Raytheon.

Powered lower-body exoskeletons are designed to aid the legs and transfer loads and can be built with either rigid or soft materials. These devices assist with mobility and reduce the metabolic cost of movement. Several examples of lower-body military exoskeletons include the Compliant Universal Knee Exosuit by Ekso Bionics, ExoAtlet by ExoAtlet, Hercule by RB3D, Kinetic Operations Suit by B-Temia, prototypes by Arizona State University, prototypes by SpringActive, Wyss Exosuit by Wyss Institute, SuperFlex by SRI Robotics, Hip Actuating Exoskeleton for Running Assistance by West Point, and Power Armor by Ekso Bionics and SRI Robotics.

Passive exoskeletons are not equipped with active components such as actuators, batteries, or electronic devices and operate solely on mechanical principles. The Marine Mojo and Terra Mojo, developed by 20KTS+, are examples of passive exoskeletons that provide shock and vibration absorption to military personnel on small, fast patrol boats. Another example is the DSTO Operations Exoskeleton, which uses Bowden cables to transfer some of the weight of a soldier's heavy backpack to the ground, thereby reducing the load on the soldier's body.

Energy-scavenging exoskeletons are designed to impede the movement of soldiers to generate energy intentionally. The energy generated can be used to either recharge a battery or directly power a device. Typically, these exoskeletons extract energy from the heel strike during walking, using a compliant element that compresses and generates a small amount of energy. Two examples of such military exoskeletons are the PowerWalk by Bionic Power (which was contracted by the U.S. Army) and the SPaRK by SpringActive. The goal of these exoskeletons is to minimize the metabolic cost of carrying a rechargeable device in terms of weight and hindrance, making it lower than the metabolic cost of maintaining non-rechargeable batteries.

Stationary military exoskeletons are designed for test fire and shooting training purposes. An example of this type of exoskeleton is the MAXFAS exoskeleton (Mobile Arm Exoskeleton for Firearm Aim Stabilization). These exoskeletons are based on research on tremor suppression, intended to minimize hand movements and variations. Test subjects who have trained with these stationary exoskeletons have been able to improve their aim with a pistol.

2.9 CLOSING REMARKS AND PERSPECTIVES

In terms of state of the art, various classifications are found within the general classification when their technical characteristics and applications are analyzed in greater depth. This classification considers that multiple combinations in the subclasses can lead to hybrid exoskeleton names, so it is up to the developers how they should name an exoskeleton that meets numerous subclasses. A classification also used in the state of the art is to name some exoskeletons with the prefix pseudo-. Pseudo-passive exoskeletons have electronic components such as batteries and sensors but do not use them to provide actuation. The C-Brace by Ottobock is an example of a pseudo-passive exoskeleton that utilizes electronics to regulate a variable damper in the knee.

The industrial exoskeleton sector is growing and has a significant market opportunity. Allied Business Intelligence (ABI) Research's latest commercial and industrial robotics market data shows that the exoskeleton market was valued at US$392 million in 2020. It will grow to US$6.8 billion in global revenue in 2030 [43].

Military exoskeletons share similar challenges as their industrial counterparts, such as being comfortable to wear for extended periods and integrating with existing equipment and standards. The exoskeletons must be universal, comfortable, and fully integrated with the soldier without interfering with weapons or ability to take cover. The latest military exoskeletons have motors and actuators at the front or back of the user to address these issues. Exoskeletons must be reliable and durable and not become a liability. Using exoskeletons can help reduce the metabolic cost of carrying heavy equipment, increasing the distance soldiers can cover, making them more independent, and providing additional armor. All military exoskeletons aim to reduce metabolic costs through direct power assistance, weight transfer, or energy scavenging.

The new expectations of small exoskeleton design consider accomplishment with the homologation of design criteria and military standards. Both include simplification, modularity, indicators, and eco-design to improve usability metrics and dismiss risk through failure modes and effects analysis (FMEA).

Evaluation activity. Please answer the next quiz.
https://forms.office.com/r/Nh3x75iVvZ

1. What is the classification of robots?
   A. Industrial and military
   B. Service and military
   C. Industrial, service, and military
   D. None of the above

2. An exoskeleton can be part of three classifications of robots.
   A. True
   B. False

3. What does "wearable technology" refer to?
   A. A computer or advanced electronic device that is incorporated into an accessory worn on the body
   B. A computer or advanced electronic device that is incorporated into an item of clothing
   C. A computer or advanced electronic device that is incorporated into both an accessory worn on the body and an item of clothing
   D. None of the above

4. Choose the subcategories of the subclassification by mobilization zone.
   A. Upper and lower body
   B. Full and lower body
   C. Upper, full, and lower body
   D. Upper, full, and left body

5. Choose the conventional exoskeletons of the subclassification by technology.
   A. No interaction, HMI (PC/APP+VR)
   B. Tensegrity, mechanical, pneumatic, electric, hydraulic, HMI (PC/APP+VR)
   C. Tensegrity, mechanical, pneumatic, electric, hydraulic, no interaction
   D. Tensegrity, mechanical, pneumatic, electric, hydraulic

6. Choose the mechatronics exoskeletons of the subclassification by technology.
   A. No interaction, HMI (PC/APP+VR)
   B. Tensegrity, mechanical, pneumatic, electric, hydraulic, HMI (PC/APP+VR)
   C. Tensegrity, mechanical, pneumatic, electric, hydraulic, no interaction
   D. Tensegrity, mechanical, pneumatic, electric, hydraulic

7. Choose the subcategories of the subclassification by scope.
   A. Research, test bench, patent, and innovation
   B. Research, test bench, patent, innovation, and support
   C. Research, test bench, patent, innovation, and professional
   D. Research, test bench, patent, and teaching

8. Choose the subcategories of service exoskeletons.
   A. Water based, ground based, and aerial
   B. Medical, sports, and teaching
   C. Rehabilitation and assistive
   D. Care at home, medical, and sports

9. To which subcategory do the subcategories shown correspond?

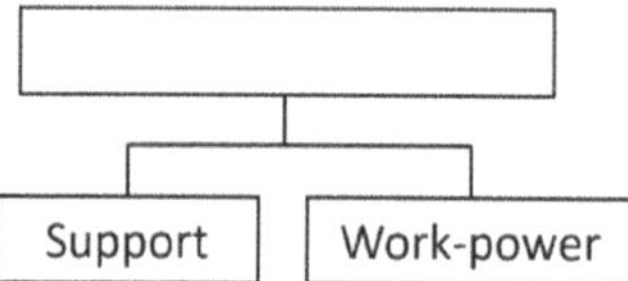

   A. Industrial exoskeletons
   B. Service exoskeletons

  C. Military exoskeletons

  D. Innovation exoskeletons

10. To which subcategory do the subcategories shown correspond?

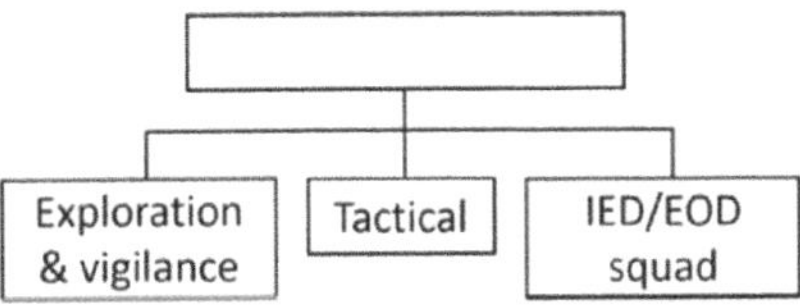

  A. Industrial exoskeletons

  B. Service exoskeletons

  C. Military exoskeletons

  D. Innovation exoskeletons

REFERENCES

1. ISO 8373, Robots and robotic devices, 2012.
2. Aviles, L.A.Z., J.C.P. Ortega, and E.G. Hurtado, Experimental study of the methodology for the modelling and simulation of mobile manipulators. International Journal of Advanced Robotic Systems, 2012.9(5): p. 192–200.
3. Qiu, S., et al., Systematic review on wearable lower extremity robotic exoskeletons for assisted locomotion. Journal of Bionic Engineering, 2022: p. 1–34.
4. Marinov, B., Soft Exoskeletons and Exosuits, 2015; Available from: https://exoskeleton-report.com/2015/08/soft-exoskeletons-and-exosuits/.
5. Gerez, L., et al., A hybrid, wearable exoskeleton glove equipped with variable stiffness joints, abduction capabilities, and a telescopic thumb. IEEE Access, 2020.8: p. 173345–173358.
6. Dávila-Vilchis, J.-M., et al., Fabric inflatable soft actuators for soft wearable devices: The MOSAR case. Machines, 2022.10(10): p. 871.
7. Davila-Vilchis, J.-M., J.C. Avila-Vilchis, and A.H. Vilchis-Gonzalez, Design criteria of soft exogloves for hand rehabilitation-assistance tasks. Applied Bionics and Biomechanics, 2020(2724783): p. 1–19.
8. Nguyen, P.H., et al., Fabric soft poly-limbs for physical assistance of daily living tasks. In 2019 International Conference on Robotics and Automation (ICRA). IEEE, 2019.
9. Althoefer, K., Antagonistic actuation and stiffness control in soft inflatable robots. Nature Reviews Materials, 2018.3(6): p. 76–77.
10. Miriyev, A., K. Stack, and H. Lipson, Soft material for soft actuators. Nature Communications, 2017.8(1): p. 596.
11. Yap, H.K., et al., Design of a soft robotic glove for hand rehabilitation of stroke patients with clenched fist deformity using inflatable plastic actuators. Journal of Medical Devices, 2016.10(4).
12. Nguyen, P.H., et al., Fabric-based soft grippers capable of selective distributed bending for assistance of daily living tasks. In 2019 2nd IEEE International Conference on Soft Robotics (RoboSoft), 2019. p. 404–409.
13. Gorissen, B., et al., Elastic inflatable actuators for soft robotic applications. Advanced Materials, 2017.29(43): p. 1604977.
14. Mosadegh, B., et al., Pneumatic networks for soft robotics that actuate rapidly. Advanced Functional Materials, 2014.24(15): p. 2163–2170.

15. Polygerinos, P., et al., Towards a soft pneumatic glove for hand rehabilitation. In 2013 IEEE/RSJ International Conference on Intelligent Robots and Systems. IEEE, 2013.

16. Hofer, M. and R. D'Andrea, Design, modeling, and control of a soft robotic arm. In 2018 IEEE/RSJ International Conference on Intelligent Robots and Systems (IROS). IEEE, 2018.

17. Paez-Granados, D., et al., Passive flow control for series inflatable actuators: Application on a wearable soft-robot for posture assistance. IEEE Robotics and Automation Letters, 2021.6(3): p. 4891–4898.

18. Nishioka, Y., et al., Development of a soft pneumatic actuator with pleated inflatable structures. Advanced Robotics, 2017.31(14): p. 753–762.

19. Oguntosin, V., et al., Development of a wearable assistive soft robotic device for elbow rehabilitation. In 2015 IEEE International Conference on Rehabilitation Robotics (ICORR). IEEE, 2015.

20. Thalman, C.M., et al., A novel soft elbow exosuit to supplement bicep lifting capacity. In 2018 IEEE/RSJ International Conference on Intelligent Robots and Systems (IROS). IEEE, 2018.

21. Passive or Active Exoskeletons—National Safety Council; Available from: www.nsc.org/workplace/safety-topics/work-to-zero/safety-technologies/passive-or-active-exoskeletons.

22. Ingber, D.E. and M. Landau, Tensegrity. Scholarpedia, 2012.7(2): p. 8344.

23. Ingber, D.E. and M. Landau, Tensegrity. Scholarpedia, 2012: p. 8344.

24. How does the AIRFRAME™ work? 2020; Available from: www.levitatetech.com/2018/01/28/how-do-exoskeletons-work/.

25. Larry, L.H., S. Magleby, and B. OLsen, Handbook of Compliant Mechanisms. John Wiley & Sons Ltd, 2013.

26. Perez-Vidal, A., Soft exoskeletons | Encyclopedia MDPI.

27. Zhang, J.-F., et al., 5-Link model-based gait trajectory adaption control strategies of the gait rehabilitation exoskeleton for post-stroke patients. Mechatronics, 2010.20(3): p. 368–376.

28. Ashraf, M., et al., (β, γ)-Skew QC codes with derivation over a semi-local ring. Symmetry, 2023.15(1): p. 225.

29. Bleuler, H., et al., Exoskeletons as a mechatronic design example. In New Trends in Medical and Service Robotics: Advances in Theory and Practice. Springer, 2019.

30. Mubin, O., et al., Exoskeletons with virtual reality, augmented reality, and gamification for stroke patients' rehabilitation: Systematic review. JMIR Rehabilitation and Assistive Technologies, 2019.6(2): p. e12010.

31. Marinov, B., Exoskeletons for Gaming and Virtual Reality, 2017; Available from: https://exoskeletonreport.com/2017/02/exoskeletons-for-gaming-and-virtual-reality/.

32. Secco, E.L. and A.M. Tadesse, A wearable exoskeleton for hand kinesthetic feedback in virtual reality. In Wireless Mobile Communication and Healthcare: 8th EAI International Conference, MobiHealth 2019, Dublin, Ireland, November 14–15, 2019, Proceedings 8.2020. Springer.

33. Gupta, A. and M.K. O'Malley, Design of a haptic arm exoskeleton for training and rehabilitation. IEEE/ASME Transactions on mechatronics, 2006.11(3): p. 280–289.

34. Cybergrasp; Available from: www.cyberglovesystems.com/cybergrasp.

35. Papetti, S., et al., Vibrotactile sensitivity in active touch: Effect of pressing force. IEEE Transactions on Haptics, 2016.10(1): p. 113–122.

36. Kara, D., Industrial exoskeletons: New systems, improved tech, increasing adoption; Industrial exoskeletons is an enormous market, as are the rewards for solution providers that can deliver real business value, 2018; Available from: www.therobotreport.com/industrial-exoskeletons/.

37. Marinov, B., 22 Exoskeletons for work and industry into 6 categories. In Exoskeleton Report, 2016.
38. Müller, C., B. Graf, and K. Pfeiffer, World Robotics 2022—Service Robots. I.S. Department, 2022.
39. Neuhaus, P.D., et al., Concept designs for underwater swimming exoskeletons. In IEEE International Conference on Robotics and Automation. Proceedings. ICRA'04. IEEE, 2004.
40. RoboGolfPro, in Exoskeleton Report, 2016.
41. Marinov, B., 42 Medical Exoskeletons into 6 Categories. In Exoskeleton Report, 2016.
42. Wille, M., Archelis' exoskeleton makes working on your feet as easy as sitting, 2022; Available from: www.inverse.com/input/tech/archelis-exoskeleton-makes-working-on-your-feet-as-easy-as-sitting.
43. Exoskeletons in 2020: A technology still finding its feet. August 23, 2022; Available from: https://www.abiresearch.com/market-research/insight/7778603-exoskeletons-in-2020-a-technology-still-fi/.

3 Design Methodologies

3.1 INTRODUCTION

Today, more than ever, medical devices should be safe and reliable. For this, their design requires tools that include state-of-the-art technological levels. Apart from those features, exoskeletons should be accepted in the market and meet different requirements. The evolution of exoskeletons' design tools has driven the creation of new methodologies for defining user requirements. It should consider the speed of their establishment not to affect exoskeletons' development times.

Product design is the process designers and engineers use to solve real problems and satisfy market needs. This process has evolved enormously in recent years with the occurrence of modern tools. The current trends in the development of products focus on multidisciplinary teams. The development process begins with the design strategy and methodology, which outline the aspects and methods that will be included in the product design. This chapter addresses the beginning of the product design using several design methodologies, such as product lifecycle management, quality function deployment, axiomatic design, design for assembly, and platforms products. A case study based on implementing a toolkit of product design methodologies is presented here, which concerns the design of a product family of exoskeletons. Different parameters involved in the operating principle of exoskeletons are considered for such a product family.

3.2 PRODUCT LIFECYCLE MANAGEMENT

The design is understandable in a simple way as the activity for sketching forms of ideas; however, creating products in the year 2023 is more complex than only forms. Fast fabrication is the base of the new meaning for the design word, so reaching the design target requires the strategy and organization of the work team. The recent trends in the development of products focus on multidisciplinary teams.

Product lifecycle management (PLM) is achieved with multidisciplinary teams working based on concurrent engineering using technologies platforms, including servers and clients who have access as authors or visualizers. In a collaborative environment, the PLM software interacts with developers and suppliers, as well as with developers and customers. Both interactions support product development, so developers meet customer requirements based on user complaints and satisfaction letters; likewise, suppliers participate during industrial design and development [1], interacting with developers to supply appropriate manufacturing resources, and with customers for design concept tests and prototype testing surveys [1]. The PLM software manages the collaboration with engineering resources product (ERP) software, the product data management (PDM) software, and the Industrial Internet of Things (IIoT) software [2].

DOI: 10.1201/9781003261995-3

The PDM software and ERP software collaborate using the bill of materials (BOM); this BOM includes the materials stock of developers and the materials stock of suppliers; by means of the PLM, the suppliers allow access to their material inventory for it to be used in the product development.

The IIoT software allows collaboration in the Internet cloud, such as among the design workstations, machinery, quality control, production monitoring, other factories, developers of the test bench, and suppliers [3].

The PDM includes computer-aided design (CAD) software, computer-aided engineering (CAE) software, and computer-aided manufacturing (CAM) software. Currently, most CAD, CAE, and CAM include PDM connections. Figure 3.1 shows the interaction among the informatics technologies inclusive in the PLM.

The evolution of technology has motivated the updating of definitions according to emergent approaches and techniques used for new product development (NPD); today, the stages for NPD are research, development, and innovation [4].

The product lifecycle begins with the product's conception in the research stage, and it continues interacting with the development and later with the innovation. Hence, it reaches the product's first generation. Figure 3.2 presents the cycle where the exoskeleton is introduced to the market, grown, reaches maturity at the top of the curve, and begins the generational replacement with the product of the next generation.

The design process requires interaction in the cloud of technological tools that accelerate and control the development of a new product. Technological platforms manage the planning, lifecycle, development phases, prioritization of participation in the project, intellectual property, and product maturity until it is commercialized; then they plan the next generation of the product. The second block describes tools that allow interaction among software, emphasizing the elements that make up modeling and prototyping. Prototyping is related to the emulation of systems on the

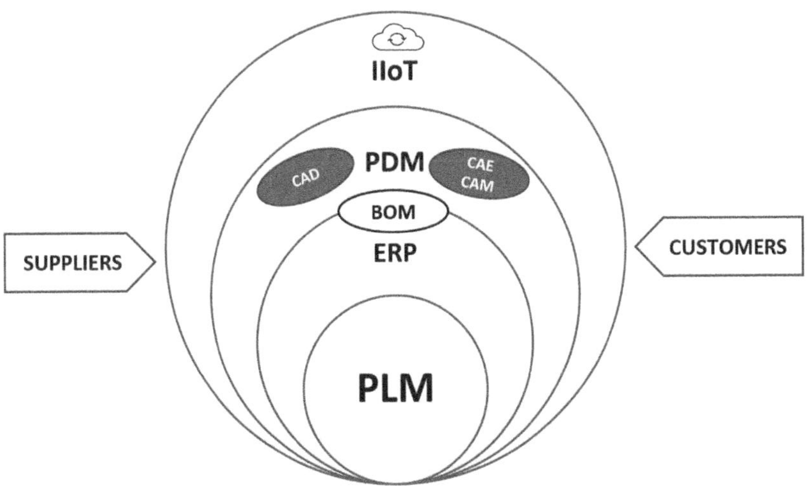

FIGURE 3.1 Framework of PLM in the exoskeleton design.

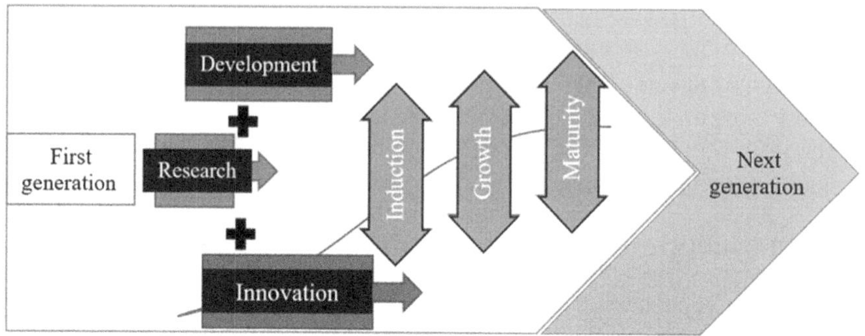

FIGURE 3.2 Cycle of product development.

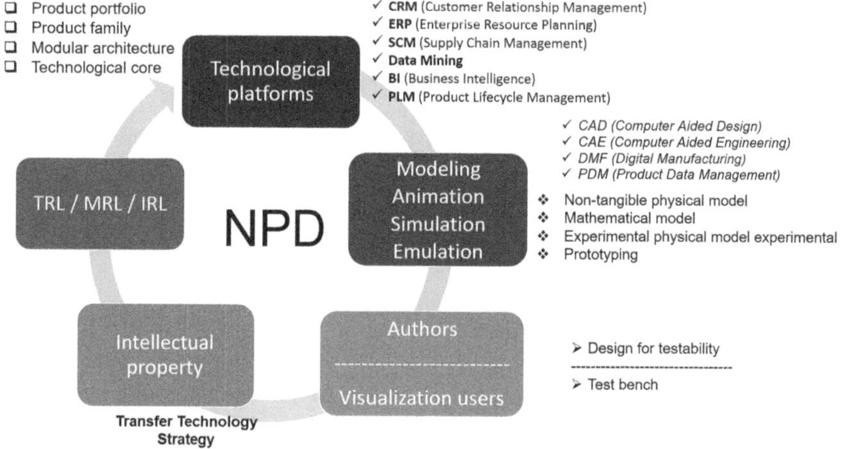

FIGURE 3.3 Interaction of key technological tools for new product development.

test bench, that is, in a laboratory environment with experiments conducted under controlled conditions. A hierarchy is used to facilitate the interaction of all the technological tools and give privileges to the authors, who generate information, and to the visualization users, who cannot modify the models but can use the information to structure the tests. On the test bench, simulations are performed, and engineering drawings and process sheets are generated. Figure 3.3 shows the participation and interaction of key technological tools and highlights some critical aspects, including the product portfolio, which today follows the development of products to satisfy different market segments.

In this book, the design process is limited to the phase of the product formulation, which starts from a creative process of idealization concerning a work environment, criteria (conditions, problem/opportunity, SWOT, budget, risk mitigation plan), and specifications (parameters and constraints), for which a methodological strategy is established concerning the timeline to deliver a prototype.

3.3 DESIGN METHODOLOGIES

Several design methodologies emerged from World War II, some of which have been consolidated and complemented based on concurrent engineering trends. The product design methods (PDMs) toolkit is presented here, which considers several design methods and aspects used as design guidelines. The methods included in the PDMs toolkit are the market pull, technology push, and quality function deployment (QFD). In addition, a tool group based on 40 principles and 39 innovation parameters to solve problems is the theory of inventive problem solving (TIPS), whose Russian acronym is TRIZ. In addition, this toolkit includes the axiomatic design, the product platforms, the design for X, and a methodology for modeling and simulation based on homogeneous transformation graphic (HTG).

The PDMs toolkit has been improved over 20 years of design practice to develop new products; this toolkit considers 11 aspects and nine methods (Table 3.1).

3.3.1 EXPECTATIONS FOR INNOVATION USING THE MARKET PULL

One of the approaches to innovation is to start the generation of a new product based on market demand. It is expected to provide solutions based on the market need. The design team's capabilities are assessed by evaluating the complexity of the product and establishing the scope as incremental innovation or disruptive innovation. The former includes adaptation and improvements within paradigms; the disruptive or radical innovation includes out-of-paradigm improvements, invention, or discovery [5]. Later, the strategy is developed either by open innovation (collaboration among universities, startups, and others) or closed innovation (typically when the development process is confidential), so the design, manufacturing, marketing, and sales begin [6].

TABLE 3.1

Aspects and Methods Included in PDMs Toolkit

Item	Aspect	Method
1	Expectation for innovation	Market pull
		Technology push
2	Design criteria	
3	Design attributes	
4	Requirements	QFD
5	Functional requirements	QFD and TRIZ
6	Design parameters	QFD and axiomatic design
7	Constraints	
8	Communality index	Product platforms
9	DFA index	Design for X
10	Modeling and simulation	HTG methodology
11	Implementation	PDMs frameworks

In principle, one might think that the pull of the market is open innovation; however, companies like Google, Microsoft, and Apple prevent other companies from benefiting from their products, developing confidentially [7]. Different companies use open innovation collaboration to determine market needs. Bayer, through start-ups, studies the need for medical systems by integrating the stakeholders involved in the rehabilitation process (doctor, physiotherapist, and patient); the market needs can be better feedbacked through networking with the hospitals [8].

3.3.2　The Expectation for Innovation Using the Technology Push

Another approach to innovation is to start the generation of new products based on the evolution of technology. It is expected to give solutions, usually as improvements to existing operating principles or from the results of basic science, such as the case of the increase of mechanical properties of some material. Subsequently, the technology implementation is evaluated, establishing the scope as incremental or disruptive.

The technology push generally contrasts with the pull of the market; it is how technology comes out and creates value in society [9]. Someone has devised a technology that often works from a scientific perspective, for example, some development of a system that moves air in larger quantities with less power; however, there is no guarantee that it will fit in the market, who the client will be, and how it will add value. Thus, it is necessary to make a lot of effort to bring technology to the community. Other examples are the car, the camera, the Internet, the touch screen, and the cell phone; all these things that nobody asked for, but the developers came up with based on new technology, and it could be pushed to the market, as well as assimilate and adopt it [10].

Ideas are often brought to market and tailored based on feedback. Therefore, there is a combination of technology push and market pull back and forth to create a long-term product reaching a minimally viable product. But it must be brought to market, quickly learned from customers, and improved. As the technology push approach relates to patent/technology licensing, it is done with a way of thinking of open innovation. It is negotiated in a market; if it does not fit, it moves to other markets or is licensed to those who can use the technology in other ways. This technology licensing is why intellectual assets are used to transfer rights in multiple contexts simultaneously. Each intellectual asset is a portfolio of possibilities, both for one market and another, as long as they do not overlap. It is a relatively easy value proposition; licensees want to collaborate to implement the technology, but some do not want to pay much [11].

The capabilities needed for a successful technology push approach are understanding the technology deeply using the intellectually active management framework, where the licensees can capture the different technological elements that allow the operation of the solution. Finally, a comparison must be made to analyze the position in the market and work toward success [12]. Some others resort to closed innovation, sensing the market. Another example of a technology push with open innovation is BMW, with an idea platform where any user could contribute ideas, concepts, and patents on new technologies, where 3% are a reality. Others, such as Metalsa, Enel AstraZeneca, and Ford, through the inocentive.com platform, propose their innovation challenges together with an economic incentive [13]. The National Aeronautics and Space Administration (NASA) is investigating the ability of the technology to fold wings during flight. The solution proposes the technologies to solve problems without focusing on demand, but on the technological advance reached after the improvements have been implemented [14].

3.3.3 DESIGN CRITERIA

Each application environment is different, so the product design must be congruent with the market segment, the application sector, and the development area. Thus, the solutions must be pertinent concerning references to the application environment; then, said reference serves as a design guideline and involves the design trend, the sector of use, standards that regulate its use, its tests, and its validation. The design criteria are conditions that must be accomplished for design approval; an example is the congruence criterion, where two triangles are congruent if two of their indicated angles have the same value [15]. Suppose the use of axiomatic design as a design tool. In that case, the axiom of independence, among others, should be fulfilled; the axiomatic design is defined as the process of seeking the uncoupled solution in the relationship between functional requirement (FR) and design parameter (DP). Then, the independence axiom will be fulfilled for a given key under the axiomatic design approach, which is a design criterion [16]. As has been observed, the design criteria are an obligatory step when starting the product design.

3.3.4 DESIGN ATTRIBUTES

The term attributes refers to qualities that differentiate a product from those known in the market through a value offered. This contribution can be an adaptation, an improvement within paradigms, an improvement outside paradigms, or an invention. Price and quality are often the most used at the beginning of the search for different aspects of the products. However, it is not the most recommended when starting a new product design. When the operating principle and the minimum viable product are reached, it is recommended to work on the quality strategy to meet customer expectations through certifications as well as comply with standards that occur at a level of technological maturity TRL8, which represents the product as a reliable option. With this technological readiness level, the pricing strategy can be generated, sometimes through a high price and high investment in promotion; subsequently, its cost will be reduced to reach the rest of the consumers, known as a skimming strategy. Other times, a penetration strategy is used, where a reduced initial price is introduced to attract the maximum number of consumers and win the market. This strategy is usually used in products with fewer attributes or different aspects and as a test method to publicize the product in its initial stages [17].

As explained, the price and quality can be confusing when starting the product design, so it is preferable to focus on other attributes at the beginning so that the value of the product is sustained, for instance, on factors like modularity, scalability, robustness, portability, wearable, gadgets, styling, and customizing. For this, it is essential to perform a benchmarking to identify and differentiate the product from that of competitors and define the client's requirements or clients in the displayed market segments.

3.3.5 REQUIREMENTS

The user requirements, also called the voice of the customer (VOC), consolidate needs and improvements expected in the new product. Today, there are multiple methodologies to understand the requirements that must be met in the product. An example is design thinking, where empathizing with the user is essential in addition to defining the needs and perceptions of users; another methodology is the user-centered design, which seeks to find the definition of the problem and, from this problem, build a value offer [18].

However, first, the user and the customer are defined, understanding that there may be different types of users, but only one customer, who is the one who pays for the product. For this reason, the house of quality (HOQ) is used to build the list of requirements. HOQ is part of the QFD methodology, where user requirements are listed and prioritized in conjunction with improvements to products already in the market. Then, a survey is conducted aimed at stakeholders who are part of a select group of users, such as suppliers, distributors, and users with proven experience.

3.3.6 FUNCTIONAL REQUIREMENTS

User requirements are analyzed, and using the first house of quality (HOQ1), technical solutions are proposed to meet those requirements; these solutions are called functional requirements (FR). For instance, suppose that a VOC is to have hot water when washing dishes that are self-regulating so as not to have to compensate between hot and cold water, then the FR would self-regulate the water temperature at $35 \pm 3\,°C$. In the QFD methodology, the user requirements are called whats, while the FRs are called hows. Every FR can meet one or more VOCs, although sometimes the FRs contradict each other. Take as an example high speed versus low weight. The TRIZ methodology is used to solve this contradiction, which includes 39 parameters and 40 innovation principles. When the parameters come into contradiction where one improves and the other worsens, they are resolved by the matrix of contradictions with some inventive principle; then the relationship of each FR with each VOC is evaluated, comparing the proposed technical solutions with the solutions of the competitors for each VOC [19].

3.3.7 DESIGN PARAMETERS

The FRs help us to consolidate the design target in a numerical way. In the second house of quality (HOQ2), the FRs are taken as input; now, the whats are the FRs, and the hows are the DPs. First, the FRs are analyzed in numerical form, following the previous section's example; suppose that an FR is to have a water temperature of $35\,°C \pm 3\,°C$. The DP would use a thermostat with digital temperature control with an error of $\pm 1\,°C$. In HOQ2 the QFD methodology is used, where each DP corresponds to an FR. Once the DPs are numerically defined, the relationships of each DP with each FR are evaluated concerning the axiomatic design equation, specifically the axiom of independence (Equation 3.1).

$$\{FR_1 \vdots FR_n\} = (X \cdots 0 \vdots \cdot \cdot \vdots 0 \cdots X)\{DP_1 \vdots DP_n\} \tag{3.1}$$

The list of FRs is used as a vector equal to the product of the design matrix by the vector of DPs. There are three possible design matrices; one of them is a coupled design matrix, where there are multiple relationships between the DPs and the FRs, which is not desirable since it means that while one FR is fulfilled, another FR is damaged. Another matrix is a decoupled design matrix, where the design improves by decreasing the relationships; this option usually presents a triangular matrix. Finally, the ideal design concerning the axiomatic design is represented by an uncoupled matrix, a matrix with minimal or null relationships, which presents a diagonal matrix [20].

3.3.8 Constraints

The product's technical specifications (tech specs) include the design parameters and the design constraints; these constraints can be external or internal. External constraints consider the operating environment and the coupling of subsystems in the product or the coupling of the product in a system that incorporates or integrates it. The internal restrictions condition the operation of the product, that is, the interactions in a mechanism, the assembly means, or the contacts between components [21].

3.3.9 Commonality Index

Product platforms include modular architectures and integral architectures. Modular architectures include modules and connectors or buses to be interchangeable and achieve modularity or scalability of the product. Integral architectures are typically dedicated to systems that do not allow the interchange of components, for example, an electronic board, a control system, a mechanism, etc. The communality index (CI) is used as a measure of the product's modularity, which must be greater than 60% to achieve an acceptable CI [22].

3.3.10 DFA Index

The design for X methodology, also known as design for excellence (DFX), is a group of methods where the X is a variable that can have one of many possible values [4]. The DFX includes the design for assembly (DFA), which is measured by an index that allows determining the assembly faster by simplifying the product's structure and selecting essential as well as non-essential components. The acceptable DFA index must be greater than 60%, which reduces the number of parts required to be assembled [23].

3.3.11 Modeling and Simulation

Modeling and simulation are the central stages of the design and development of the product. After having generated the idealization and the design concept, the modeling phase is reached, which includes three kinds of models: the computational, iconic, digital model, and virtual in CAD software; the mathematical model that is made based on the HTG; and the experimental physical model (EPM) [24]. The simulation is developed based on the modeling and includes three kinds: the simulation in CAE software for structural evaluation, computational fluid dynamics, and motion assessment; the numerical simulation using mathematical software such as Matlab, using the multibody systems module in along with the mathematical model; and the CAM simulation that performed by taking the CAD components of the modeling phase, which are generated in the assessment for the manufacturing and are refined according to the machining times and the manufacturing process. The simulation in CAE software is usually validated with at least two solvers, obtaining a permissible correlation index; the numerical simulation is validated with the position in the workspace through a graphical user interface (GUI). The simulation is subsequently validated by comparing it with the emulation carried out on a test bench, for which a permissible error is taken. A machining test for the validation of CAM simulation is also carried out. However, when machining complex workpieces (high accuracy), waste is expensive and can break the tool by features of new material (e.g., sintering materials), due to the machinability properties of new materials. It is necessary to use techniques based on kinematics and dynamics simulation [25].

3.3.12 PDMs Frameworks

The design methodologies included in the PDMs toolkit are implemented based on five frameworks. Figure 3.4 shows the first framework consisting of seven stages for product generation development. The design concept stage is where the solution is formulated. The animation stage is distinguished by the fact that there is no physical force feedback, but rather the operation system is proposed; animation software like Unreal Engine, Unity, 3D Max, Maya, Character Studio, and Poser are used for this task. The modeling stage includes three kinds of models; the first is the CAD model (non-tangible physical model), distinguished by the fact that CAD software is used to allow the feedback of physical force (SolidWorks, Solid Edge, Inventor, among others); the second is the math model, which is referred to in kinematics and dynamics model as ; the third model is the EPM, which is used to validate the operating principle of the system. The simulation stage is identified because CAE software is

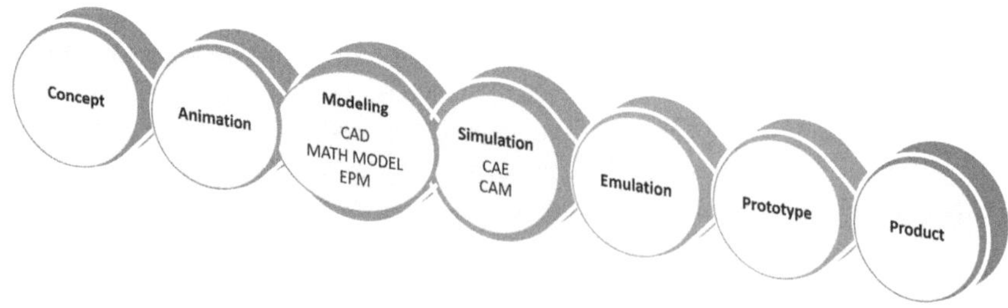

FIGURE 3.4 Stages for the generation of new products for exoskeletons.

used to verify the system behavior in the computational environment. Simulation is validated, obtaining a correlation index among this behavior and its behavior of EPM in the test bench. The emulation stage is characterized by the use of instrumented test benches to perform emulation tests of the system behavior in a real environment. The prototyping stage is dedicated to obtaining a prototype, the first replicable type with which it is expected to have field tests; once the prototype is controlled and released, the consolidation stage of the product can be reached [26].

Figure 3.5 presents the second framework where the interaction among technology readiness level (TRL), manufacturing readiness level (MRL), and investment readiness level (IRL) is shown. As mentioned in the first framework, the design starts with the design concept corresponding to TRL1 and TRL2 levels. The EPM alpha, where the design concept is validated and the TRL3 level is reached, is related to the MRL1 and MRL2 levels, which correspond to initial materials. The TRL4 level is reached when there is an EPM validated in a laboratory environment, which is related to an IRL1 level where a preliminary market analysis is started (complete first-pass business model canvas or lean model canvas). TRL5 level is reached when there is a beta prototype; TRL5 is related to MRL3, where an experimental lot is manufactured, as well as to IRL2 in which the market analysis is defined (market size: total available market [TAM], serviceable available market [SAM], and target market). TRL6 level is reached when there is a prototype operating in relevant environment testing; it is related to the MRL4 level, where the manufacturing technologies are determined, as well as to IRL3, where there is the solution validation. TRL7 is reached when there is a prototype operating in real testing; it is related to MRL5, where most of the materials and tooling are refined, as well as to IRL4, where there is a valuable minimum product (VMP) of low fidelity. TRL8 level is reached when there is a certified product. It is related to MRL6 and MRL7, where all materials are defined and tested in the pilot production lines, and IRL7, a VMP of high fidelity. TRL9 level is reached when there is a commercial product. So, in MRL8 is released the initial production and in MRL9 is carried out the process statistical control. In IRL8, there is a value delivery, and IRL9 is focused on metrics-based growth [27].

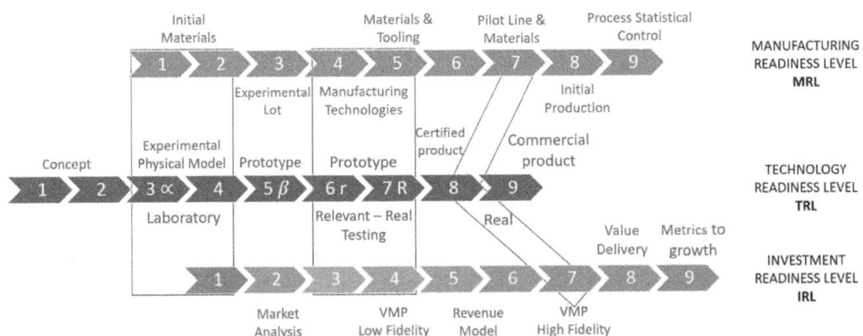

FIGURE 3.5 Interaction among TRL, MRL, and IRL for exoskeletons.

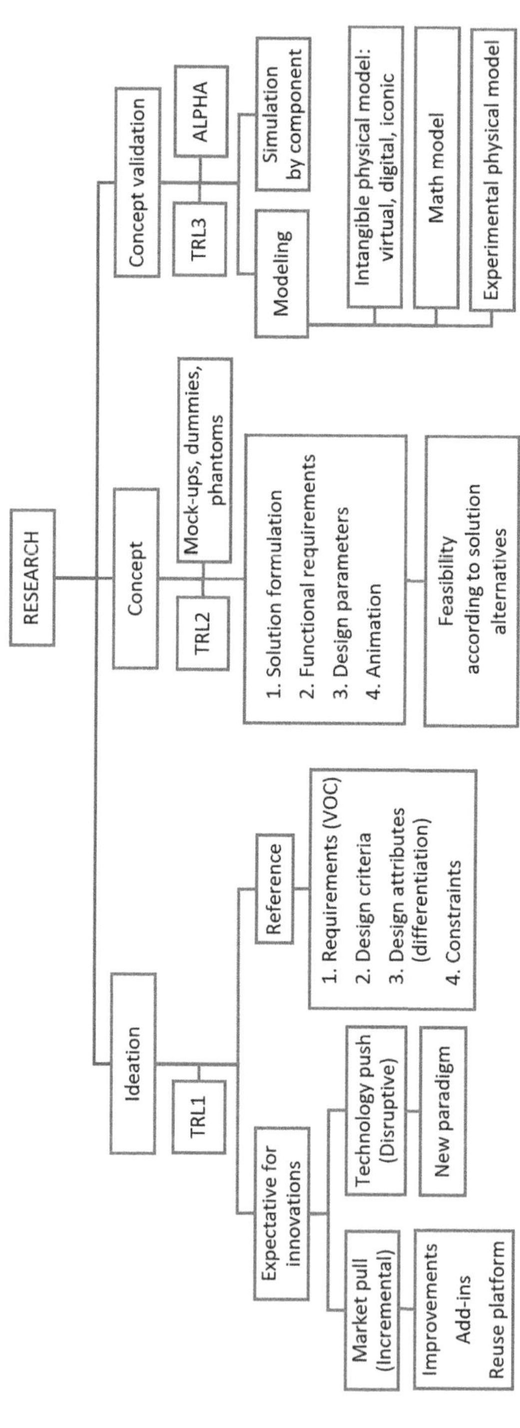

FIGURE 3.6 Phases of research in the TRL for exoskeletons.

Figure 3.6 shows the third framework corresponding to the TRL's research phases. The premise is to create a value offer based on a clear differential concerning competitors. However, this task is not so easy. Suppose the market demand (users) is analyzed, and based on this, an expected fast solution is proposed; it is best to think of it as an incremental innovation, in which case it will be an enhancement to a reuse platform plugin or app. Since a solution that implies a greater differential is based on new technology, this is not so trivial, requiring more scientific research time since the uncertainty is higher. Then the approach would initially be to use the technology push and later make the pertinent modifications to adapt the product to an application that is in demand in the market; therefore, we will be making a mixture of the two approaches. It should be considered that this procedure is recommended in designs made by universities and entrepreneurs with limited experience in the industrialization of products to obtain disruptive innovations. Companies or entrepreneurs with extensive experience in the industrialization of products use the technological surveillance of the competitors based on the technology push and take the technological trend as a reference. Solutions are created with a risk mitigation plan since the more different the products are, the higher the risk; however, it is a constant task that consolidates their reputation as creators of disruptive innovations [28].

The fourth framework in Figure 3.7 shows the TRL's development phases. Since it is preferable to improve something tangible, the product's refinement revolves around small-scale manufacturing. This manufacturing allows statistically evaluating the occurrence of failures and the repeatability of the operating principle to have controllable operating ranges and allowable errors both of tolerances and system adjustments, such as security in interaction with users. For this, usability metrics are used, which will ensure the product's performance [29].

Figure 3.8 shows the fifth framework in the phases of deployment in the TRL. In the development phase, we were able to observe how important it is to repeat the operating principle in experimental demonstration and industrial environment to reach the necessary maturity of the product so that it can be implemented and

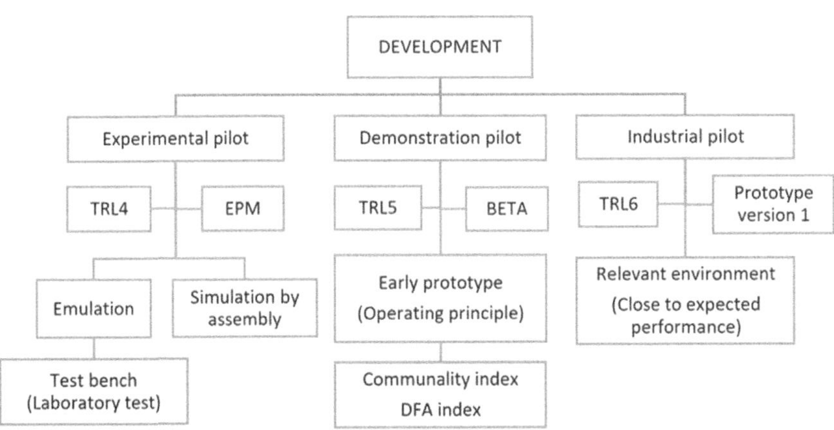

FIGURE 3.7   Phases of development in the TRL for exoskeletons.

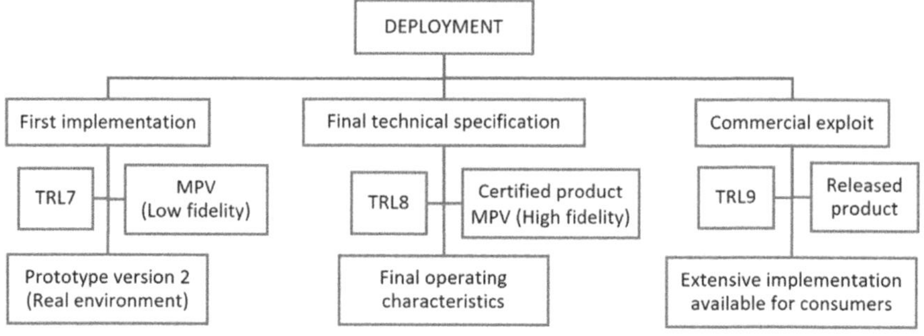

FIGURE 3.8 Phases of deployment in the TRL for exoskeletons.

commercially exploited based on the tech specs validated both in test benches and with users [30].

3.4 A CASE STUDY BASED ON PDMS TOOLKIT

3.4.1 Exoskeleton Description

A two-degrees-of-freedom continuous passive mobilizer, configurable for right or left knee rehabilitation, with the capability to switch between lying, sitting, and standing therapy position modes. It includes 21 components, grouped into three subsystems: main base; configurable mobilizer assembly; and adaptable mechanism for children, adolescents, and adults. In lying therapy mode, the belt rotates on the hip base pin and keeps the patient's abdomen and back on the bed. In seated therapy mode, the belt rotates on the hip base pin, supporting the patient's abdomen, considering that the patient's buttocks rest on the bed or wheelchair. In standing mode, the patient walks, propelling the feet on a conveyor belt, and the hip base supports the patient's weight through support, which is depicted in Figure 3.9.

3.4.2 Market Pull Analysis

Briefly, an analysis of the TAM for medical devices is carried out; for this, the exoskeleton market size was selected. The global exoskeleton market size was valued at USD 254.8 million in 2022 and is forecast to reach USD 1.4 billion by 2032 at a compound annual growth rate (CAGR) of 17.2%. These exoskeletons differ according to their structure, mechanisms, control, and actuators. Several factors, including the aging population and the increasing adoption of medical equipment in various industries such as defense, construction, and automobiles, are driving the exoskeleton market growth. Additionally, there has been an increase in the incidence rate of strokes and spinal cord injuries (SCIs) globally. According to the National Spinal Cord Injury Statistical Center (NSCISC), the number of SCI cases for 2019, 2020, and 2021 was 17,730, 17,810, and 10,900, respectively, and a further 296,000 Americans have suffered from SCIs [31].

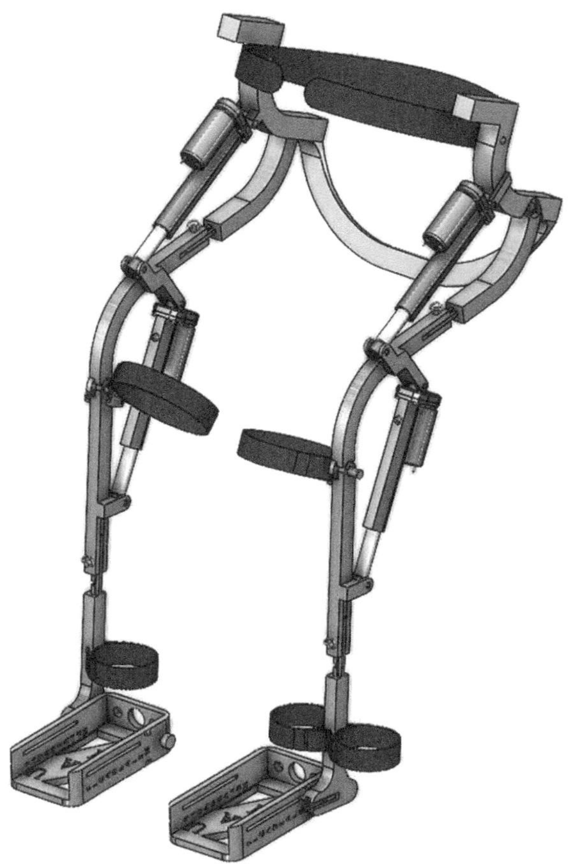

FIGURE 3.9   Exoskeleton for knee rehabilitation.

In the projected future, there will be a high demand for technological advancements and diverse products, creating significant potential for innovative companies. The materials used in the industry include steel, aluminum, carbon fiber, polycarbonate, and other polymers. The polymer subsegment is expected to grow the fastest due to its higher manufacturing efficiency using 3D printing techniques. Further development is expected in the healthcare industry in North America, especially in the United States, owing to its leading investment in medical devices. North America (Canada, USA, Mexico) is the region that has grown the most annually; therefore, it is the market chosen to compete in. Figure 3.10 shows the market analysis for the North American area.

3.4.3   Design Criteria

Most of these criteria are considered to define a robust exoskeleton design. The standard is used to evaluate the design concerning norms like FDA, ISO, ASME, IEEE,

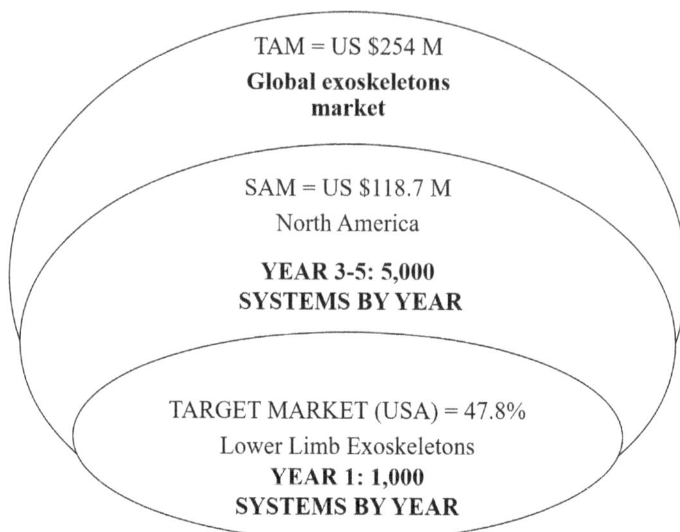

FIGURE 3.10   Market analysis of exoskeletons for North America.

TABLE 3.2

Criteria for Exoskeleton Design

Item	Name	Item	Name
1	Mobilization zone	12	Usability
2	Structure	13	Maintainability
3	Action type	14	Safety
4	Standard	15	Elegant design
5	User interaction	16	Styling
6	Required capacitation	17	Customizing
7	Pathologies	18	Scalability
8	Interaction virtual axis	19	Reliability
9	Kutzbach-Grubler	20	Profitability-viability-feasibility
10	Standardization	21	Quality
11	Portability	22	Sustainability

---

and IEC standards. The standard includes the rules according to the approved body, while standardization is used as a technique aiming to reduce the number of different parts within a product. In other words, standardization is part of having more common parts than unique ones, which is represented by the commonality index (CI). Table 3.2 shows the criteria taken into account for exoskeleton design.

In order to design an exoskeleton, different requirements and specifications that affect the performance and ergonomics of the hand exoskeleton should be considered. Some primary design characteristics are [32] as follows: Transparency; in other words, a haptic device that can be worn as an exoskeleton should provide a seamless connection to remote and virtual environments. This means that the user should experience a sense of touch when interacting with virtual objects as if they were interacting with real objects. The degree of stiffness that can be achieved by the exoskeleton depends on the mechanical rigidity of the system and the controller's stability. The performance of the device is crucial to the overall effectiveness of the haptic display, regardless of the control algorithm used. In essence, the maximum stiffness of the exoskeleton is determined by the system's mechanical rigidity and controller's stability, and the device's performance plays a vital role in the performance of the haptic display. The performance of a system is heavily influenced by its actuation method, as well as the type of actuation and transmission systems employed. A range of actuation technologies is available, including electric motors, hydraulic, pneumatic, magneto-rheological, electro-rheological, electroactive polymers, and shape memory alloys. However, the selection of an actuation method may impact the portability of the system. For a haptic device to provide high force fidelity, its force feedback system must have the capability to render a maximum range or limits of force, velocity, and acceleration. However, when interacting with hard contacts that require high forces or fast deceleration to display impulsive forces, the performance of an active force feedback control may suffer from actuator saturation. In other words, the haptic device's ability to apply high forces may be limited, which could impact its ability to accurately render the sensation of interacting with hard surfaces. When designing a haptic device for wearability, it is important to consider several factors. First, the kinematic design should be such that it can accommodate different hand sizes with minimal adjustment required. The actuation system should be lightweight, portable, and compact, making the device easy to carry around. Additionally, the device should be comfortable to wear, and the way it is attached to the fingers should not impede hand motions. Typically, there are two ways to attach such a device—through single-point attachment or multi-phalangeal attachment; single point attachment is simpler and provides haptic transparency by reducing unwanted internal forces between the mechanical structures and the finger phalanges; multiple attachments to the phalanges provide an easier way of articulation of the finger and provide direct feedback forces to the attached phalanges—such a design considers the number of DOF achievable by the hand and the size of the workspace reachable by the human hand [33].

Proper alignment of the exoskeleton joint and hand joint must be preserved during the use of these devices. Various reasons lead to improper alignment of the exoskeleton joints from the finger joints. The first one is the inherently compliant mounting of the exoskeleton onto the hand, which leads to inaccurate positioning of the exoskeleton joints during movements. The other one is that the intersubject variability of the anatomical structure, size, and shape of the hands requires an adjustable mechanism to align the joints.

3.4.4 Requirements

The user requirements to design the new portfolio products were defined from an analysis of scientific communications and patents. This portfolio includes two product families, a platform, and a modular architecture.

3.4.5 Functional Requirements

The FR are detailed numerical solutions that are proposed to meet user requirements. When these FR are in contradiction, using the TRIZ methodology—in this case, supposing the integral architecture is an FR that is in contradiction with the commonality index—then the recommended principle is the modular architecture. Table 3.3 shows the relationship between user requirements (VOC) and functional requirements (FR).

3.4.6 Design Parameters

The design parameters (DP) are detailed numerical solutions that are proposed to meet functional requirements based on the axiom of independence from axiomatic design. Table 3.4 shows the relationship between functional requirements (FR) and design parameters (DP).

3.4.7 Constraints

Design constraints are conditions that delimit the formulation of solutions and the principle of operation in the design problem. They can be described in a mathematical way when related to the operating environment or coupling with other systems; in this case, they are called external constraints. Internal constraints intervene in

TABLE 3.3

User Requirements and Functional Requirements

VOC	FR
Lightweight	Polymers and sintered materials
Customization	Modular architecture
Scalability	CI >60%
Standardization	CI >60%
Elegant design	DFA index >60%

TABLE 3.4

Functional Requirements and Design Parameters

FRs	DPs
Polymers and sintered materials	70% of components
Modular architecture	Methodology of product platforms, creating two product families
CI >60%	Methodology of product platforms, creating two product families
DFA index >60%	DFA algorithm to select the essential and non-essential parts

---

TABLE 3.5

External and Internal Constraints

Constraints	External	Internal
Anthropometry and ergonomics	X	
Ergonomic	X	
Operating mechanisms		X
Accessory rails	X	
Overall tolerances of 0.1 mm		X

---

the relations of movement, position, force, moment, time, and others. Examples of internal constraints are perpendicularity, concentricity, symmetry, collinearity, parallelism, and proportionality. Table 3.5 shows the external and internal constraints in the design of exoskeletons.

3.4.8 COMMONALITY INDEX

The example that follows shows a platform of products with two product families, A and B, each with common and unique components (Figure 3.11).

The calculation of the commonality index C (Equation 3.2) shows that the more common components there are, the larger the commonality index.

$$C = \frac{100\,x}{x+u} \tag{3.2}$$

$$C = \frac{100(2)}{(2)+(1)} = 66.7\%$$

$$C = \frac{100(2)}{(2)+(2)} = 50\%$$

3.4.9 DFA INDEX

The following example shows the original components of the operating mechanism before simplification. Table 3.6 shows the minimum part criteria related to the essential parts, where the DFA index (Equation 3.3) is 53%.

$$DFA = \frac{100\,N_m t_m}{T_P} \tag{3.3}$$

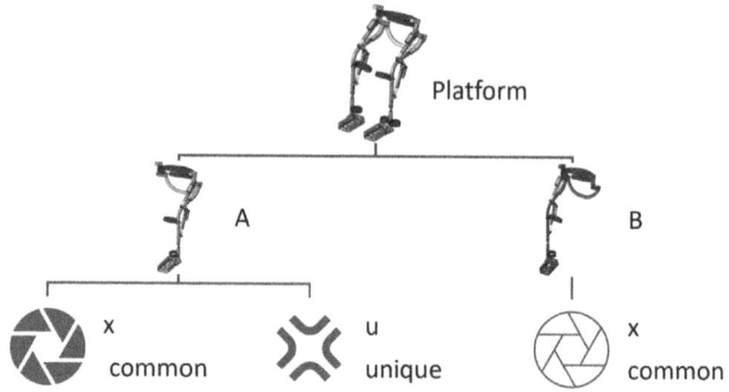

FIGURE 3.11   Modular architecture of an exoskeleton.

TABLE 3.6
Components of Operating Mechanism Before DFA Simplification

Item	Part	Quantity	Minimum Part Criteria
1	Bushing of link	1	None
2	Body of link	1	Movement
3	Body of slider	1	Movement
4	Bushing of slider	1	None
5	Base casing	1	Base
6	Bushing of selector	1	None
8	Right selector lever	1	Assembly
9	Left selector lever	1	Assembly
10	Pin	3	Assembly
11	Pin of selector	2	Fastener
12	Disconnector	1	Movement
13	Automaticity plunger	1	Movement
14	Spring	4	None
Total		19	3 meet the theoretical minimum

DFA: Design for assembly index

N_m: Number of minimum part criteria

t_m: Minimum assembly time by part

T_P: Total of parts

$$DFA = \frac{100(3)(3)}{(17)} = 53\%$$

TABLE 3.7

Components of Operating Mechanism After DFA Simplification

Item	Part	Quantity	Minimum Part Criteria
1	Link	1	Movement
2	Slider	1	Movement
3	Base casing	1	Base
4	Right selector lever	1	Assembly
5	Selector coupling	1	Assembly
6	Pin of selector	1	Fastener
7	Pin	3	Assembly
8	Disconnector	1	Movement
9	Automaticity plunger	1	Movement
10	Spring	4	None
Total		15	3 meet the theoretical minimum

After DFA simplification using the minimum part criteria, a DFA index of 60% is obtained:

$$DFA = \frac{100(3)(3)}{(15)} = 60\%$$

It can be seen in Table 3.7 that the smaller the number of components concerning the minimum part criterion, the greater the DFA index.

3.4.10 PRODUCT PORTFOLIO

The following product portfolio is composed of a platform with a modular architecture with two product families. The design concept of the platform begins with the exoskeleton; each subsystem does commonality and DFA indexes as the modular architecture so that the product family can be scaled. Figure 3.12 shows the exoskeleton of the product family A.

This product family is an exoskeleton; sometimes, it is convenient to generate a brand per platform and a brand for each family product (Figure 3.13).

3.5 CLOSING REMARKS AND PERSPECTIVES

The design strategy and methodology are the best way to start the development process. In this sense, both parts allow for outlining the aspects and methods that will be included in the product design. Currently, innovation trends focus on the market pull: the user-centered design (UCD), which implies empathizing with the user and using tools to identify user preferences such as storytelling, mapping travel, and empathy mapping. However, the technological push is transcendental in terms of disruptive

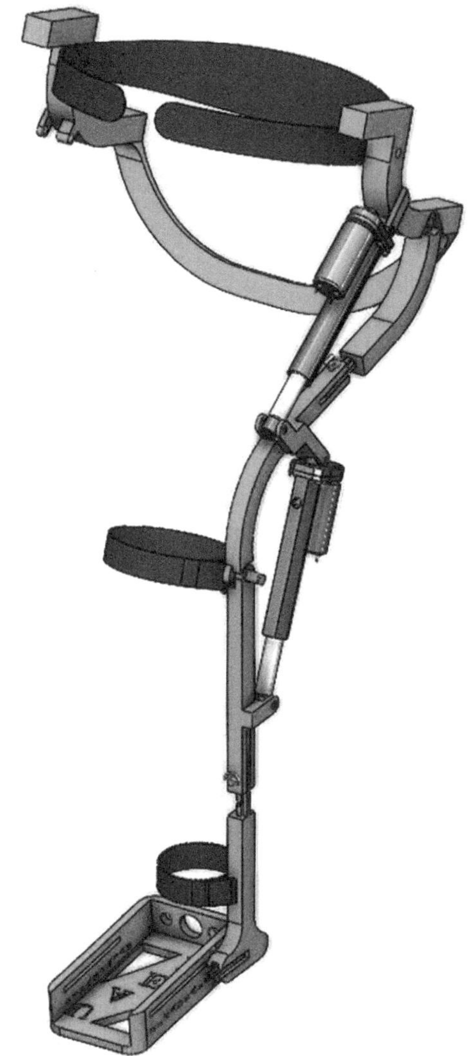

FIGURE 3.12   Exoskeleton of the product family A.

innovation. Think of cars or motorcycles; perhaps the pull market could be used when talking about comfort, luxury, clothing, and color. However, push technology would be used when talking about motors, which are not requested or perceived by customers, but designing more efficient and eco-friendly engines is part of the offer that, as cluster technology, marks a trend in design technology. This technology push is later adapted to the market, assimilated, and adopted by the users, mainly when the usability includes this exoskeleton, and then the rest of the users perceive the reliability of the systems.

The new expectations of exoskeleton design consider accomplishment with the homologation of design criteria and medical standards. Both include simplification,

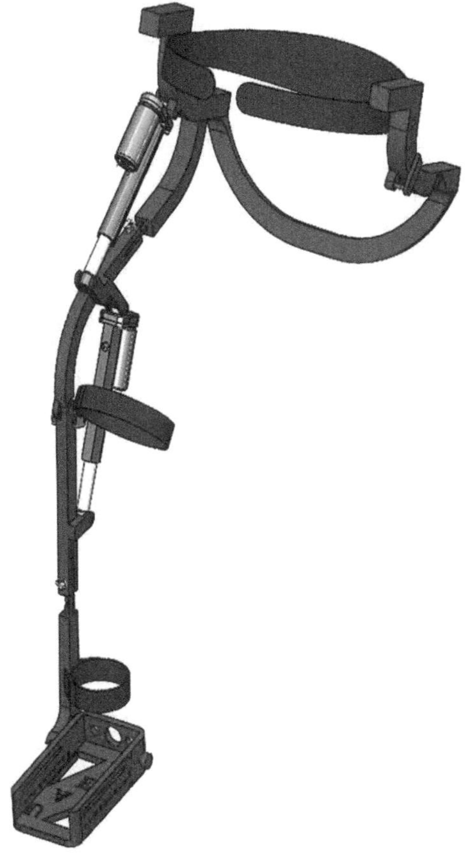

FIGURE 3.13   Exoskeleton of the product family B.

modularity, indicators, and eco-design to improve usability metrics and dismiss risk through failure modes and effects analysis (FMEA).

Evaluation activity. Please answer the next quiz.
https://forms.office.com/r/vfmnTrrv0L

1. What are the stages of NPD according to the current definition?
   A. Research, development, and implementation
   B. Research, design, and production
   C. Research, development, and innovation
   D. Research, development, and marketing

2. What is the main function of technological platforms in the design process?
   A. To manage the planning and development phases of a new product
   B. To control the commercialization of a new product
   C. To manage the prioritization of participation in the project
   D. All of the above

3. What is the main difference between open innovation and closed innovation?
   A. Open innovation is focused on collaboration, while closed innovation is focused on confidentiality.
   B. Open innovation is focused on market pull, while closed innovation is focused on technology push.
   C. Open innovation is focused on incremental innovation, while closed innovation is focused on disruptive innovation.
   D. Open innovation is focused on networking, while closed innovation is focused on product development.

4. What does the term "attributes" refer to?
   A. Qualities that make a product different from others in the market
   B. The price and quality of a product
   C. The operating principle of a product
   D. The level of technological maturity of a product

5. What is the purpose of benchmarking in the product design process?
   A. To identify and differentiate the product from competitors
   B. To determine the client's requirements in the displayed market segments
   C. All of the above
   D. None of the above

6. What are the technical solutions proposed to meet user requirements called in the HOQ1?
   A. VOCs
   B. Functional requirements (FR)
   C. Whats
   D. TRIZ

7. The design parameters (DP) are detailed numerical solutions that are proposed to meet functional requirements, based on the axiom of independence from axiomatic design.
   A. True
   B. False

8. What are the three types of models included in the modeling phase?
   A. Computational, iconic, and experimental physical
   B. Virtual, mathematical, and physical
   C. Computational, mathematical and the experimental physical model
   D. Iconic, mathematical, and digital

9. What are the three types of models included in the simulating phase?
   A. CAE, numerical, and CAM
   B. Structural evaluation, computational fluid dynamics, and motion assessment
   C. CAM, CAD, and CAE
   D. None of the above

10. A prototype is the first replicable type that is expected to have field tests.
    A. True
    B. False

11. What are the stages for the generation of new products?
    A. Concept, animation, modeling, simulation, emulation, prototype, and product
    B. Concept, animation, modeling, simulation, prototype, and product
    C. Concept, modeling, simulation, emulation, prototype, and product
    D. Concept, animation, modeling, simulation, emulation, prototype, and manufacturing

12. What does TRL mean?
    A. Technology readiness level
    B. Technology region level
    C. Technological rigor level
    D. Technology research laboratory

13. When is TRL8 level reached?
    A. When there is a certified product
    B. When there is a valuable minimum product
    C. When there is a prototype operating in real testing
    D. When there is a prototype operating in relevant environment testing

REFERENCES

1. Ullman, D.G., The Mechanical Design Process. McGraw-Hill, 1992.
2. Sodhro, A.H., S. Pirbhulal, and A.K. Sangaiah, Convergence of IoT and product lifecycle management in medical health care. Future Generation Computer Systems, 2018.86: p. 380–391.
3. Bowland, N., J. Gao, and R. Sharma, A PDM-and CAD-integrated assembly modelling environment for manufacturing planning. Journal of Materials Processing Technology, 2003.138(1–3): p. 82–88.
4. Kahn, K.B., et al., An examination of new product development best practice. Journal of Product Innovation Management, 2012.29(2): p. 180–192.
5. Brem, A. and K.-I. Voigt, Integration of market pull and technology push in the corporate front end and innovation management—Insights from the German software industry. Technovation, 2009.29(5): p. 351–367.
6. Chesbrough, H., W. Vanhaverbeke, and J. West, Open Innovation: Researching a New Paradigm. Oxford University Press on Demand, 2006.
7. Cusumano, M.A., Staying Power: Six Enduring Principles for Managing Strategy and Innovation in an Uncertain World (Lessons from Microsoft, Apple, Intel, Google, Toyota and More). Oxford University Press, 2010.
8. Lazzarotti, V. and R. Manzini, Different modes of open innovation: A theoretical framework and an empirical study. International Journal of Innovation Management, 2009.13(04): p. 615–636.
9. Di Stefano, G., A. Gambardella, and G. Verona, Technology push and demand pull perspectives in innovation studies: Current findings and future research directions. Research Policy, 2012.41(8): p. 1283–1295.
10. Herstatt, C. and C. Lettl, Management of" technology push" development projects. International Journal of Technology Management, 2004.27(2–3): p. 155–175.
11. Moogk, D.R., Minimum viable product and the importance of experimentation in technology startups. Technology Innovation Management Review, 2012.2(3).
12. Nemet, G.F., Demand-pull, technology-push, and government-led incentives for non-incremental technical change. Research Policy, 2009.38(5): p. 700–709.

13. Jovanović, T., et al., The crowdfunding idea contest of BMW. In Proceedings of the 26th International Association for Management of Technology Conference, Vienna, Austria, 2017.
14. Sadin, S.R., F.P. Povinelli, and R. Rosen, The NASA technology push towards future space mission systems. In Space and Humanity. Elsevier, 1989. p. 73–77.
15. Dávila-Vilchis, J.-M., J.C. Ávila Vilchis, and A.H. Vilchis-González, Design methodology for soft wearable devices—The MOSAR case. Applied Sciences, 2019.9(22): p. 4727.
16. Suh, N.P., Axiomatic design theory for systems. Research in Engineering Design, 1998.10(4).
17. Sauser, B., et al., From TRL to SRL: The concept of systems readiness levels. In Conference on Systems Engineering Research, Los Angeles, CA. Citeseer, 2006.
18. Consolvo, S., et al., Design requirements for technologies that encourage physical activity. In Proceedings of the SIGCHI Conference on Human Factors in Computing Systems, 2006.
19. Thompson, M.K., A classification of procedural errors in the definition of functional requirements in axiomatic design theory. In 7th International Conference on Axiomatic Design (ICAD 2013). Worcester, MA, USA, 2013.
20. Kulak, O., S. Cebi, and C. Kahraman, Applications of axiomatic design principles: A literature review. Expert Systems with Applications, 2010.37(9): p. 6705–6717.
21. Thompson, M.K., et al., Design for additive manufacturing: Trends, opportunities, considerations, and constraints. CIRP Annals, 2016.65(2): p. 737–760.
22. Kota, S., K. Sethuraman, and R. Miller, A metric for evaluating design commonality in product families. Journal of Mechanical Design, 2000.122(4): p. 403–410.
23. Prakash, W.N., V. Sridhar, and K. Annamalai, New product development by DFMA and rapid prototyping. ARPN Journal of Engineering and Applied Sciences, 2014.9(3): p. 274–279.
24. Zúñiga-Avilés, L., et al., Htg-based kinematic modeling for positioning of a multi-articulated wheeled mobile manipulator. Journal of Intelligent & Robotic Systems, 2014.76: p. 267–282.
25. Živanovic, S., et al., Machining simulation and verification of tool path for CNC machine tools with serial and hybrid kinematics. In Proceedings of VIII International Conference Heavy Machinery-HM, 2014.
26. Cruz Martínez, G.M. and L. Z.-Avilés, Design methodology for rehabilitation robots: Application in an exoskeleton for upper limb rehabilitation. Applied Sciences, 2020.10(16): p. 5459.
27. Fernandez, J.A., Contextual Role of TRLs and MRLs in Technology Management. Sandia National Laboratories (SNL), Albuquerque, NM, and Livermore, CA . . ., 2010.
28. Ross, S., Application of System and Integration Readiness Levels to Department of Defense Research and Development (Postprint). Air Force Research Lab Kirtland AFB Nm Kirtland AFB United States, 2016.
29. Engel, D.W., et al., Development of Technology Readiness Level (TRL) Metrics and Risk Measures. Pacific Northwest National Lab (PNNL), 2012.
30. Puig, L., A. Barton, and N. Rando, A review on large deployable structures f1. Global Exoskeleton Market Size, Share, Trends | Forecast 2023–32, in Market.us.
31. Global Exoskeleton Market Size, Share, Trends | Forecast 2023–32, in Market.us.
32. Secco, E.L. and A.M. Tadesse, A wearable exoskeleton for hand kinesthetic feedback in virtual reality. In Wireless Mobile Communication and Healthcare: 8th EAI International Conference, MobiHealth 2019, Dublin, Ireland, November 14–15, 2019, Proceedings 8.2020. Springer.
33. O'Hare, G.M., et al., Wireless mobile communication and healthcare. In 8th EAI International Conference, MobiHealth 2019, Dublin, Ireland, November 14–15, 2019, Proceedings. Vol. 320.2020. Springer.

<h1>4 Design of Exoskeletons</h1>

4.1 INTRODUCTION

The speed in the development of exoskeletons largely depends on the synergy between the design experience and the interaction of technological tools. For this, it is essential to have a team trained to continuously adapt to technological changes in product lifecycle management. This design team must overcome obstacles such as having experience dealing with outdated software. A competitor acquires the modeling and simulation tool and modifies it; the software is no longer compatible with some type of hardware or requires add-ons and updates; besides that, its mode of operation and user interface (UI) are different.

The challenges posed by using technologies for modeling and simulation have to do with the constant training of the design team and the collaboration with engineering consulting companies and universities as part of the concurrent development. Additionally, exoskeleton developers sometimes prefer traditional tools rather than investing in technological tools that could represent a hiatus in product development due to training or hiring skilled personnel. This chapter addresses the implementation of CAD and CAE tools in exoskeleton design, considering the evaluation environment and its performance validation. Several case studies are presented in the chapter to exemplify the potential of different simulation software. In addition, this chapter describes the kinematics and dynamics, controllers, and metabolic cost.

4.2 MODELING AND SIMULATION

Computational modeling and simulation are one of the fastest-growing areas in engineering. They are used in a wide range of areas to predict or explain the behavior of a product or a system. They are also used for gaming entertainment, which is probably by far the largest market. The fundamental aspects of using these tools are predicting product performance through simulation, already at the design stage, with higher precision and fidelity.

So now, these tools have the potential to reduce product development time drastically and are a fundamental part of what is called the base model design. In recent years, there has been a rapid development in system simulation, primarily due to hardware development, so no other area of technology has had such a drastic sustained increase for decades. Likewise, advances in software have also been significant, such as in the case of compilers and algorithm development [1].

One consequence of this is that the behavior of much larger and more complex systems can be analyzed, and this advantage has prompted the development of a new generation of simulation software with graphical interfaces that are much easier to

DOI: 10.1201/9781003261995-4

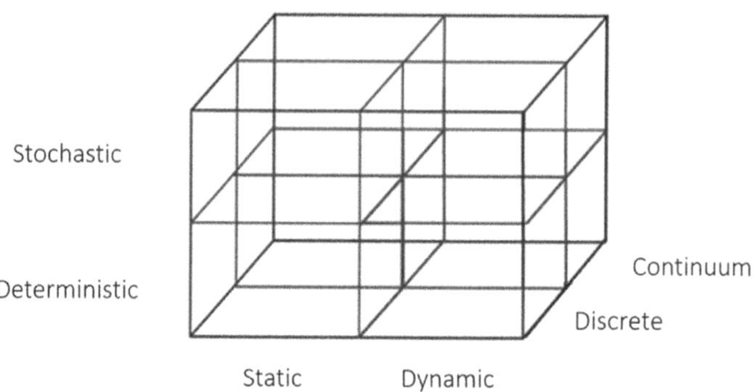

FIGURE 4.1 Dynamical systems.

use. The new graphical interfaces make it more effective to work with heavier systems. Large systems that integrate several physical domains are currently simulated in multi-domain software [2].

Modeling and simulation are tools that support the planning, design, and evaluation of systems. Their importance will continue to grow at a remarkable rate; this growth is also a consequence of the increasing availability of important computing resources and the human capacity that allows taking advantage of this computational power. However, any practical use of a tool, especially a multifaceted tool such as modeling and simulation, implies an increasingly rapid learning curve.

In the modeling phase, the system to be analyzed is classified, determining the required simulation's characteristics. Depending on the model type, it can be deterministic when its behavior is known or stochastic when its behavior can be measured and approximated. According to the variability of time, a system can be static when time is not a variable in the model; further, it can be a continuum dynamical system when it evolves or a discrete dynamical system when it occurs in time steps [3]. According to the variables involved in the mathematical model, the system classification is visualized based on the diagram shown in Figure 4.1.

The software for modeling and simulation is included in the 3D computer graphics software, and due to its evolution and the new requirements of immersion, interaction, and imagination, today, it is related to virtual reality software. This software is classified as shown in Figure 4.2, where the usability testing and training focus on the user model, and the exoskeleton and test bench refer to the environment model.

4.3 CAD MODELING

A model constitutes a representation of a particular aspect of reality. On the one hand, its structure involves the elements that characterize the modeled reality and, on the other, the relationships between them. A CAD model is a physical, non-tangible representation carried out in CAD software. There are three types of models (Figure 4.3): wireframe, surface, and solid. The surface is divided into polygon mesh and non-uniform rational B-spline (NURBS), and the solid is divided into parts and

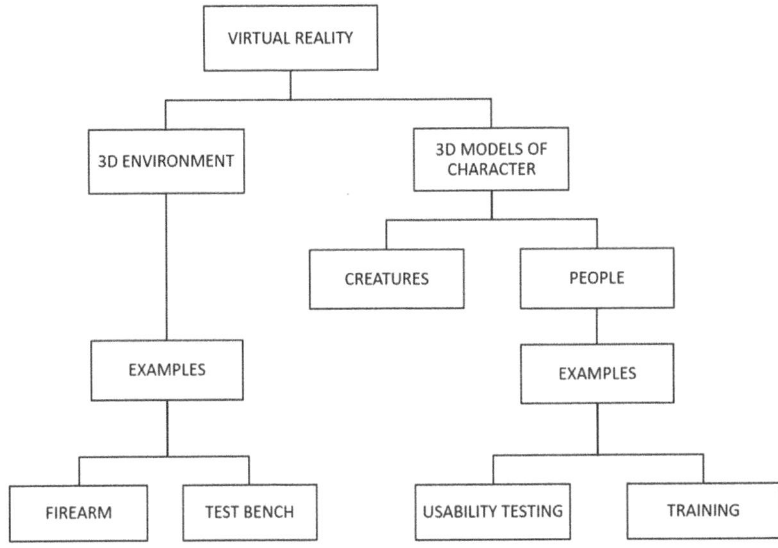

FIGURE 4.2 Virtual reality software used in exoskeleton design.

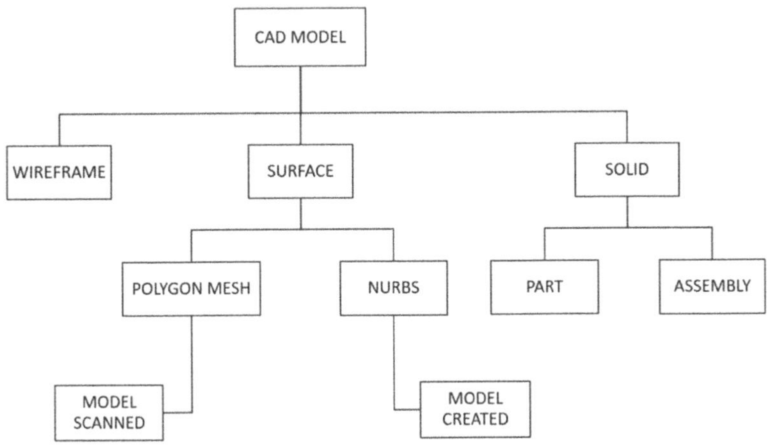

FIGURE 4.3 Types of CAD models.

assembly. A surface model is created using NURBS, while 3D scans are exported as a polygon mesh.

Each type of model is created using a specific modeling technique (Figure 4.4). The wireframe is a skeletal description; it consists only of curves, lines, and points. The polygon mesh consists of small triangles. NURBS are mathematical representations that describe complex 3D organic freeform objects consisting of points connected by curves. Surface modeling focuses on the external faces, and the solid model is a parametric graphic that includes the feature operations realized from the

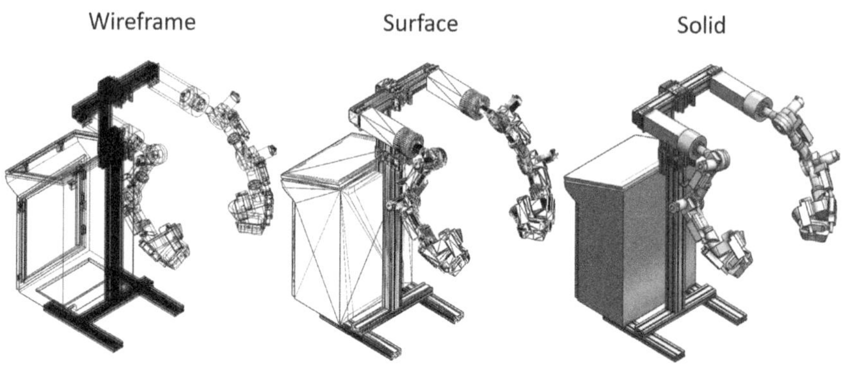

FIGURE 4.4   Comparison of the kinds of CAD models for an exoskeleton.

sketch. Solid modeling is widely used in sketching, engineering analysis, animation, simulation, prototyping, and rendering [4].

4.3.1   Obtaining a Digital Model

Digital modeling is the process of getting non-tangible models using several modeling techniques, such as 3D sculpting and photogrammetry, as well as box, polygon, procedural, NURBS, and curve modeling. As shown in Figure 4.3, the CAD model can be obtained either by model creation in CAD software or by model scanning. 3D scanning is suitable for obtaining data and shapes of exoskeleton components made of plastic or worn metal parts. The process begins with data acquisition by 3D scan, later importing the objects to analyze the data with software such as GOM Inspector Pro. The objects can then be imported into CAD software to handle the surfaces by means of an operation detection tool or remodeling using solid tools [5].

4.3.2   Materials Database Storage

In the design process in CAD-CAE software, it is required to include physical properties, which depend on the materials. CAD and CAE software have a material database, called the material library, where the properties of materials are stored; this database is necessary to design and evaluate the behavior of the system. A new exoskeleton design requires considering the real parameters of the materials; therefore, they are added to the material library as custom materials once they are characterized. The accuracy of the evaluation is highly dependent on the parameters of the materials. For this reason, the parameters of materials are obtained by testing laboratories.

4.3.3   Bill of Material Property Manager

CAD software includes a tool to manage the materials used in the exoskeleton design. This bill of material property manager considers each material of every component that belongs to the exoskeleton assembly. These material data is used to prepare the

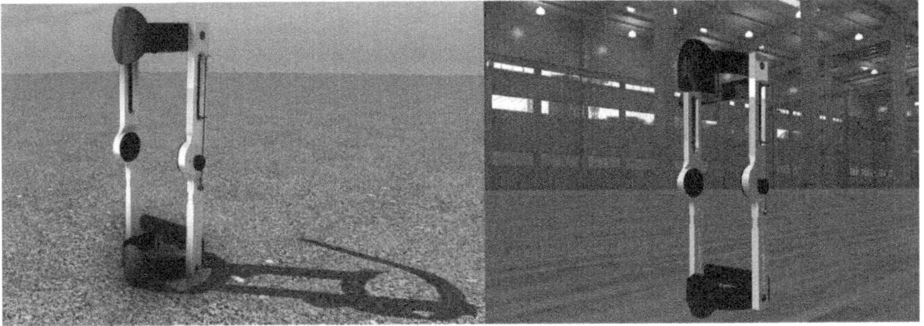

FIGURE 4.5 CAD animation using extended reality tool from Solidworks.

experimental lots, detailing the preliminary manufacturing process, the logistics to organize the assembly zones, suppliers, rules to purchase, and standards for exoskeleton operating.

4.3.4 CAD ANIMATION

The CAD software has tools to animate the exoskeletons, giving movement to their components and recording events, the main characteristic of this tool being to show the virtual functioning and rendering appearance.

As reviewed in Chapter 3, the animation is suitable for proposing a design expectation, which requires compatibility to translate between CAD format and animation software format. Animation software has a better rendering capability than CAD and incorporates better textures, illumination, and materials. At present, some software such as SolidWorks, Unreal Engine, Maya, and 3D Max include virtual reality (VR) tools to improve imagination, immersion, and interaction. A SolidWorks tool called extended reality allows, for instance, to generate an exoskeleton in CAD, saving the file in extended reality (*.gltf) or extended reality binary (*.glb). These extended reality files can be linked in PowerPoint to animate slides, in the smartphone App eDrawings using the augmented reality (AR) icon, and in eDrawings PC with virtual environments using the VR icon. Figure 4.5 shows an animation example of an exoskeleton.

4.3.5 INTERFERENCE DETECTION

During the modeling process, it is necessary to ensure proper movement of the parts to achieve the required interaction among the components, verifying the principle of operation. A task to evaluate the design is detecting interference in assemblies, which highlights the overlap and measures the overlapped surface. Figure 4.6 presents a mechanism as an example where the bushing interferes with the gear.

Another task to evaluate the design is the clearance verification in assemblies. This verification marks the clearance in a defined position showing a measured gap. Such interference detection as clearance verification aims to estimate the permissible gap. Figure 4.7 shows the clearance verification between the gear and support.

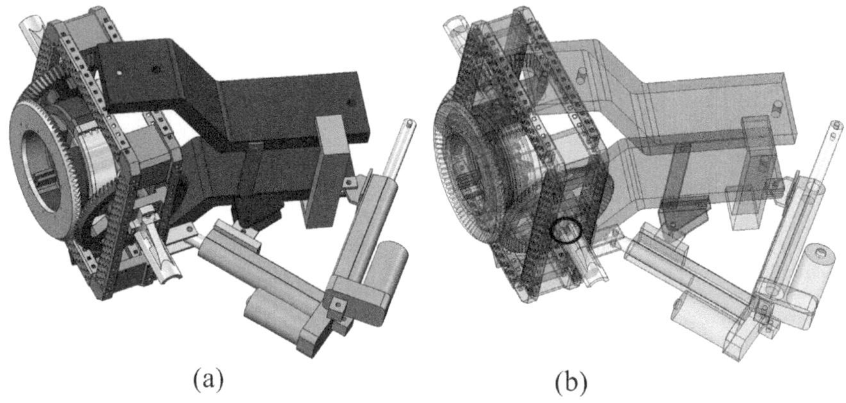

(a)   (b)

FIGURE 4.6   Wrist exoskeleton: (a) Without CAD evaluation and (b) interference detection.

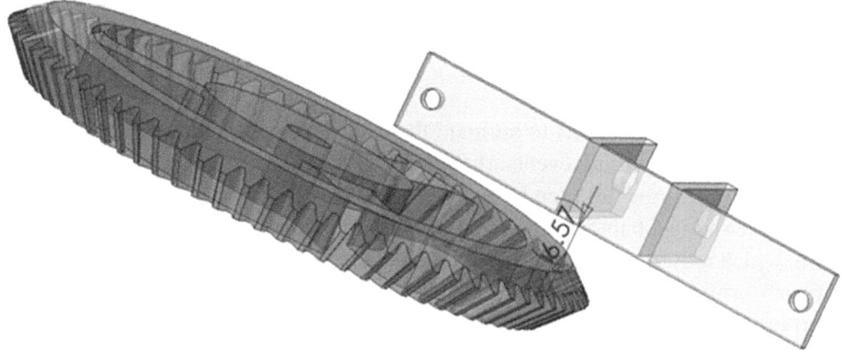

FIGURE 4.7   Clearance verification between the gear and support.

Considering the tolerances of manufacture, calibration, controllable and critical dimensions, interference detection, and clearance verification are analyzed to decide permissible measures.

4.3.6   TOLERANCE STACK-UP ANALYSIS

Fits and tolerances are controlled through several statistical methods to maintain the permissible error that allows the operating ranges of an exoskeleton. Fit refers to dimensions between two parts to engage and achieve the defined functioning in an assembly. Tolerance is the acceptable error between maximum and minimum dimensions, which is searched to avoid cumulative tolerances using tools for tolerance stack-up analysis. The six main methods (Figure 4.8) are described next.

The root sum squared (RSS) method assumes that the normal distribution describes the variation of dimensions. The bell-shaped curve is symmetrical and fully described with two parameters, the mean μ, and the standard deviation σ. Adding the means and taking the root sum square of the standard deviations provide an

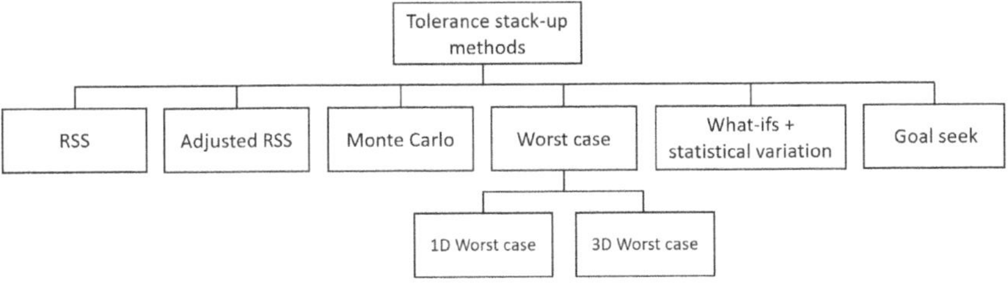

FIGURE 4.8 Tolerance stack-up methods.

estimate of the normal distribution of the tolerance stack-up. This method can be used for 3D tolerance analysis. Adjusted RSS is an RSS value multiplied by 1.5 as an established factor, which is added and subtracted from the nominal distance to find the minimum and maximum [6].

The Monte Carlo method (MCM) uses random numbers and probability to solve problems. The MCM includes a diagram showing the components and operations sequence for evaluating measurement uncertainty [6]. Worst-case tolerance analysis is a method that derives from setting all the tolerances at their limits to make a measurement the largest or smallest possible by design. This process does not use statistical probability and focuses on whether the product falls within its specification limits. 1D worst-case assumes that all tolerances have a one out of one effect on the measurement, while 3D worst-case considers geometric effects and angular variation. Complex assemblies require a combination of what-ifs tolerances and statistical variation modeling software, so iterations are performed until a combination of tolerance components is achieved to obtain an acceptable result. Goal Seek of Excel is a function that allows determining the tolerance value. The analyst can set the desired mounting tolerance value and have the program iterate to find the exact solution [6].

Opening tolerances is a technique for changing mates, such as swapping butt joints for lap joints or changing the geometry of the surface to make misalignment less obvious using shims to reduce the number of parts than the cumulative total. The tolerances opening and tolerances stack-up tool work together to reach suitable tolerances for functioning and manufacturability.

TolAnalyst is a tolerance analysis tool used to study tolerance effects and assembly methods that have one-dimensional stack-up between two features of an assembly [7]. The result of each study is a minimum and maximum tolerance stack, a minimum and maximum RSS tolerance stack, and a list of contributing features and tolerances reported in an Excel sheet. A tolerance study uses four steps: 1. define the measurements as linear distances between two DimXpert features; 2. use the assembly sequence to establish a tolerance chain between the measurement features; 3. use assembly constraints to define how the part is placed or constrained; and 4. use analysis results, where the minimum and maximum worst-case tolerance stacks are evaluated and reviewed. This tool uses type plus and minus or geometric tolerances (Gtols) concerning three datums named A, B, and C. It is essential to mention that setting tolerances so close increases the manufacturing cost; for this, the tolerances analysis must consider the tolerances that a defined manufacturing process can reach for each component.

4.3.7   CAD DRAWINGS

Communication with other areas, such as manufacturing, experimental testing, quality control, intellectual property, technology transfer, and resources material, is done through engineering plans, drawings, or drafting. Currently, drawings can be visualized in apps, including a solid model in AR. Design teams usually define their template and the information control, classifying it as confidential only for testing, experimental issue, or prototype. Drawings require the signature of approval tolerances, materials, and components in case of assembly drawings.

4.4   CAE SIMULATION

The simulation technique comprises an extensive collection of methods and applications whose objective is to reproduce the actual behavior, generally on a digital computer with the appropriate software. Computer simulation studies a wide variety of models applying numerical techniques and creating a computerized model of the system under study to carry out experiments that improve the knowledge of the system behavior in a set of working conditions [8]. Analysis objectives, modules, types of analysis, output, solution method, workflow, and components in the simulation environment integrate CAE simulation. Analysis objective refers to the problem conditions by solution, as in the case of noise, vibration, and harshness (NVH) analysis. A modal mass is a property of natural vibration, a piece of the dynamic behavior of vibration systems (modal analysis). A modal mass can be understood as a mass that is activated in specific modes of vibration. A vibration mode is a property of the structure described by a natural frequency, a damping factor, and a modal shape, which describes the dynamics of the structure. A mode can be normal or complex. The modal analysis allows for defining at which frequencies the structure can be excited in resonance and reduce unwanted effects [9].

The modules consist of linear finite element analysis (FEA), nonlinear FEA, computational fluid dynamic (CFD), multibody dynamics (MBD) as the case of Simscape, multiphysics of multi-domains such as Ansys, acoustic, crash, co-simulation, and correlation. The types of analysis can be classified into static, dynamic modal, dynamic transient, and dynamic harmonic. In the static analysis, inertial loads are ignored, which is valid when the loads are applied slowly, so the results are time-independent. In dynamic modal analysis, vibration modes are analyzed. In dynamic transient analysis, inertial loads are taken into account for fast loads and rigid body motions, with time-dependent results. In dynamic harmonic analysis, the inertial loads are considered, but external loads are assumed to be sinusoidal. Output refers to simulation responses, which are, in an overall way, the temperature, pressure, reaction forces, displacement, stresses, and strains. The solution method can be implicit or explicit. The implicit method is used when the events are slower since the effects of strain rates are minimal and can be considered a static equilibrium. The explicit method is used in exoskeleton design, where a dynamic equilibrium or otherwise is assumed [10]. This method is used for crash and impact tests; in these cases, the material models must consider stress variation and strain rate.

The workflow of CAE simulation has three stages: 1. preprocessor, geometry treatment, material properties, meshing, loads, and boundary conditions (BC);

2. solver, equation solution, and nodal loads; and 3. postprocessor, which refers to analysis result evaluation in graphs and animations. Some components of CAE simulation are the nodal force vector, nodal displacement vector, degree of freedom (DOF), materials, meshing, loads, field variables, field problems, governing equations, initial conditions, domains, and stiffness matrix, which are shown in Equation 4.1, where is the global stiffness matrix (an overall expression of linear problems), is the nodal forces vector, and is the nodal displacement vector (unknown) [11].

$$[K]\{u\} = \{F\}$$

(4.1)

Other components are BCs, governing equations, and shape function, which interpolates the solution between the discrete values obtained at the mesh nodes. Low-order polynomials are typically chosen as shape functions, which can be nonlinear or linear shape functions [12]. Governing equations are shown as follows for an axially loaded elastic bar (Equation 4.2), a Poiseuille flow in a pipe (Equation 4.3), a 1D heat flow (Equation 4.4), and a 1D diffusion (Equation 4.5).

$$\frac{dy}{dx}\left(AE\frac{du}{dx}\right) + b = 0$$

(4.2)

Where: $u = displacement,\ A = area,\ E = Young's\ modulus,\ b = axial\ loading$

$$\frac{dy}{dx}\left(A\frac{D^2}{32\mu}\frac{d\rho}{dx}\right) + Q = 0$$

(4.3)

Where: $p = pressure,\ A = area,\ D = diameter,\ \mu = viscosity,\ Q = fluid\ supply$

$$\frac{dy}{dx}\left(Ak\frac{dT}{dx}\right) + Q = 0$$

(4.4)

Where: $k = Thermal\ conductivity,\ A = area,\ T = temperature,\ Q = heat\ supply$

$$\frac{dy}{dx}\left(AD\frac{dC}{dx}\right) + Q = 0$$

(4.5)

Where: $c = iron\ concentration,\ A = area,\ D = difussion\ coefficient,\ Q = ion\ supply$

Figure 4.9 shows a framework of CAE simulation. Some simulations are named according to the elements used in the framework. For instance, explicit dynamic transient simulation comes from the fact that it contains an explicit solution method and belongs to the type of dynamic transient.

Implicit and explicit problems are expressed through partial differential equations (PDEs) in matrix equations; they can be linear (Equation 4.1) or nonlinear, expressed in Equation 4.6.

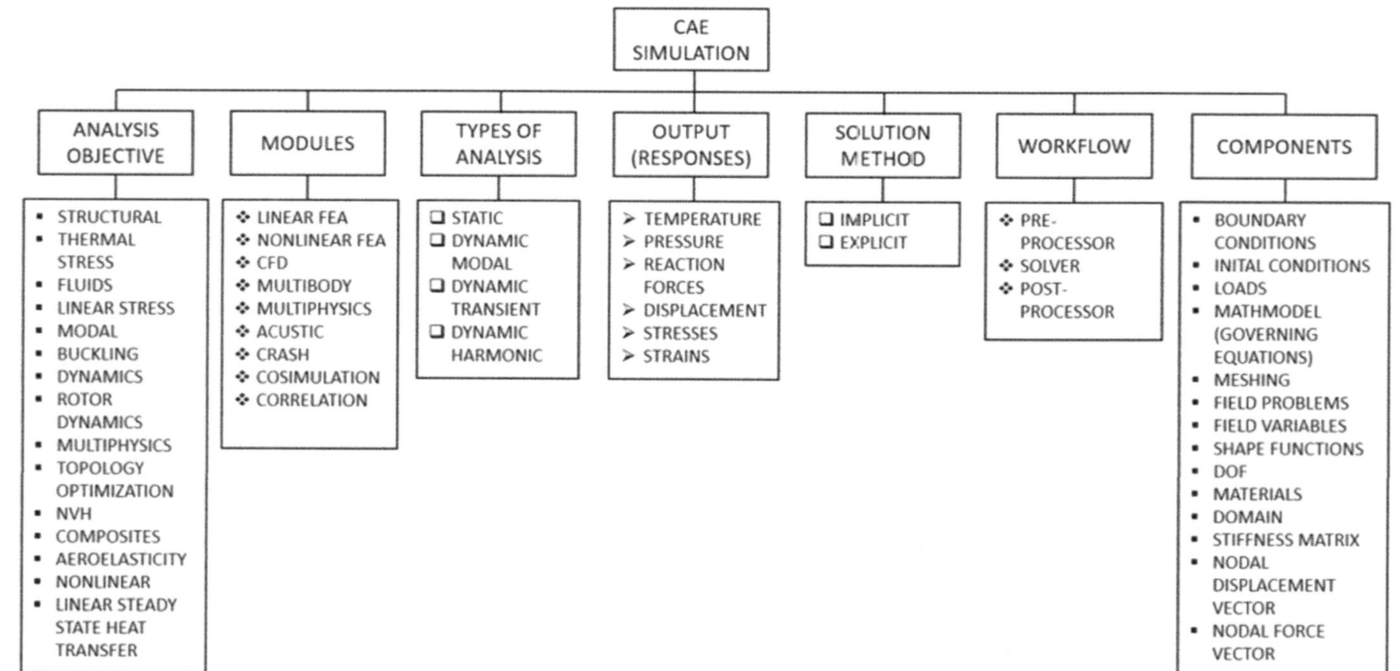

FIGURE 4.9 Framework of CAE simulation.

$$\left[K(u) \right]\{u\} = \{F\} \tag{4.6}$$

The nonlinear equations can be of a different nature: material nonlinearity, where deformations and strains are large, as in the case of polymeric materials; geometric nonlinearity, where strains are small, but rotations are large, thin structures; and boundary nonlinearity, as, for instance, in contact problems [13]. For dynamic problems, Equation 4.7 is used, where M denotes the mass matrix, U is the displacement, is the velocity, is the acceleration, C is the damping matrix, K is the stiffness matrix, and F is the loading vector.

$$M\ddot{U} + C\dot{U} + KU = F \tag{4.7}$$

Figure 4.10 shows how loads, mesh, materials, and BCs interact. Preprocessing defines the loads and can be concentrated, distributed, or shear. The mesh can be classified into adaptive (refining method of a simulation mesh based on the solution) and grid (types of mesh: structured, unstructured, and hybrid); the materials can be classified into form and properties. BCs are also defined in the preprocessing stage. Meshing is part of the discretization necessary to provide a solution through the simulation process, and this discretization generates a set of points and cells [14].

BCs define the interactions of systems (exoskeletons) with the environment and include the BC types (thermodynamics, solid mechanics, and fluid dynamics), BC assignments (assigned to the domain boundary), and BC values (pressure, temperature, force, velocity). Thermodynamics include fixed-value temperature, convective heat, surface heat, and volume heat flux. Solid mechanics include pressure, force, nodal load, fixed value, surface load, volume load, centrifugal force, remote force, symmetry plane, remote displacement, fixed support, rotating motion, elastic support, and bolt preload. Fluid dynamics include velocity, pressure, natural convection, wall, periodic, symmetry, and wedge [15].

BCs depend on constraints applied to the governing equations of an exoskeleton. These are the following (Figure 4.10): **Dirichlet BC**, which specifies the value that the unknown function needs to take along the boundary of the domain (for instance, a no-slip condition in fluid mechanics where the value of the velocity is set to zero, in solid mechanics prescribing a particular load or displacement, and in heat transfer setting the temperature at a surface); **Neumann BC**, which specifies the values that the derivative of a solution is going to take on the boundary of the domain (for instance, fluid mechanics is the fully developed condition at an outlet where the gradient of flow variables is set to zero, traction conditions in solid mechanics, and insulated surfaces in heat transfer); **Robin BC**, when in a differential equation $\left(mu + n\left(\dfrac{\partial u}{\partial x} \right) = y; m \text{ and } n \neq 0 \right)$, a linear combination of the values of a function (y) and the values of its derivative $(\dfrac{\partial u}{\partial x}; u$ is the unknown solution defined on Ψ domain) on the boundary $(\partial \Psi)$ are specified; **Cauchy BC**, which is a condition on both the unknown field and its derivatives (implies the imposition of two constraints, **Dirichlet + Neumann**); and mixed BC, which consists of applying different types of boundary conditions in different parts of the domain [16].

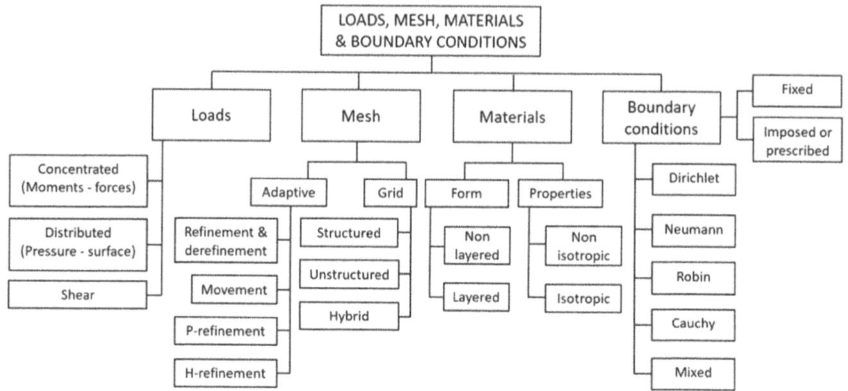

FIGURE 4.10   Interaction scheme of loads, mesh, materials, and BCs.

Topology optimization is a technique encompassed within the field of structural analysis. It is based on the mechanical analysis of a component or structure, and its main objective is structural lightening while maintaining the mechanical functionalities of the target component [17].

4.4.1   CAD Model Treatment

A CAD model is prepared according to the experience of the design team and capabilities of the CAE software, considering simplification, model layers, small chamfer, and rounding. Sometimes, this treatment requires the experimental protocol using case studies and tasks as well as suppressing sharp edges and softening curves.

4.4.2   CAE Analysis by FEA

FEA is the simulation of any given physical phenomenon using the finite element method (FEM) numerical technique. Engineers use FEA software to complement the product design and experiments and to optimize components, improving the solution certainty. FEA focuses on individual parts (microscopic behavior); the structural performance of a part; small motion; stress, strain, and deformation of individual parts; and static or dynamic transient analysis for a very short duration [18].

4.4.3   CAE Motion

Exoskeletons are composed of several mechanisms such as augmentation, action, safety, or configuration or use mode mechanisms. The Motion program provides complete, quantitative information about the kinematics, including position, velocity, and acceleration, and the dynamics, including joint reactions, inertial forces, and power requirements, of all the components of a moving mechanism. Motion verifies interferences in real time and provides the exact spatial and time positions of all mechanical components as well as the exact interfering volumes [19].

Sometimes, the motion simulation is configured by applying torque to moving parts in contact until the simulation time is reached, measured in the angular displacement.

4.4.4 FLOW CFD

Several packages can perform CFD, including CAE software, and Ansys has various CFD packages. For example, Ansys Fluent is a CFD software that includes a solver of high-performance computing (HPC) technologies; Ansys CFX contains multi-stage CFD modeling, transient blade row methods, and harmonic balance methods; and Ansys Chemkin-Pro is for modeling complex, chemically reacting systems [20].

4.4.5 CAE MULTIBODY DYNAMICS

MBD consists of solid bodies (links) connected by joints that restrict their relative motion. This study describes the mechanism movements due to forces relative to forward and reverse dynamics. MBD focuses on the entire exoskeleton (macroscopic behavior), performance, relatively large motion, calculation of displacement, velocity, acceleration, loads of several components, and transient analysis for a long duration [21]. For instance, Simscape from Matlab is capable of representing the joints and links from CAD assembly imported from SolidWorks using the code to import the model into Matlab (smimport, 'exoskeleton.xml'). Figure 4.11 shows a block diagram of an exoskeleton.

4.4.6 CAE CO-SIMULATION

Co-simulation, or cooperative simulation, is a methodology applied to simulation that allows individual components to be simulated with different tools running simultaneously and exchanging information collaboratively. The environment in the co-simulation must receive at least two inputs that interact with each other and automatically generate an output [22]. Two main characteristics are required in co-simulation. The first is flexibility, which is a tool available to be adaptable to modifications that may occur during the design, such as in the external or technological environment: modularity and scalability. The second is precision, which must allow the designer to choose the accuracy levels; depending on these, it can be divided into validation time and functional validation [23].

4.4.7 CAE MULTI-DOMAIN

Multi-domain, also known as multiphysics, is defined as the coupled processes or devices involving more than one simultaneously occurring physical field [24]. There are several multiphysics packages, such as COMSOL, Matlab, and Ansys Multiphysics. The latter allows simulating the interaction among structural mechanics, heat transfer, fluid flow, acoustics, and electromagnetics within a single unified simulation

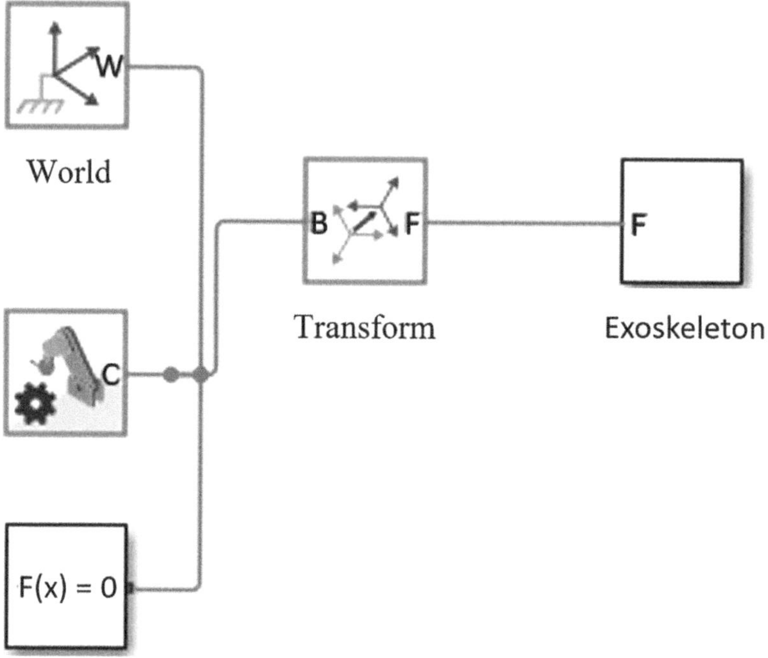

FIGURE 4.11   Block diagram for an exoskeleton in Simscape.

environment or through add-ins to create a collaborative environment [25]. Complex industrial problems such as exoskeleton design, testing, and production require solutions that span a multitude of physical phenomena, which often can only be solved using simulation techniques that cross several engineering disciplines simulating a unified or collaborative UI [26].

4.4.8   CAE EMULATION

The dataset in CAE comprises the input and output (results) data. The output data is analyzed in data technologies that focus on using bulk and complex data, employing data mining (existing datasets to find patterns) or machine learning (making sense of data and predictions about new datasets). The improvement of these datasets makes a difference between simulation and emulation.

The simulation tries to accurately reproduce (or predict) the behavior of the real system, but only approximates it. Emulation, unlike simulation, does not approximate real system behavior, but rather copies the real system behavior. For this, MSC Nastran has spread the slogan 'Simulating reality, delivering certainty' [27], which emphasizes the accuracy of the dataset. Furthermore, several companies of CAE software such as NX Nastran and Ansys can take datasets as a datasheet in CAE software; an input file in CSV from Excel; and equations of displacements, velocities, accelerations, temperatures, and pressure tabulated in Excel.

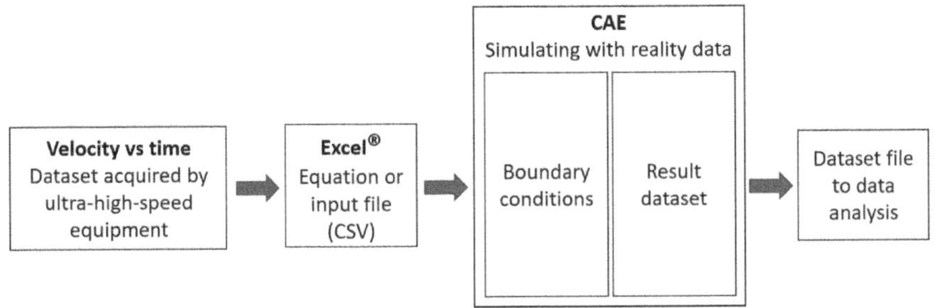

FIGURE 4.12 Dataset sequence in CAE emulation.

For instance, in a CAE analysis of the dynamic behavior of the exoskeleton mechanism, the dataset is acquired from ultra-high-speed equipment on a test bench, tabulated in Excel, and used like an input equation in the CAE software, as shown in Figure 4.12.

4.5 CAD-CAE DOCUMENTATION AND REPORT

Formerly, there was a documentation section in the software CAD, which allowed the generation of a Word document to explain important aspects of design. Today, CAD software such as SolidWorks includes tools to insert notes and markups on a CAD model. A report is a document that details results and diagnosis. A CAD report shows the results of interference, sustainability, or geometric comparison reports, while a CAE report describes the simulation results. The location of this file depends on each software, but, in general, the reports are saved in the report manager. In some cases, the report manager is called the report generator, as is the name in Ansys. NX Nastran and Femap call it user-defined report generation. The customization of the report is fundamental to formalizing the results, clearly displaying the results, and integrating the company logos.

4.6 KINEMATICS AND DYNAMICS

The kinematics and dynamics of an exoskeleton can be obtained by Denavit-Hartenberg parameters and Lagrangian formulation, by analysis and synthesis of mechanisms plus Lagrange-Euler, and by instrumentation such as OptiTrack (motion capture systems) and dynamometers.

4.6.1 GAIT PATTERNS

Typical gait patterns in CP can be divided into spastic hemiplegia (drop foot, equinus with different knee positions) and spastic diplegia (true equinus, jump, apparent equinus, and crouch) [28]. In the spastic hemiplegia, four groups of gait patterns based on kinematic data in the sagittal plane were identified. The key feature of Group I is the foot drop throughout the swing phase, which results in a lack of the first rocker at the initial walking ability distribution for 8-year-old children with CP across the United States in 2010 [29]. The gait pattern of Group II is characterized by a drop foot in the swing phase and a permanent plantarflexion in the stance phase. This pattern is associated with knee hyperextension. Group III has all the deviations of Groups I and II plus reduced knee flexion during the swing phase, an increased lumbar lordosis, and hyperflexion of the hip. In addition to deviations from Groups I to III, patients in Group IV have limited motion at the knee and hip [28–30]. In spastic diplegia, based on the ankle, knee, hip, and pelvis kinematics in the sagittal plane, four main groups were addressed: true equinus, jump gait, apparent equinus, and crouch gait. True equinus is characterized by the ankle in plantarflexion during the stance phase and the hips and knees extended.

The jump gait pattern is defined by ankle equinus, knee and hip flexion, anterior tilt, and increased lumbar lordosis. The apparent equinus pattern addresses a regular range of dorsiflexion at the ankle, but the knee and hip are in excessive flexion across the stance phase, causing the patient to walk on the toes and giving a sense of equinus. Crouch gait is characterized by excessive dorsiflexion at the ankle and excessive flexion at the hip and knee joints [28].

In clinical routines, gait analysis makes it possible to identify certain normal or pathological movements. Based on a simplified model of the structure of the human body, this analysis is performed at different levels and with complementary techniques that evaluate different aspects of neuromuscular function, such as those described next [31–33]:

- Kinematic variables describe the body's movement by registering the angular variations of the joints and the relative movements of the body segments in space. In the same way, they record the length of the stride and the speed of the movement [34].
- Kinetic variables quantify the relationships between the action-reaction forces, the moments, and the powers measured for each body segment. The kinematic variables, in turn, make it possible to describe the vertical oscillation of the center of gravity (CoG) and to analyze relations of generation or absorption of mechanical energy in the joints produced by muscular action [35].
- Muscle activation variables evaluate the electrical activity of muscle activity during the gait cycle. These variables are recorded by EMG signals (superficial dynamic electromyography) [35–37]. In addition, other variables recorded by monitoring cardiorespiratory expenditure allow for obtaining a relationship between energy consumption during movement [38].

The human gait can be described and analyzed through a set of dynamic patterns obtained in a gait laboratory based on statistical analyses performed on large population groups that have defined normal ranges of motion. In the same way, gait cycle abnormalities have been defined in some diseases [38], including:

- Diplegic gait: Pathology of neuromuscular origin, characterized by an evolution in the communication of neuromotor commands. The result is a gait with uncoordinated movements and a high degree of spasticity in the lower extremities. The hips and knees are flexed during gait, and the ankles maintain extended adduction and internal rotation, while the trunk typically remains tilted [34].

- Parkinsonian gait: This movement is the product of a degenerative disorder of the central nervous system, characterized mainly by muscle rigidity, evident tremor, and slow movements of each body segment. During gait, patients lean forward, gait initiation is slow, stride length is small, and the feet are often shuffled [34].

Despite the wide range of pathologies and abnormal movements that can be described with dynamic patterns recorded in a gait laboratory, these descriptions are insufficient in the early stages of some diseases. In the Trendelenburg gait, characterized by the inclination of the trunk toward the supporting side, patterns are observed that indicate weakness and paralysis of the gluteus medium. These patterns may also describe a hip dislocation due to mechanical factors that reduce the leverage of the abductors [34]. On the other hand, it is important to note that the acquisition in normal patterns is large enough to hide the alterations that occur in the early stages of Parkinson's or in pathological gaits of psychiatric origin. Next, different models of human movement are described with different levels of detail and degrees of precision [31].

4.6.1.1 Structural Models

A first approximation to the movement of the human locomotor system consists of the study only of the structural relationships: body mass, lengths, and angles. Two different currents have used these relationships. The first assumes that the CoG describes a linear trajectory, while the second, built based on models that include an inverted pendulum, defends the idea of a CoG with a cyclical trajectory [31]:

- Inverted pendulum model
- Model of the six determinants of gait

In clinical applications for which a detailed and precise description of gait dynamics is needed, these types of models are ineffective since they do not allow for representing the dynamic patterns related to the leg joint and ground reaction forces. In addition, the CoG trajectory resulting from the implementation of these models moves away from the "smooth" trajectory characteristic of normal human gait, where the trajectory of the pendulum model generates abrupt changes at the instants in which the heel strike occurs. Each foot (two in a complete gait cycle) is far from the smooth trajectory of the normal CoG. It is why this type of representation is widely used in humanoid robot development but with significant limitations in model development of march oriented to the development of clinical support tools [31].

In general, these models do not consider fundamental aspects of robotics related to the stability of a bipedal system, such as the zero-moment point (ZMP). Based on this concept, Kudoh and Komura propose an improved inverted pendulum model through which it is possible to generate angular moments around the CoG, managing to represent a more significant number of dynamic gait patterns [39]. This improvement to the inverted pendulum model allows the ZMP to simulate the reaction force produced in contact with the ground so that the reaction force vector is not parallel with the vector that joins the ZMP with the CoG. Thus, the continuity of the trajectory is guaranteed throughout the movement. The model independently calculates movement in the sagittal and frontal planes, applying inverse kinematics to a set of postures obtained after calculating the trajectory of the CoG concerning the ZMP. A "ballistic gait" is a gait pattern in which the feet do not have contact with the ground for some moments and give stability to the system. However, the application of these models is restricted to the field of engineering, which is why new approaches arise that consider, in addition to structural relationships, force-generating and dissipating elements, which allow the representation of both normal and pathological movements [31].

4.6.1.2 Musculoskeletal Models

In analyzing the human gait, an adequate description of muscular participation in the generation of movement is essential to identify musculoskeletal disorders [40]. In the literature, models have been proposed that introduce factors representing the force-generating elements necessary to accelerate and decelerate the body (muscles and tendons). In this way, it has been possible to simulate, using computational tools, pathological gaits such as prosthetics or hemiplegia [41, 42]. These simulations have made it possible to optimize the rehabilitation mechanisms used in these cases [35, 42, 43].

4.6.1.3 Models Based on Electromyography Recordings

Dynamic electromyography is one of the most widely used techniques for recording and evaluating muscle behavior during walking. A neuropsychological study is performed using surface electrodes that capture muscle bioelectric activity in different movement phases. This technique has made it possible to obtain a set of patterns that make it possible to identify the sequence of muscle activation and deactivation during a gait cycle [37, 44]. Based on some biomechanical relationships of movement, different representations of human gait using approximating muscles and joints and the interaction of the musculoskeletal system have been proposed [45]. The models can be divided based on mechanical and computational models according to the complexity of these models to represent the musculoskeletal interaction of the locomotor system,

4.6.1.4 Models Based on Mechanical Systems

The global contraction pattern of the muscle groups can be modeled by subsystems using simple mechanical models composed of springs, dampers, and resistances. Under the restriction, each of these subsystems emulates a small part of the muscle, and the global contraction is some linear combination of these subsystems [31].

One of the most outstanding models is the one proposed by Hill, who describes a muscle group using three essential elements: a contractile element (CE), which represents the muscle fibers, and a parallel elastic element (PEE), which represents the tissues. Connectives and an elastic element in series represent all elastic elements, such as tendons [46].

Models have shown how the force generated by each muscle group affects the acceleration of each body segment. However, these models are not accurate enough to describe the complex interaction between different muscle groups using experimental parameters for continuous adjustment [35, 36].

4.6.1.5 Computational Musculoskeletal Models

Various computational models seek to describe the interaction of each of the components of the locomotor system, using the information provided by electromyographic records or in particular biomechanical relationships [35, 40]. These models have allowed gait dynamics to be simulated, considering some non-linear behaviors of the locomotor system and describing different relationships between each of its components [31].

This model is based on the inverted pendulum theory and the Hill muscle-tendon model. The first represents structural and efficiency relationships in terms of energy, while the second serves to represent each muscle group [31].

In rehabilitation engineering, the development of gait models that allow the description, quantification, and simulation of different dynamic gait patterns associated with some pathology has been important. Approaches such as the inverted pendulum seek to describe the dynamics of the center of mass of people with some amputation [42, 47], considering prostheses as rigid bodies without muscular elements and of variable mass. These strategies have managed to describe with a certain degree of similarity the dynamics of a prosthetic gait. However, the clinical utility is still very limited because this analysis is very simple [35, 48]. The computational ones have allowed a more useful analysis, with some complementing the information obtained from dynamic biomechanical models [35, 36, 49], with which it has been possible to simulate a larger number of dynamic gait patterns.

Goujon et al. proposed a dynamic method for calculating the external forces applied to the feet during gait, achieving an approximation to the kinetics of pathological gait to analyze the behavior of prosthetic feet and the loads applied during gait [50]. These contributions have influenced the manufacturing processes of orthopedic and rehabilitation devices, adding new strategies for calculating load distribution and the applicability of existing prosthesis designs [36, 50]. Kuruvilla et al. developed a method that describes the characteristic patterns of Charcot-Marie-Tooth disease, also known as hereditary motor and sensory neuropathy, or fibular muscular atrophy, using data obtained from gait laboratories. The altered results have made it possible to considerably improve the understanding of this and the extraction of the set of dynamic patterns that characterize it, positively influencing the design of treatments specifically oriented to this pathology [51].

With this new field of application, new areas of knowledge, such as computational biomechanics, have proposed new strategies for the description of normal and pathological gait patterns, improving accuracy and highlighting the models proposed so far [35]. In this sense, one of the most representative models is the one proposed by Komura et al. [39], who, based on the inverted pendulum theory and the muscle relationships proposed by Delp et al., propose a computational model that allows the simulation of pathological movements related to the weakening of certain muscle groups. Komura assumes that the PMC is not fixed, as is generally considered [40].

The model proposed by Komura suggests that the force vector generated from the PMC does not intersect the point given by the CoG, allowing the generation of rotational and angular moments and the angular momentum at the instant. He then formulates an inverse kinematics problem based on the structural model used by Delp. Subsequently, he calculates the torques generated in each joint [31].

4.6.1.6 Neuromuscular Models

Studies of human locomotion have shown that gait stability and flexibility are produced by the interaction between the rhythmic activity of the nervous system (neuromotor commands) and the movement of the musculoskeletal system. One of the most relevant hypotheses in the development of neuromuscular models suggests the existence of a central pattern generator (CPG) in charge of the generation and control of muscle-articular movement. Discovered in 1985, the CPG may be located relatively low in the central nervous system (spinal cord). Theoretical studies on the control of the locomotor system have shown that the CPG is a complex adaptive system from where movements originate from the dynamic interaction between the nervous system, the body, and the environment in a self-organized way [31].

The discovery of the CPG motivated the development of control systems adapted to existing musculoskeletal systems and models, seeking a more detailed description of the human locomotor system during walking. Buchli [52] made important contributions in the area of robotics, inspired by the CPG, developing a control scheme through a group of neurological oscillators that synchronously induce activation in certain muscle groups that control a joint. Output signals from the CPG induce body movements by activating the muscles, such that each neurological oscillator in the CPG controls the muscles around a single joint [31].

Some researchers have made attempts to use some classical machine learning approaches, such as neural networks, to represent bipedal gait based on the CPG concept [53, 54], looking for efficient and complex control systems. The simplest models consider only the cyclic movements of one leg in the sagittal plane, assuming symmetry in gait [31].

Taga et al. proposed a neuromusculoskeletal model with which the control mechanisms are explored, responsible for generating human movement based on the emerging properties of the GCP as a basic neuronal system [53, 55]. Other approaches have attempted to model the neuromuscular system using independent oscillators and autonomous controls for each joint. These musculoskeletal models allow adjustment to different degrees of pathology, employing certain parameters that can be varied and facilitating the analysis of pathological movements. However, the set of pathologies that can be represented in this way is still limited since certain structural and neuromuscular aspects cannot be considered, such as bone deformations, deficiencies in neuromotor control derived from obstructions in the nerve channels, or cerebral motor dysfunctions (common causes of pathologies associated with the human locomotor system) [31].

Various gait models have been reported, from models based on inverted pendulum dynamics to complex computational models describing the dynamics of the neuromusculoskeletal system. However, the motivation has been almost exclusively the solution to engineering problems, with which the inclusion in clinical practice has been almost non-existent [31].

4.6.2 Kinematics of Upper Limb Exoskeletons: Case of ERMIS Exoskeleton

The ERMIS exoskeleton requires seven articulation variables that correspond to the DoF of the system. These variables represent the angle that exists between two links at the point where they articulate. All joint variables are defined by angles whose axis of rotation has been made to coincide with the Z axis of each reference system. The direction of the Z axis coincides with the axis that was used with the goniometer network. The reference systems are built proposing the direction of X, and from the definition of the orthonormal vectors, Y is defined with the Denavit-Hartenberg (DH) algorithm [56].

First, the reference systems are located in the conceptual model, representing the location of the axes of rotation of the joints. Afterward, the relationship between each anatomical movement of the human arm with the corresponding joint variable and the associated reference system is presented. The home position of the system corresponds to the natural state of the rest of the upper limb, with the subject standing with the arm aligned to a vertical axis and the palm facing forward [56].

Subsequently, the joint variables will be defined: θi (degrees) description adjunct referencing system, $\theta 1$ shoulder abduction/adduction $X1Y1Z1$, $\theta 2$ shoulder flexion/extension $X2Y2Z2$, $\theta 3$ shoulder internal/external rotation $X3Y3Z3$, $\theta 4$ elbow flexion/extension $X4Y4Z4$, $\theta 5$ pronation/supination $X5Y5Z5$, $\theta 6$ flexion/extension wrist $X6Y6Z6$, and $\theta 7$ radial/ulnar deviation $X7Y7Z7$ [56].

4.6.2.1 Forward Kinematics

The DH parameters containing the exoskeleton's physical characteristics are described in the DH table. After substituting the values of the DH table, the homogeneous matrix that leads from the global system to the end of the exoskeleton is obtained. Using Matlab's numerical simplification tools, the components of the homogeneous transformation matrix corresponding to the position vector are obtained (Cartesian references to the global reference system). In this way, the Cartesian variables are obtained from the joint variables [56].

4.6.2.2 Simulation

Simscape Multibody is a Matlab platform that can simulate environments and bodies in 3D. Models can use the Matlab platform to acquire or send variables and hydraulic, electrical, and pneumatic properties from Simulink. The simulation is supported by blocks, which indicate the properties of bodies, joints, sensors, and motors. The Simulink model uses signal connections, which define how data flows from one block to another. The Simscape Multibody model is built using physical connections, allowing bidirectional power flow between components, and physical connections allow additional stages to be added as input/output connections. The rigid bodies designed in CAD are imported with their properties into the Simulink environment; they are connected after carefully selecting their reference frames, resulting in the dynamic model of the exoskeleton [56].

All modules have two ports: the base B (base) and the follower F (follower), representing the frames of reference for a joint. The direction of the joint is defined by the movement of the follower's reference frame concerning the base's reference frame. Each solid body block contains the characteristics of mass, inertia, the center of mass, and moment of inertia [56].

4.6.2.3 Simulation of Forward Kinematics

The captured trajectory of the rudder exercise comprises seven individual and simultaneous trajectories, corresponding to the movements of each articular system of the arm. Each joint data file is linearly interpolated and imported into the ERMIS simulated model to serve as the desired behavior. In the simulation, a block is added that generates the trajectories of position, velocity, and acceleration (signal builder). Each corresponding linear actuator and motor allow for obtaining the desired behavior. These trajectories are not the same as desired, since the effect of the transmission that is coupled with the pivot of the articulation of each GDL is still missing. The transmissions for the linear actuators are rod mechanisms, and for the motors, they are a differential set of bevel gears. The simulation is configured to calculate the gain necessary for the actuators to have the force or torque to compensate for the error between the desired trajectories and the actual trajectories of each joint [56].

This section specifies the joint movement profile of each DoF of the exoskeleton. The joint trajectories that are used as inputs in the joint blocks correspond to those obtained in the characterization of the case studies. The results obtained from the model when simulating it correspond to the spatial location of the terminal element of the exoskeleton (corresponding to the patient's hand) expressed as the trajectories $x(t)$, $y(t)$, and $z(t)$, and referring to the frame of world reference. The data that will be acquired with the experimental measurement of the case study in each joint will be added. The original data is found in a file that contains an array formed by a pair of discrete data: one for angular amplitude and the other for time. Then it is changed to the data time series type. In Simulink, the font file block is added, where the demo time is configured, the type of extrapolation before the first value, and finally, the type of interpolation of the data with a zero-order retainer [56].

During the model simulation, the exoskeleton's final position that coincides with the end effector (end of the exoskeleton) reference frame is calculated. The Transform Sensor block is connected to this joint, which extracts the trajectories of the reference frame measured concerning the reference frame global.

4.6.3 HAND EXOSKELETON KINEMATICS

Understanding the kinematics of the human hand is essential to design a proper exoskeleton. For multi-phalangeal design, the joint degrees of freedom, joint ranges, and phalanx length should match the average human hand kinematic parameters. Its kinematics can be considered using a skeletal structure. The first link is the metacarpal joint, which is located in the palm. The base of each finger is connected to metacarpophalangeal (MCP) joints. Three phalanges, called the distal phalanx (DIP), the middle phalanx, and the proximal phalanx (PIP), are connected through the interphalangeal (IP) joints. The MCP joint connects the metacarpal and proximal phalanx. The PIP joint connects the proximal and middle phalanx, and the DIP joint connects the middle and distal phalanx. The thumb has only one IP joint.

The motion of each finger includes flexion and extension, as well as abduction and adduction [57].

The index finger can be considered a three-link mechanism with four-DOF motion. However, human anatomy studies show that the motion of the DIP is naturally coupled with the PIP motion. Levangie et al. [58] show that the maximum range of the index finger joints is 90° for the MCP, 100°–110° for the PIP, 80° for the DIP in flexion and extension movements, and 40° for the adduction and abduction movements. These motion ranges vary for different fingers and users according to the hand's bone geometry and tendon and muscle structure. The thumb's kinematics are different from the other fingers. Unlike the index finger, the thumb has only three joints: the first two joints, MCP and DIP, have revolute joints, whereas the metacarpus (MC) joint of the thumb can execute three-DOF motion [57].

A simplified kinematic model of the finger is used to study the kinematic properties and trajectories of the hand. The index finger mechanism provides three rotary joints that allow extension and flexion of the finger. Accordingly, a planar model with three revolute or rotational joints (RRR) has been used as the kinematic model of the index finger. The thumb also considers a planar model with two R joints. All the joints in the design use revolute pin connections. Extension and flexion are possible for both the index and the thumb mechanisms, whereas abduction and adduction movements are locked [57].

The revolute joints R1 and R2 mimic the PIP and DIP joints, respectively, while the third joint, R3, refers to the MCP joints. All three joints have parallel rotation axes forming a planar mechanism. The model follows the precise articulation of the index finger. The exoskeleton's joint position carefully matches the human hand's joint position on the lateral side. The last MC joint uses two links to allow both rotation and translation of the finger assemblies concerning the palm. Each joint is coupled with passive pulleys, which correspond to the R joints. In addition, the exoskeleton is designed to keep the fingertip and the palm area free from additional tactile feedback. This also helps reduce the overall system's weight [57].

Each finger of the exoskeleton can be modeled as a planar and serial three-link mechanism, where the mount on the hand's dorsum is considered the ground link. The planar method ignores lateral movements of the finger, namely the adduction, and abduction. Therefore, the overall exoskeleton device can be considered an independent three-link (index) and two-link (thumb) mechanism. A separate thumb kinematic analysis is unnecessary, as the two-link kinematic model of the thumb can be easily calculated by setting the first link length and the joint value of the index kinematic model to zero [57].

These angular ranges are chosen to match the effective anthropomorphic articular ranges of the human hand. The position and orientation of each fingertip are calculated using the forward kinematics equation. The position and orientation of the fingertip concerning the MC link (ground) can be expressed using the 3×3 2D homogeneous transformation matrix, which consists of the rotation of each link concerning the previous link and the translation of each joint from the previous joint. It holds the 2D position and orientation of the fingertip, which can be extracted from the previous transformation matrix. Precisely, the fingertip contact point C (x, y, z) can be expressed by transforming the joint coordinates.

The forward kinematic equation can be generalized as $x = f(q)$, where x is the position and orientation of the fingertip and q is the Lagrange joint variable. The derivative of this equation returns the Jacobian matrix, $J(q)$. Accordingly, the linear velocity is expressed as a function of the Jacobian and joint velocities. And finally, the rotational velocity can be expressed as a function of the fingertip velocities [57].

4.6.3.1 Workspace

When exploring a free space in a remote or VR environment, the haptic device should not restrict the human user's motion. Thus, the DOFs of the haptic device should match the natural ones of the human hand. According to Gruebler's formula, the mobility of the overall mechanism can be calculated as $F = 3(n-1) - 2l - h$, where F is the total DOFs of the mechanism, n is the number of links (including the frame), l is the number of lower pairs (i.e., one DOF), and h is the number of higher pairs (i.e., two DOF). According to the kinematics, the results of the equation provide a three-DOF mechanism for the index and a two-DOF for the thumb. Enough workspace for the haptic device is also needed to achieve the desired motion possible with natural hand movement.

4.6.3.2 Actuation and Force Transmission

An underactuated mechanism has been chosen to match the requirements, such as compact size, low weight, and low power system. The underactuated system allows having a number of actuators lower than the number of DOFs performed with the hand. It also enables the exoskeleton mechanism to adapt passively to the finger structure [57]. Both exoskeleton fingers are activated via a cable transmission system, which is routed from the actuators on the palm to each finger joint up to the fingertip. The cable transmission systems provide adequate power to reduce the weight and inertia of the moving parts and allow remote actuation from the palm [57].

Angular joint trajectories of the index finger mechanism are calculated from the fully open configuration to the fully closed one. All revolute joints are driven by applying a tension force F to the cable, which is wrapped around the finger joints of radius r. Assuming that the friction force is negligible and that the cables are ideally rigid, the applied torque on each joint can therefore be expressed as a function of the radius of the pulleys and the tension force. Finally, an underactuated mechanism with a cable force transmission system couples the joint torques with the cable tension F. The tension forces are also assumed to be constant for the same cable. This happens considering that the tension torque on the pulleys is negligible and the torque due to the pulley inertia is small. Unlike the rehabilitation exoskeleton—which requires two cables for the extension and flexion movements—the haptic exoskeleton requires a single cable to restrict the extension movement. The flexion can be passively performed not to restrict the natural movement of the finger [57].

A DC motor actuation system pulls the cable. The haptic system needs either active control of the cable position or should be back-derivable so that the user can pull the cables with less force. The haptic system should also be capable of delivering a maximum force that matches the human hand output force. Here, thanks to the motors used, the maximum thumb and finger force output are in the order of 35 N.

The CyberGrasp, a commercial force feedback device, can apply a 12 N maximum output force, enough to provide a realistic force feedback sensation. Consequently, in this design, a 10–12 N maximum force is considered [57].

The system has an underactuated kinematic structure that enables the exoskeleton to act as an adaptive finger stimulator. The exoskeleton has sensors for motion detection and control. The proposed architecture offers three main advantages. First, the exoskeleton enables accurate quantification of subject-specific finger dynamics. The exoskeleton configuration can be fully reconstructed using measurements from three angular position sensors placed on the kinematic structure. In addition, the actuation force acting on the exoskeleton is recorded. Thus, the range of motion (ROM) and each finger joint's force and torque trajectories can be determined. Second, the adaptive kinematic structure allows the patient to perform various functional tasks. The force control of the exoskeleton acts as a safeguard and limits the maximum possible joint torques during finger movement. Last, the system is compact, lightweight, and does not require extensive peripherals. Due to its safety features, it is easy to use in the home [57].

4.6.3.3   Hand Exoskeleton Dynamic Model

With the use of the contact forces between the exoskeleton and the finger, a dynamic model can be derived. The model consists of the three finger joints moving in a plane and connected by revolute joints. The minimum coordinates of the dynamic model and the contact forces are known. Then, the dynamic model can be solved for the unknown torques in the case of unrestrained motion [59].

For each body in the system, the sum of forces and moments is calculated and projected in the directions compatible with the kinematic constraints via the transposed individual Jacobian matrices for translation. Actions on each body are described concerning the inertial reference frame, while the moments are described in body fixed coordinate frames. Since the moving masses in the system and their velocities and accelerations are small compared to the external forces and moments acting on the system, the model can be approximately described quasi-statically [59].

4.6.4   Gait Kinematics by OrthoTrak

The following case study is extracted from the scientific communication "Elbow Kinematics During Gait Improve with Age in Children with Hemiplegic Cerebral Palsy". Children with hemiplegic cerebral palsy (hCP) exhibit a typical posture of elbow flexion during gait. However, the change in elbow kinematics and symmetry during gait across age span in both hCP and typically developing (TD) children are not well described. This study aimed to quantify the change in elbow kinematics and symmetry across age span in hCP children compared with TD children [60].

Methods: Upper extremity kinematic data were extracted and analyzed from a database for gait studies performed between 2009 and 2015. A total of 35 hCP and 51 TD children between the ages of 4 and 18 (mean age: TD = 11.2 ± 0.6, hCP = 9.8 ± 0.5) met inclusionary criteria. The groups were further subdivided into ages 4–7, 8–11, and 12+ years old. Elbow angles were extracted, and peak elbow flexion, the overall range of motion during gait, and asymmetry indices were calculated. A one-way analysis of variance was performed on each group with post hoc Tukey honestly significant difference pairwise comparisons [60].

Results: Peak elbow flexion during gait increased with age in TD children (P <0.05) and decreased with age in hCP children on the affected side (P <0.05). There was no change on the less affected side of hCP children. TD children demonstrated significantly less elbow flexion (mean = 51.9±2.1 deg.) compared with the affected side in hCP (mean = 82.1±3.8 deg.) across all age categories (P <0.05). There was no change in elbow asymmetry index (0 = perfect symmetry) across age in either controls or hCP children; however, there were differences between hCP and TD groups in younger age groups (TD = 28, hCP = 62, P <0.05) that resolved by adolescence (TD = 32, hCP = 40) [60].

Procedure: Gait analysis data were extracted from a database of gait studies. All gait studies utilized a 12-camera motion capture system (Motion Analysis Corporation, Santa Rosa, CA). Thirty-five retroreflective markers were placed on each subject's UEs, trunk, pelvis, and LEs using the Cleveland Clinic Marker set and were captured at 100 Hz. Joint kinematics were calculated in OrthoTrak (version 6.55; Motion Analysis Corporation). An average of 10 representative gait cycles were collected as subjects walked at the self-selected walking speed [60].

Analysis: Gait cycles were normalized to time, and peak elbow flexion, extension and overall range during each cycle were calculated. Peak elbow flexion was defined as maximum elbow flexion achieved during gait testing. Elbow range (i.e., the total arc of motion) was defined as elbow range of motion excursion during gait and was calculated as the difference between maximum elbow flexion and maximum elbow extension during gait analysis. An asymmetry index was used to quantify differences between the two limbs. Elbow asymmetry indices (ASI) were calculated according to the following formula: an ASI closer to 0 indicates the more symmetrical movement of the UEs during gait. All statistical analyses were performed using IBM SPSS Statistics; Armonk, NY (version 19.0) [60].

Conclusions: During gait, hCP children have greater peak elbow flexion on the affected side than TD children. Peak elbow flexion angle converged between the two groups with age, decreasing in hCP children and increasing in TD children. Furthermore, elbow symmetry during gait improves with age in hCP children, approximating the symmetry of TD children by adolescence [60].

4.7 SENSORS

Recent technologic advancements have enabled the creation of sensors with the potential to alter the clinical practice of rehabilitation. The application of wearable sensors to track movement has emerged as a promising paradigm to enhance the care provided to patients with neurologic or musculoskeletal conditions. These sensors enable the quantification of motor behavior across disparate patient populations, and emerging research shows their potential for identifying motor biomarkers, differentiating between restitution and compensation motor recovery mechanisms, remote monitoring, telerehabilitation, and robotics [61].

4.7.1 Gyroscopes

A gyroscope measures the rate of change of angular motion by detecting the Coriolis forces that act on a moving mass in a rotating reference frame. These forces are proportional to the rate of angular rotation of the limb. Gyroscopes are secured to body segments in line with the plane of movement that is being measured [62], and tri-axial gyroscopes allow three-dimensional measurements. The strengths of gyroscope sensors are that their measurements are not influenced by gravitational forces [63], and vibrations during heel strikes do not distort the signal [64].

4.7.2 Accelerometers

An accelerometer measures body movements based on the rate of change of speed. A mass-spring system commonly explains the measurement principle underlying accelerometry [65]. Based on the displacement of the mass element, the resultant acceleration is derived [65]. Although there are several classes of accelerometers, the most used in rehabilitation research are strain gauge, capacitive, piezo-resistive, and piezoelectric [65]. Accelerometers used in rehabilitation commonly have one to three sensing axes, which allow motion detection in one- to three-dimensional space. Accelerometers are commonly used for continuous monitoring of gait, mobility, and activities of daily living.

Accelerometer signals can be used to compute position or velocity; however, drift from integration decreases data quality [64]. Additional limitations associated with the use of accelerometers include poor reliability when measuring non-dynamic events [66] and the influence of gravity on the acceleration signal [67]. Various signal-processing strategies are being developed to improve data quality [67]. Magnetometers are devices that detect the Earth's gravitation vector. Their measurements provide compass heading information and a reference measure for body orientation relative to gravity [67]. Because magnetometers are insensitive to acceleration during dynamic movements, their use alongside accelerometers allows the separation of gravitational components from kinematic acceleration data. Moreover, given the qualities and limitations of gyroscopes, accelerometers, and magnetometers, these sensor types are often combined in self-contained devices called inertial measurement units (IMUs) to optimize measurement capabilities [61].

4.7.3 Force-Based Sensors

Force-based sensors offer additional insight into a wearer's interaction with the environment and have been used alongside IMUs. By and large, limitations in the quality of individual sensor signals can be addressed with advanced processing and intelligent algorithms [68]. The following section provides an overview of the applications of these sensors across neurologic and orthopedic domains. State-of-the-art clinical application wearable sensors are portable, low-cost, and unobtrusive tools that provide objective, quantitative, and continuous information about motor behavior in a range of environments. Clinically, wearable sensors have been used for assessment, including the instrumentation of common mobility tests [69], identification of pathologic movement [70, 71], characterization of disease stage [72], falls management [73, 74], and activity recognition (AR). They also have been used to augment treatments, such as enabling biofeedback-based gait training [75–77]. Below are some clinical applications of cutting-edge technology, where the following concepts are abbreviated: Timed Up and Go Test (TUG), Parkinson's Disease (PD), Huntington's Disease (HD), Berg Balance Scale (BBS), Knee Adduction Moment (KAM), OsteoArthritis (OA) [61].

- Assessment.
  - o Clinical instrumentation, using IMU sensor. Finding: High reliability and low measurement error for most measures used for instrumented TUG in individuals after stroke [69].
  - o Falls management, using phone-based IMU sensor. Finding: Can identify differences in kinematic gait variables in those after a stroke with and without a history of falls [73].
  - o Falls management, using IMU sensor. Finding: Can identify differences in dynamic gait stability between stroke and control cohorts and variables that could play an important role in increased fall risk [74].
  - o Identify pathologic motor features, using IMU sensor. Finding: High test-retest reliability and sensitivity in measuring bradykinesia, hypokinesia, and dysrhythmia in those with PD [70].
  - o Identify pathologic motor features, using iPod-based IMU sensor. Finding: Can detect significant differences in trunk control during static activities in people with HD compared with controls; it found amplitude of thoracic and pelvic trunk movements was significantly greater in participants with HD [71].
  - o Activity recognition, using IMU sensor. Finding: Ability to classify (90.4%) basic activities common to daily life in individuals after stroke [78].
  - o Activity recognition, using Step Watch Activity Monitor sensor. Finding: Able to characterize activity levels without relying on self-report data or clinician opinion [79], assess real-world performance [80], and guide community-based treatments using goal setting for individuals after stroke [81].
  - o Activity recognition, using Phone-based IMU sensor. Finding: Good sensitivity and specificity in detecting immobile (standing, sitting, lying) vs. mobile (walking) states, but poor ability to classify more complicated movements (walking up stairs) in people with stroke.
  - o Characterization of disease stage, using IMU sensor. Finding: High correlation between disease severity and turning velocity, duration, and step number in those with PD tracked over 7 days [72].

- Treatment.
  - o Biofeedback, using force sensor smart shoes, custom made IMUs smart pants, custom made. Finding: Significant improvements in balance, mobility, strength, and range of motion comparable to improvements

seen with therapist cueing only; suggesting potential use in at-home training for those with PD and after stroke [75].

o Biofeedback, using IMU sensor. Finding: Improved BBS score and decreased mediolateral sway during standing in participants with PD who received biofeedback with gamepad during training [76].

o Biofeedback, using Force sensor and pager motor. Finding: Decreased KAM by 14.2% in people with OA [77].

4.7.4 Technology for Stroke

Advanced signal processing approaches have enabled IMU instrumentation of popular clinical tests such as the 10-meter walk test [74] and the Timed Up-and-Go Test [69], providing clinically relevant data on movement quality in addition to the traditional outcome of "time to complete". Moreover, advanced AR algorithms have enabled IMU data to be used to identify and quantify gross movements with high sensitivity and specificity [78]. Data extracted from IMUs located in mobile phones have differentiated stroke survivors who are fallers from those who are not based on an estimate of stride variability [73]. However, these analyses have been limited when quantifying more complex movements, motivating further work in this area [82].

Accelerometer-based step activity monitors have also been used to monitor physical activity in the home and the community, providing ecologically valid mobility data for developing treatment-based classifications [79], to assess real-world performance [80], and to guide community-based treatment programs [81].

Wearable sensors also have enabled novel gait training approaches, such as biofeedback-based interventions. For example, a custom body-worn sensor system composed of force sensors and IMUs was used to provide kinematic biofeedback during gait training, leading to improvements in balance, mobility, strength, and range of motion that were comparable to the treatment benefits obtained through therapist-directed gait training [75]. These results demonstrate the potential for wearable sensors to provide effective gait intervention without direct oversight by a clinician (e.g., in real-world settings) [61].

4.7.5 Technology for Parkinson's Disease

As in stroke, AR algorithms have enabled IMU data to be used to identify pathologic motor features characteristic of PD. For example, in levodopa-treated individuals, periods of motor fluctuations between mobile and immobile states (i.e., on-off periods) were detected using IMU data analyzed with an advanced AR algorithm [83]. Other studies have demonstrated how IMUs can be useful in tracking primary physical symptoms of PD, such as tremors [84], dyskinesias, and bradykinesia [70], and in tracking disease progression [72]. IMUs have differentiated between tremor-dominant and non-tremor-dominant patients with PD [35]. Mancini et al. [72] tracked features of turning performance (e.g., velocity, duration, and step number) for 7 days and found a high correlation between disease severity and turning mobility. Additional studies have shown that IMU-enabled continuous monitoring of baseline gait metrics can predict disease progression and gait decline 1 and 2 years later [85]. Moreover, a recent study of 190 patients with PD and 101 age-matched controls showed the feasibility of large-scale clinical trials to use IMUs to robustly track spatiotemporal parameters of gait [86].

As in stroke, sensor-enabled biofeedback interventions have gained popularity as noninvasive training tools in PD rehabilitation. Wearable sensors have been used to facilitate the delivery of rhythmic auditory or haptic cues during gait training, an approach shown to enhance motor learning in persons with PD [86]. Similarly, IMUs have been used effectively to provide haptic and visual biofeedback related to kinematic data during balance and gait training in persons with PD [76].

4.7.6 Technology for Knee Osteoarthritis

Wearable sensors have been used to understand population-level behavior in individuals with OA. Based on the Osteoarthritis Initiative, a large epidemiologic study on knee OA that used wearable sensors to track physical activity in 1,111 adults, only 12.9% of men and 7.7% of women with knee OA met aerobic physical activity guidelines [87]. The study showed that in people with knee OA, more sedentary behavior was associated with worse physical function [88] and a greater risk of future functional decline [89]. The Multicenter Osteoarthritis Study, another large epidemiologic study enabled by wearable activity trackers, showed that disease severity and knee pain were not predictive of physical activity levels [90]. Older adults with a high risk of knee OA did not meet physical activity guidelines despite walking at least 10,000 steps per day [91]. These wearable sensor-enabled studies have yielded critical insights into the factors related to decreased physical activity in persons with knee OA and the effects of decreased physical activity on health.

For people with OA of the knee, the most common therapeutic application of wearable sensors is to alter the kinematics to decrease the load on the knee joint during walking. People with medial tibiofemoral OA walk with greater medial compartment loading compared with individuals with knee OA [92]. Greater medial compartment loading is implicated in more rapid disease progression [93]. Thus, there is significant interest in interventions that can decrease medial compartment loading. The knee adduction moment (KAM) during walking, measured using three-dimensional motion capture, is commonly used as a surrogate for medial compartment loading [92]. There are several examples in the literature of wearable sensors being used to decrease KAM. Dowling et al. [77], for example, developed an active feedback system fitted inside a shoe. The system delivered haptic feedback if the pressure on the shoe's lateral aspect exceeded a specific threshold, intending to produce a subtle medial shift in weight bearing to decrease KAM [61].

The use of this innovative biofeedback system led to a mean decrease of 14.2% in KAM. Although encouraging, this study was performed in healthy individuals, in a controlled laboratory environment, using expensive motion analysis instruments, and with a prototype version of the device. Significant work is needed to translate these systems to free-living conditions for people with knee OA [61].

4.7.7 TECHNOLOGY FOR RUNNING

Up to 79% of runners are injured each year [94]. There is emerging interest in impact mechanics' role in running injuries. Accumulating evidence shows associations between impact loading, as measured with a force plate, and injuries in runners. Indeed, vertical load rates during the impact phase of running are associated with tibial stress fractures [95]. Runners with diagnosed injuries also have higher vertical load rates than those who have never been injured [96]. Similarly, vertical load rates are related to other common running injuries such as patellofemoral pain and plantar fasciitis [96]. Although vertical load rates are related to running injuries, peak tibial acceleration during landing is related to these load rates [97]. Therefore, peak tibial acceleration, which can be measured with an accelerometer, has become a surrogate measure for vertical load rates [61].

Wearable sensors also can assist in examining other gait characteristics that might contribute to running injuries, such as cadence and strike patterns. Among elite runners, achieving cadences near 180 steps per minute is believed to optimize performance [98]. Increased cadence has other benefits, such as decreases in hip and knee energy absorption, patellofemoral stress, and hip adduction [99, 100]. Further, increasing habitual cadences have demonstrated small decreases in vertical load rates [101]. In contrast, strike pattern influences ground reaction forces applied to the body [61].

Rearfoot strike results in a very distinct impact peak in the vertical ground reaction force that is absent during a forefoot strike [102]. Transitioning to a forefoot strike pattern has been shown to resolve chronic patellofemoral pain [103] and chronic anterior compartment syndrome [104]. These distinct impact features can be seen in accelerometer data and can be used to differentiate a rearfoot strike from a forefoot strike pattern [61].

Wearable sensors present an exciting opportunity in the prevention and treatment of running-related injuries by affording the ability to provide real-time feedback to the runner. Many commercial IMUs provide information on cumulative loads, which can be extremely helpful in preventing overload injuries in runners. Given the range of gait characteristics that can be measured (e.g., strike pattern, lower extremity angles, and tibial shock), a wide variety of gait deviations can be addressed. Once the physical therapist identifies the faulty aspect of the gait, the runner can be instructed on how to alter the gait pattern [61].

Then the therapist can set audible signals to remind the patient to attend to the gait when it begins to degrade beyond a certain threshold. Then feedback can be gradually removed with time. Runners can first practice these gait changes in the clinic; however, wearable sensors allow runners to translate the gait changes from the clinic into their natural running environment. This provides greater ecological validity to the treatment and can decrease the number of clinical visits needed, lowering overall healthcare costs [61].

IMUs have important limitations to note when assessing running. Impact magnitudes during running can often exceed 16g, the limit of some commercial devices. Similarly, accelerations during running include high-frequency components that require adequate sampling frequencies (500–1,000 Hz). These factors need to be considered when choosing IMU-based devices for running studies [61].

The use of wearable sensors to inform neurologic and orthopedic rehabilitation practice warrants careful consideration of their clinometric properties, which vary among devices [105], conditions, measures, and environments [106]. Information on reliability, validity, and sensitivity is available for some devices, but not all. For example, wearable sensors used for running have been shown to provide acceptable, valid, and reliable values for some measures [107]; however, IMU-derived measures of tibial acceleration magnitudes and determinations of strike patterns require validation. For PD, a recent review of sensor characteristics concluded that only 9 of the 73 devices considered could be recommended based on the availability and acceptability of their clinometric properties [105]. Continued examination of the clinometric properties of wearable sensor measurements could improve data processing standardization, variable definitions, and the development of population-specific algorithms [105, 106].

Emerging clinical applications using existing sensor technologies include their use (i) to identify biomarkers of disease onset and progression, (ii) to differentiate between restitution and compensatory mechanisms of motor recovery, (iii) to provide opportunities for telerehabilitation and big data collection, and (iv) in next-generation robotics [61].

4.7.8 BIOMARKERS

Tracking disease onset and progression is particularly valuable for those with chronic diseases. As such, there is increasing research effort directed toward the identification of biomarkers. A biomarker is a measurable characteristic that represents a normal biologic process, a pathologic process, or a response to an intervention [108]. For example, there is emerging research on identifying motor biomarkers in genetic neurodegenerative diseases. The discreet nature of wearable sensors and their ability to measure subtle changes in mobility in ecological settings make them a highly promising tool for detecting subclinical motor changes that can signal disease onset and progression. Evidence for this emerging application follows [61].

PD is characterized by dopamine depletion in the basal ganglia, which results in motor disturbances such as tremors, postural instability, bradykinesia, and gait impairment. Although most cases of PD are idiopathic, a subset can be explained by genetic factors, of which the most common mutation is leucine-rich repeat kinase 2 (LRRK2) plus G2019S [109]. Accelerometers fixed on the low back have been used to identify increased stride time variability [110], arm swing asymmetry, and trunk axial jerk in asymptomatic carriers of the LRRK2-G2019S mutation (i.e., at risk for PD) during dual-task walking compared with healthy controls [111].

Identifying motor biomarkers in HD is also an emerging area in which wearable sensors have strong potential. HD is an autosomal-dominant neurodegenerative disease that is characterized by a combination of hyperkinetic and hypokinetic motor features [112].

Pharmaceutical and rehabilitative interventions are being developed to delay the clinical onset or slow down the progression of HD [113]. However, these efforts are attenuated owing to limited knowledge of optimal clinical endpoints needed for clinical trials [61].

There is emerging evidence for the use of wearable sensors to identify alterations in motor control, which could serve as a worthwhile endpoint. As in PD, an IMU fixed on the low back of individuals with pre-manifest HD and healthy controls was effective in detecting subclinical decrements in the sensory modulation of postural control [114] and variability in trunk movement during walking [115]. Similarly, wearable iPod sensors (IMU-based) fixed on the trunk and low back detected abnormal trunk movements in persons with manifest HD compared with controls [71]. Despite these exciting preliminary findings that support the use of wearable sensors to identify and monitor biomarkers of disease onset and progression in movement disorders, larger, multisite, and longitudinal studies are needed to catalyze this application [61].

4.7.9 Motor Restitution Against Compensation

An emerging clinical application of wearable sensor technologies is in differentiating restitution from compensation when assessing the nature of motor recovery [116]. Restitution refers to the reappearance of movement patterns present before the injury. In contrast, compensation refers to the emergence of a new set of movement patterns after an injury resulting from substitution or adaptive mechanisms [116]. Elucidation of the mechanisms by which recovery occurs during rehabilitation allows for the development of computational models that can organize biological and behavioral data to inform clinical decision-making [116].

Researchers have also begun using wearable sensor technologies and analytical techniques to look beyond gross functional and biomechanical recordings, focusing on the neural control of movement. An example is the use of surface electromyography (sEMG) in the examination of motor modules during functional activities [117] to identify neuromechanical differences between healthy and pathologic movement [118] and to evaluate the effects of neurorehabilitation intervention [119] and assess changes in neuromotor control resulting from robotic intervention [120]. Although more research is needed, this is a promising application of commercially available sensor technology. By differentiating between restitution and compensation mechanisms of recovery after neuromotor injury or dysfunction, sEMG analyses have the potential to influence the prescription and evaluation of rehabilitative treatments [61].

4.7.10 Telerehabilitation

As the population ages and chronic disease rates and healthcare costs continue to rise, there is demand for increased access to healthcare services and decreased costs. Telerehabilitation is a relatively new branch of telemedicine that prioritizes developing and optimizing telecommunication technologies for rehabilitation services (e.g., evaluation, monitoring, and treatment) [121].

The emerging use of wearable movement sensors to enable telerehabilitation services is exciting and timely. It is not the goal of telerehabilitation to replace health professionals; rather, it is to elevate the level of care [122]. The remote monitoring afforded by wearable sensors allows for real-time movement tracking in real-world settings. This enables the continuous sampling of activity rather than a finite series of collections taken during periodic clinic visits. Clinicians could use continuous remote monitoring of movement data to map progress and develop personalized interventions [61].

The transmission of these data to clinicians through wireless communication systems could increase patient access to clinicians by bypassing the need to travel to a clinic physically. Similarly, for those with progressive neurologic conditions, personalized biofeedback or teletherapy can be administered in the comfort of home or community settings. These data, coupled with supported human-computer interactions, also could enable an assessment of the quality of task practice and patient engagement and compliance with home-based interventions (e.g., exercise programs). There is limited moderate evidence showing that telerehabilitation results in comparable improvements to conventional therapy. Additional research is needed to extend the evidence base [123]. Research is also needed to determine the reliability and validity of the wearable sensor data that might be used through telerehabilitation [121]. Furthermore, challenges in privacy and security of information exist, warranting consideration of enhanced security protections based on policy, regulatory protocols [124], and security protocols [125].

4.7.11 ROBOTICS

Wearable sensors have played an important role in enabling the development of next-generation assistive and rehabilitation robots [61]. For example, during the past decade, portable rigid exoskeletons have emerged as an exciting tool to enable individuals who cannot walk to walk again [126]. These powerful systems use sensors such as encoders or potentiometers to measure their movement and estimate limb movement information that is used to modulate the forces delivered to the wearer. However, such sensors are incompatible with a new class of wearable robots made from soft and compliant materials [127]. IMUs and force sensors are more easily integrated into these soft robotic exosuits, enabling their emergence for different biomedical applications, including decreasing the energy used during healthy walking [128] and running [129] and restoring more normal walking after a stroke [130, 131].

4.7.12 NEXT-GENERATION WEARABLE SENSORS

Extending the discussion of sEMG-enabled assessment of motor module analyses, complementary sensor modalities are emerging that enhance movement measurement by monitoring underlying neural control mechanisms. Indeed, motor impairments arise from changes in neural control and degradation of the mechanical properties of muscles, and the relative contribution of each could be unique for everyone [61].

Inherent to the control of movement are the firings of individual motoneurons that propagate toward the neuromuscular junction, where their activation and rate coding regulate muscle contraction force and quality of movement. Deficits in motoneuron control are known to underlie neurologic [132, 133] and musculoskeletal [134] conditions. However, they have been difficult to discern using traditional techniques based on needle EMG recordings [135], which are invasive, yield the firings of relatively few motoneurons, and are not practical beyond monitoring highly constrained activities from isometric muscle contractions. With the advance of neural sensors and their underlying artificial intelligence concepts, methods for extracting motoneuron firing behavior from noninvasive sEMG during isometric contractions [136] and, more recently, during functional activities of everyday life have been made possible [137].

Recent work in this area has shown that groups of motoneurons are regulated differently when multiple muscles function in synergy to perform a functional task [61] and that abnormal motoneuron firing behavior underlies motor impairments after stroke [132, 133]. Assessing motoneuron recruitment patterns across neurologic and orthopedic populations could provide valuable insight into determining whether rehabilitation efforts that target abnormalities in movement also have a measurable effect on reversing underlying deficits in motoneuron firing behavior [61].

Another emerging application of this technology includes assessing activation patterns of motoneurons specific to different training interventions. For example, a recent study showed that subjects could selectively activate different populations of motoneurons and thereby exercise components of the muscle with greater fatigue-resistance capabilities. Subjects could increase the activation of relatively larger motoneurons that control higher forces concerning relatively smaller motoneurons that control lower forces, in some cases by as much as 40%. Research is continuing to expand on these exciting preliminary findings to provide a basis for new strength-training protocols to mitigate muscle weakness in patients with muscle atrophy from normal aging, musculoskeletal injury, or long-term bedrest [138].

4.7.13 Hybrid Sensors for Monitoring Muscle Activity and Movement

Recent technologic advancements have enabled the integration of miniaturized sensor components into electronic chip systems with ultralow power consumption [61]. This has fostered the development of hybrid wearable sensors that combine in a single encapsulation (i) motion sensing and (ii) EMG sensing of muscle activity. Hybrid sensors can be particularly advantageous for monitoring the quality of movement when assessing and treating motor impairments. Indeed, the ability to measure characteristics of the wearer's movement and the underlying muscle activity responsible for regulating the movement provides a more holistic assessment of movement dysfunction. Hybrid sensors currently used for movement monitoring include an EMG recording component and a motion component, such as an accelerometer or IMU [139, 140].

The feasibility of this technology was initially evaluated for automated detection of functional activities of daily living in individuals with stroke [141]. Using a minimal subset of four hybrid sensors (combined sEMG and accelerometer sensors located on the two upper arms, one on the forearm, and one on the thigh), activities related to feeding, grooming, dressing, transferring, locomotion, and toileting were detected with a mean sensitivity of 95.0% and a mean specificity of 99.7%. Significant improvements in sensitivity and specificity resulted when sEMG and accelerometer data was included, highlighting the value of a hybrid sensor approach for this application. Preliminary work in stroke demonstrated that a hybrid sEMG and accelerometer sensor could differentiate voluntary from spastic contractions [142].

Hybrid sensing also is effective for the automated detection of involuntary movements associated with PD during unscripted activities of daily living [139, 141]. Indeed, the use of one hybrid sensor (sEMG and accelerometer) per symptomatic limb was sufficient in achieving 94.9% sensitivity and 97.1% specificity for autonomous tracking of tremor and dyskinesia in that limb in response to levodopa treatment [61].

Hybrid sensors that combine sEMG and IMU sensing hold even greater opportunities for wearable activity monitoring of movement disorders. The availability of angular velocity measurement in such a hybrid sensor proved highly effective in providing the first whole-body bradykinesia detector for PD (with an average accuracy of 95.0% for combined walking and non-walking activities) during unconstrained activities of daily living before and after levodopa therapy [141]. Similar technology is effective when assessing the quality of movement in stroke [143] and monitoring athletic performance to prevent injury [144].

4.7.14 SOFT SENSORS

Advances in materials science have enabled explorations into the development of soft sensors and their applications to rehabilitation. Soft sensors can be placed in locations not possible with current movement monitoring devices. For example, stretchy sensors can be placed on the arch of runners with plantar fasciitis [61].

Because runners with plantar fasciitis often have weak intrinsic foot muscles [145], there is resultant flattening of the arch and increased strain on the plantar fascia. Stretchy sensors can provide feedback to runners when their arch is lowering too much, reminding them to engage those muscles [61].

Because the placement of sensors could be a source of imprecision in measurement [146], the prospect of soft textile-based sensors that could be worn like clothing is very attractive. For example, ultrathin, ultralight, and stretchable sEMG sensors that resemble a temporary tattoo and are mechanically unnoticeable to the user are being tested to evaluate exercise performance during rehabilitation [147]. In addition, soft elastomeric sensors have been integrated into a wearable sensing suit to measure hip, knee, and ankle kinematics [148]. Such sensing garments could be used for continuous kinematic monitoring in the community. More recently, an alternative stretchable capacitive sensor has been developed with conductive knit fabrics as the electrode layer and a dielectric layer made from a silicone elastomer [149]. These sensors can be rapidly customized through a layered manufacturing process using a film applicator and laser cutting has demonstrated scalable, fast, low-cost production and arbitrary shaping of strain [149] and pressure [150] sensors. The textile-based nature of these sensors makes them much more suitable for integration into apparel than existing sensor technologies. It has been demonstrated that these sensors can be integrated into a glove for measuring finger movements [149] and grip force [150]. Additional promising initial results with other textile-compatible sensors have demonstrated the ability to measure tension [151] and applied pressure [152] in wearable devices. Apart from making the transduction mechanism compatible with apparel, developments have focused on creating conductive traces within textile materials to eliminate wiring and enable systems to be washable. Highlights adaptations of this early work to develop an insole for measuring contact pressure [61].

4.7.15 LIMITATIONS

First, this review does not provide a comprehensive systematic review of the literature, but rather a focused discussion of the current and emerging sensor technologies and their clinical applications. Therefore, studies presenting similar technologies and clinical applications might not have been included. Second, the clinical applications discussed are limited to stroke, PD, HD, OA, and running populations. Although these are only a few conditions that use and can benefit from wearable movement sensors, the conditions chosen illustrate the large spectrum of individuals with varying capabilities who could benefit from existing and emerging sensor technologies [61].

The central goal of physical rehabilitation is to facilitate the reacquisition of movement abilities after injury or onset of disease. Motor behavior is viewed as an output of the movement system based on its encompassing interaction with cardiovascular, pulmonary, endocrine, integumentary, nervous, and musculoskeletal systems [153]. Thus, movement data has a high potential in examining health and disease across systems. Wearable sensors are a promising rehabilitation technology because of their precision, non-invasiveness, and easy deployment compared with other methods. Their complementary kinematic motion, neural activity, and muscle dynamics measurements offer a targeted approach for assessing and treating different neurologic and orthopedic conditions. In addition, more widespread monitoring of movement in clinical and ecologic settings and across different rehabilitation timescales could serve as a pathway to developing computational recovery and precision medicine models. Moreover, advancements in materials science are allowing for the development of next-generation sensors that can record biological movements from device interfaces that are more fully transparent to the wearer [61].

4.8 CONTROLLERS TO LOWER LIMB EXOSKELETONS

The control diagram of the human–exoskeleton environment-coupled system in terms of bioelectrical signal sensors include electroencephalogram (EEG) [154, 155], electromyography (EMG) [156], and electrooculography (EOG) [157].

One of the most popular control system categories for exoskeletons, the lower limb exoskeleton (LLE), is a hierarchy-based control Sarajchi et al. system divided into three levels of supervisory level, high level, and low level [158–161]. In LLEs, the supervisory level controller (e.g., finite state machine [FSM]) detects and, in some applications, predicts human gait phases to provide the high level of a control system with a joint reference trajectory. The high-level controller (e.g., impedance control) is responsible for torque control of human-exoskeleton interaction according to the signals received from the supervisory level to generate a reference torque for the low-level control system. The low-level controller (e.g., position/ torque control) intends to control the position or torque of actuators based on the reference torque of the high-level or reference joint trajectory of the supervisory level [159–161]. In LLEs, this hierarchy-based control system is also known as gait pattern control [161].

4.8.1 SUPERVISORY-LEVEL CONTROLLER: FINITE STATE MACHINE (FSM)

Due to the transitional nature of the gait cycle, especially the stance and swing phases, it is usually helpful to divide the controller into separate control states based on the phase of the gait cycle [162]. In LLEs, FSMs are frequently used to define controller states, such as between the stance and swing phases. More divisions of the gait cycle are sometimes employed, such as specifying a late-stance phase for powered plantar-flexion or splitting up the swing into several separate phases for swing flexion (early) or swing extension (mid/late). Although not all controller architectures have an FSM, many do [162]. Many of the states of FSMs are highly dependent on the interactions with the environment. For instance, foot contact with the ground indicates the stance and swing phases of the gait cycle [159].

4.8.2 HIGH-LEVEL CONTROLLER: IMPEDANCE CONTROL

It is critical to ensure that patients actively participate in the therapy and never resist the applied movement. To this end, impedance control is commonly used to implement rehabilitation therapies and takes advantage of patients' residual movement under the philosophy "assist as needed" [163–165]. A robot manipulator with impedance control is presented by an equivalent mass-spring-damper with tunable parameters [154]. Hogan introduced impedance control in 1985. The impedance of a system, $Z(s)$, is specified as the relationship between the force of the system, $F(s)$, and its movement, where f is force, I is inertia, B is damping, k is stiffness of the system and θ, $\dot{\theta}$, and $\ddot{\theta}$ are the position, velocity, and acceleration of a robot, respectively. Adaptive impedance control is employed to overcome uncertainties in the dynamic parameters of robotic exoskeletons [154].

4.8.3 LOW-LEVEL CONTROLLER: POSITION/TORQUE CONTROL

The low-level control is the closest level to the actuators; hence, it is necessarily device-dependent [166]. Position and torque controls are the most common control strategies for low-level controllers. Position control or trajectory tracking guides the patient's lower limb to fixed reference gait trajectories based on the joint angles as feedback. It comprises an internal control loop using the error between the joint reference angle trajectories and measured angles by sensors on each LLE joint [164, 165]. For position control, defining the reference trajectory is critical, while prerecorded gait trajectories from healthy subjects and mathematical models of normal gait trajectories are commonly employed [167, 168]. A positive point of this control strategy is the imposition of a predefined joint angle trajectory resulting in limited kinematic error, an influential factor in driving human motor learning [167]. Position control is especially appropriate for individuals with neurological disorders who cannot move their lower limbs due to a lack of muscle strength [162, 167]. Nevertheless, it gives patients the least control and interaction with LLEs, limiting its overall applicability [162].

Although position control is common in robotics, it is not appropriate for all tasks, particularly when robots need to interact physically with the environment [169]. Torque control can be beneficial in achieving versatile and robust behavior as well as dependable and safe tasks in the presence of humans [169]. Therefore, torque control is widely employed in exoskeletons [170]. The low-level torque control tries to effectively track a reference torque using the actuator's electric current as the system input [171]. This control method uses the error between the reference torques and measured torques by sensors on each actuator. Since torque control closely interacts with actuators, it delivers a simple way of controlling the flow of energy from the exoskeleton to the user, which is helpful in biomechanics research [172]. Moreover, this control method plays a critical role in implementing a rigid-body inverse-dynamics control strategy [173].

FSMs and impedance control are the most common supervisory-level and high-level controllers. In contrast, the most popular low-level controllers are torque and position control based on PID or PD.

4.8.4 TRAJECTORY TRACKING

The purpose of trajectory tracking is to perform movement tasks without assuming any motor ability of the human, making the actuated joints follow a predefined trajectory. Among many control strategies for rehabilitation LLEs, one of the simplest approaches is trajectory tracking, which is to replay a predefined position or velocity prole on the actuators. It often incorporates offline trajectory definition, online trajectory regulation, and real-time trajectory tracking [174]. The offline trajectory definition can be accomplished by manually setting the position prole, such as a sinusoidal curve [175], or modified from gait data of healthy subjects [176]. But these simple definition does not guarantee balance without crutches. Some methods also used offline optimization techniques to consider individual information and balance maintenance [177]. PID control is a common choice for real-time trajectory tracking and is often built into the low-level motor driver [178]. Other choices include sliding mode control, LQR, or model-based controller with disturbance rejection. Many commercialized exoskeletons have adopted the trajectory tracking control, such as ReWalk [179], Ekso [180], and ExoMotus. Moreover, it is also widely used in the powered exoskeleton race session of a unique competition, the Cybathlon [181].

4.8.5 ADMITTANCE SHAPING

The purpose of admittance shaping is to make the LLE compliant to interaction torque or voluntary muscle torque, reshaping the intrinsic admittance of the LLE. Admittance shaping has been extensively applied to robots interacting with the external environment. From the perspective of humans, especially those with muscle weakness, it can alter the dynamic response of the wearable devices and even render them assistive to intended motions. Methods for admittance shaping include admittance control and impedance control [182]. Admittance control refers to control structures that use a virtual admittance that takes effort as input and then outputs the desired flow. The desired flow is further tracked by an impedance (trajectory tracking controller) to generate effort on the intrinsic admittance of the controlled object. At the same time, impedance control refers to controllers which directly generate effort on the controlled object using an impedance model. Despite the similarity, admittance control has been widely adopted for LLEs because of its good performance in soft-contact environments [183].

4.8.6 Controllers Utilizing Back-Drivability

One of the properties of the exoskeleton joints is back-drivability, which measures how much torque a person needs to apply on the joint to reverse it. Back-drivability of joints can be achieved by either the actuator's unique mechanical design or specific controllers such as admittance shaping and zero-torque control. But the problem of limited bandwidth has been shown for controller-implemented back-drivability [184]. Recent years have witnessed several LLEs with back-drivable actuators, including the Vanderbilt exoskeleton [185], a knee exoskeleton by Wang et al. [186], and a knee-ankle exoskeleton by Zhu et al. [187]. Among them, a common choice to obtain back-drivability is a quasi-direct drive actuator, which is compliant through the lack of inertia of the motor.

Interestingly, back-driving the motor results in harvesting energy and prolonging the battery life [174]. Given that the expected users of back-drivable s still have partial abilities to move the affected leg, one of the simplest approaches in this category is using FSM to assist only when necessary and allowing the user to move the limbs for the rest of the time voluntarily. Murray et al. have proposed a control strategy for patients with lower limb hemiparesis [188]. The controller consists of three behaviors: gravity compensation; feedforward movement assistance, especially when reversing or initiating lower limb movements during the swing phase; and knee joint stability reinforcement. The assistance strategy was designed without specifying spatiotemporal trajectories such that users should help themselves to maintain balance and select step length [174].

4.8.7 Virtual-Field-Based Control

The purpose of virtual-field-based control is to provide gait guidance and assistance by imposing a virtual field to the configuration space of LLE. This control allows step-by-step variance and encourages voluntary walking. Virtual-field-based control explicitly guides patients to a suitable gait trajectory [189, 190]. The torque field is equivalent to a spring-damper system that connects an arbitrary point in the configuration space perpendicularly to the desired path. Thus, it will always pull the leg generally to the path. The damping and stiffness coefficients are adjustable. When the damping coefficient is zero, the control scheme can be regarded as an artificial potential field, where torque is the field's gradient.

In contrast, the flow field offers guidance and assistance and combines them into one component. The flow field is designed so that the leg would be dragged by an flow force when the configuration point is immersed in a viscous fluid. Thus, the force exerted on the leg depends on comparing the real velocity in the state space and the reference velocity [189].

4.8.8 Energy Shaping

Energy shaping aims to provide partial assistance to voluntary human movement by imposing desired dynamics on the controller plant system. It allows free movement of the wearer through task invariant assistance [174]. Energy shaping is another control strategy that relies on back-drivable actuators, and it imposes desired behavior on the controller-plant system. In contrast with admittance shaping, which can only reshape the apparent dynamics of one DoF, energy shaping extends to reshape the whole actuated DoFs. This strategy has been explored in underactuated robotic systems such as bipeds [191]. Locomotor Control System Laboratory recently assessed the feasibility of using this strategy in the control of LLE with back-drivable motors [192, 193].

In this control strategy, a relatively accurate dynamic model underactuated model is needed for describing the exoskeleton side. The floating base's three-dimensional position and the unpowered joints' angle are typically underactuated degrees of freedom. However, finding the optimal generalized coordinates can sometimes be complicated when deriving the dynamic equation from the Lagrangian approach. Interestingly, this process can be simplified by defining holonomic constraints to eliminate redundant generalized coordinates [174].

4.8.9 Virtual Constraint

The purpose of a virtual constraint is to perform movement tasks without assuming any motion ability of humans, using input-output feedback linearization to track an optimized time-invariant trajectory. This control guarantees stability along the trajectory and self-balance without crutches [174]. The virtual constraint was developed in the late 20th century to control bipedal robots, largely thanks to Byrnes et al. [193]. Impressive results have been achieved by implementing this control approach to bipedal robots [194] and prostheses [195]. LLEs and bipedal robots share many challenges, e.g., having many underactuated degrees of freedom, especially from the posture of the floating base, and state variables undergoing discrete jumps when the foot contacts the ground. Like energy shaping control strategy, an underactuated hybrid dynamics model that captures full-body motion is needed. First, assuming that the human and the machine are rigidly connected, then the Euler-Lagrange method is used to derive equations of motion (EOMs) of the human-machine system. Within the EOM, the term of contact force is calculated using holonomic constraints like that in energy shaping. When the preimpact state meets the switching surface, it will be transitioned to the postimpact state by a precalculated reset map. Specifically, it is imposed by designing a set of outputs as desired trajectories with a relative degree of two and desired speed with a relative degree of one. The term partial hybrid zero dynamics (PHZD) means that the zero dynamics manifold is contact invariant and is derived by ignoring the output function with relative degree equals one. It is important to study PHZD because the stability of the designed trajectory can be examined on the reduced dimensional internal dynamics [177]. The problem of how to design a trajectory for walking with an exoskeleton that is both stable and natural is in the domain of trajectory optimization [174].

4.8.10   Oscillator-Based Control

The purpose of oscillator-based control is to synchronize the assistance of LLE with actual human walking and adaptively learn the periodic characteristics of walking. The oscillator-based control method features a set of or a single oscillator(s) that are used to synchronize the phase of the controller with the periodic-assuming gait phase. Oscillators are used to generate a limit cycle that synchronizes itself to the phase of actual walking. When the actual gait deviates from the prior orbit, the oscillator parameters will be adapted to maintain synchronization [196]. The first scientific communication applying the adaptive frequency oscillator (AFO) to LLE was by Ronsse et al. [197]. Afterward, that oscillator-based approach was mainly designed for the hip joint exoskeleton [198]. Recently this method was further validated on single knee [199] or ankle [200] joint actuation and multidegree-of-freedom exoskeletons [201]. Because the oscillators are robust to perturbation and can reduce the dimension of control input, in addition to assistive robots, they have been used for autonomous robot locomotion. Oscillators are closely related to the notion of central pattern generators (CPGs). CPGs have been widely found in animals to render rhythmic motion [202], and based on the same principle, they have been created for robotics control [203]. This method utilized a pool of oscillators, each of which learned each sinusoidal component's phase, amplitude, and frequency. In this way, the online Fourier decomposition was performed to estimate the real-time hip joint angle. This approximation was further improved by kernel-based non-linear filter (NLF) adopted from [204] to output the estimated joint angle trajectory [174].

While most of the oscillator-based controller is for single joint actuation, Seo et al. use it to control GEMS exoskeleton with multidegree-of-freedom actuation [201]. First, IMUs and the dead-reckoning method were used to obtain the real-time foot-to-foot distance, which was later sent to the oscillator as a forced input. Second, one of the techniques for improving the converging performance is to use a particularly shaped adaptive oscillator (PSAO), which means the basic function of the online Fourier decomposition is mainly shaped using prior information. Third, another technique is adding a coupling term of actual gait frequency detected by FSM to the equation of frequency learning rate. The torque output was based on the estimated gait phase and the offline trajectory function, which was regulated by environment class and walking speed [174].

4.8.11   Surface Electromyography (sEMG)-Based Control

The sEMG is a non-invasive technique for assessing the myoelectric output of a muscle. The purpose of this strategy is to control the LLE according to human intent decoded from the sEMG signal. Controllers based on sEMG utilize the measuring of electrical activities for stimulating muscles to estimate human intention and further control the exoskeleton to aid. There are many advantages of controlling with sEMG. First, the time lag between the onset of muscle movement and that of the exoskeleton assistive motion can be drastically reduced because of the avoidance of electromechanical delay (EMD) [205]. It is in favor of forming a real-time neuro-feedback loop [206] and further enhancing motor learning according to neuroplasticity [207]. Second, for those with muscle weakness (e.g., patients with incomplete SCI or hemiparetic stroke), motor intention can still be read through the residual sEMG signal. Third, compared with interaction force, sEMG can predict voluntary joint torque without overcoming the limb's inertia and gravity. Fourth, this type of neural signal can implement continuous mapping to joint torque, joint angle, etc. However, there are also disadvantages of sEMG-based control. First, from the perspective of EMG generation, the redundancy of muscle activation solution induces complexity of EMG signal decoding. Second, extra complexity was added by confounding factors from different conditions of capturing the sEMG signal, including electrode shift, limb position, contraction intensity, muscle fatigue, and time variation [208]. Third, due to the lack of robustness of sEMG, the exoskeleton controlled solely by sEMG input is still unsafe for assisting patients with motor weakness in daily life.

The emergence of the human-machine interface using sEMG signals dates to the 1970s [209]. Since then, sEMG has been extensively applied to prostheses [210], teleoperation [211], rehabilitation robots [212], etc. Over decades of development, the sEMG-based control can be divided into the sEMG signal decoding and control parts. The simplest approach is on-off control, which relies on pattern recognition to separate human intention into several classes [213]. The predefined trajectory is replayed when a class is detected. In addition to discrete classes, the decoding process can also map the sEMG signal into continuous output. Three alternative methods can do this: 1. proportional estimation that the predicted joint torque is computed by multiplying a gain to a single channel of filtered sEMG signal [212, 214]; 2. non-linear model that uses relatively complicated methods; and 3. musculoskeletal model proposed by Hill [215] that estimate joint torque upon a biological understanding of internal dynamics of the human limb [216]. After continuous torque mapping, a wide range of controllers can be applied to provide aid. The impedance or admittance controller takes the estimated human joint torque as input to reshape the apparent dynamics of the exoskeleton joint to be assistive [217]. Dynamic-model-based control mainly uses dynamic models adopted from humanoid robotics [218] on which assistive torque calculation was based [219]. Another uncommon method includes ambulation speed regulation based on sEMG signal and synergy-based control [220].

4.8.12 Electroencephalography (EEG)-Based Control

The purpose of EEG-based control is to control the LLE according to human intent decoded from the electroencephalography signal. Various control methods based on human intent are decoded from the signal of brain activities. Advantages include direct volitional control, wearers with severe paralysis can still command the LLE, and the potential to decode rich information from EEG [174].

EEG-based control manipulated the LLE according to the command from the brain-machine-interface (BMI) with EEG input. Unlike other brain signals such as ECoG [221], EEG utilizes non-invasive electrodes and has a global view of the brain signal. The term BMI was coined by Professor Miguel Nicolelis, who led the Walk-Again project that showcased the EEG-controlled exoskeleton in the 2014 Brazil World Cup. Like EMG, EEG is also a biological signal generated by the human body. The current EMG-based control can perform direct neural control supported by prior knowledge of continuous kinematic information decoding, such as the musculoskeletal model. Yet most of the current EEG-based exoskeleton controllers still must resort to pattern recognition to decipher the brain signal into discrete classes. The result is that the exoskeleton controller must provide a set of commands based merely on the abstraction of intent. Therefore, how to decode the human intent from the EEG signal and how to control the exoskeleton based on the output of the BMI become two major challenges of the EEG-based control strategy. The general structure of an EEG-based controller is as follows: First, the BMI captures brain signals to estimate human intent, which is then output as an intent abstraction. Second, motor control algorithms generate command signals to the exoskeleton to provide assistive torque on the human limbs. And finally, the sensorimotor feedback to the human closes the loop by enabling the wearer to regulate the brain signal to better receive active assistance. Because the exoskeleton aims at assisting patients whose corticospinal connection or descending tracts to the muscles are cut due to lesions, the future brain-controlled exoskeleton should function as the substitution for the spinal cord and the musculoskeletal system so that the wearers can control the human-machine system using the same neural signal to control their intact limb [174].

4.8.13 CONTROL OF HYBRID EXOSKELETONS

The purpose of this control is to generate a walking gait by controlling robotic actuators and functional electrical stimulation at the same time. Robotic actuators and muscles contribute the required joint torque for walking. Advantages include improved cardiorespiratory fitness, significant reanimated muscle function, and lighter exoskeletons are needed due to muscle torque contribution [174].

The hybrid exoskeleton is a kind of rehabilitation device that combines functional electrical stimulation (FES) with robotic exoskeletons [222]. Control of lower limb hybrid exoskeletons requires modulating torque generated by muscle stimulation and by robotic actuation to achieve a desired walking gait [223]. It was believed to be more beneficial than using FES or robotic assistance only [136]. For example, the weight of the robotic actuators in LLE can be reduced due to the significant torque contribution of muscles. Also, regular FES-induced muscle recruitment will facilitate cardiorespiratory fitness enhancement [174].

As a special device that controls both humans and robots, hybrid exoskeletons can be categorized according to whether the robotic actuation is semi-active or fully active and whether the FES is in open-loop or closed-loop control [224]. When controlled, semi-active robotic actuation only dissipates or stores kinetic energy created by muscle stimulation [225]. Instead, fully active robotic actuation can compensate for resisting muscle torque to perform a desired motion [226]. Open-loop control of FES replays a predetermined pattern of stimulation triggered by FSM [227]. In contrast, closed-loop control of FES relies on indirect measurement of muscle performance to modulate the stimulation in real time [228]. In the spectrum of hybrid exoskeletons, the ones with fully active robotic actuation and closed-loop FES control have been the focus of research in recent years. However, three challenges must be addressed for these devices. Some designed a control strategy that can allocate torque contribution between muscles and motors in an arbitrary ratio. Recently, a bioinspired synergy-based control strategy was proposed to address this challenge, which has the advantage of controlling high-dimensional systems by solving low-dimensional problems [229].

4.8.14 SYNERGY-BASED CONTROL

A hypothesis inspires synergy-based control that the central nervous system controls the overly redundant musculoskeletal system by linearly combining a small number of synergies and coherently activating a group of muscles [230]. Despite no proof of muscle synergy [231], this concept has been used in many robotic applications. Systems with redundant actuation, especially hybrid exoskeletons, can take full advantage of the synergy-based control [232].

4.8.15 SENSING TECHNOLOGIES

One of the earliest yet the most widely used approaches is the use of buttons, which are pressed by wearers or doctors nearby to select the walking mode. The buttons can be in various types, such as a joystick in Rex, a touch screen in Atalante [177], and a joystick plus trigger buttons in Mina V2 [233], even though this human input approach can only be incorporated with FSM or other high-level trajectory planning units. Its high efficacy has been proven in the Cybathlon in that persons with complete lower limb paraplegia could traverse through the complex terrain using this input approach [234].

Joint angle feedback is mandatory for exoskeleton control, especially in regulating the motor current by comparing the commanded and the real joint angle. But in terms of human intention detection, it is often used to detect the extent to which the user's limb has deviated from the desired path in an exoskeleton with a back-drivable actuator. Thus, the application includes inferencing interaction torque by displacement of the series elastic actuator [235], deducing the virtual field force by joint angle deviation [236], and calculating virtual impedance by the current angular velocity [237]. Interaction torque is another frequently used input, especially for admittance controllers, which can generate a real-time trajectory [238] or make trajectory corrections accordingly [235]. It is also used to reshape the equivalent constraint dynamics into a desired form [239].

Multi-sensor information fusion has the potential to decode human intent better, and a fusion approach is critical to exploit this potential. The first choice among these approaches is machine learning techniques. The second is an onboard musculoskeletal simulator, proposed in [240] to estimate the wearer's kinetic gait prole using sensor data from humans and robots. The third is explicitly putting multiple sensor inputs into the control law [239].

4.8.16 OPTIMIZATION TECHNIQUES

Recent years have witnessed the increasing application of optimization techniques in control of LLEs to meet better different control objectives, which can be 1. quick adaptation to different user conditions or preferences [241], 2. minimizing human joint torque or metabolic cost [242], and 3. faster, more comfortable walking [243]. These techniques have been employed to perform parameter optimization, trajectory optimization, and control law optimization (optimal control) [244].

Parameter optimization is used to find the optimal set of parameters within the designed control algorithm instead of heuristically tuning it. However, the fact that usually the cost function can only be updated after completing a few gait cycles makes the cost function a black box whose derivatives are impossible to compute. Therefore, derivative-free optimization techniques can be applied. For example, the performance of Bayesian optimization and evolution strategy were evaluated in [242] to find the best energy shaping factors that minimize the human joint torque exerted. Trajectory optimization is used to plan an optimal motion profile for the subsequent tracking controller. In the field of LLE, the complex hybrid and under-actuated dynamics make solving the optimization problem time-consuming. Thus, often only offline trajectory optimization is employed. For example, the direct collocation technique [245] is applied to the **Atalante exoskeleton**, considering a friction cone for no foot slippage, ZMP for no foot rotation, and proper foot clearance [246].

4.9 CONTROLLERS TO UPPER LIMB EXOSKELETONS

The control methods implemented on the robotic exoskeleton during the passive mode command the motors to move the patient's limb through preset standard exercises. Once some of the patient's mobility returns, the active training mode can be applied. Control strategies during the active mode take into consideration the patient's intention to move. Furthermore, during this stage, the patient is expected to initiate the move, a step that has been proven to be necessary to promote neural plasticity [247, 248]. The robotic exoskeleton control systems can be set to assist the patient in performing and completing training exercises in assist-as-needed therapy, encouraging and promoting patient engagement. Eventually, the control methods can be set to have the robotic exoskeleton resist the patient's motion for more advanced training [248]. Some of the more popular control methods for this type of application are proportional integral derivative (PID) control, impedance control, admittance control, adaptive control, and sliding mode control (SMC) [248].

4.9.1 PROPORTIONAL, INTEGRAL, AND DERIVATIVE CONTROL

PID control does not require system modeling and is relatively straightforward to implement. In the PID control law, u(t) denotes the control input, and error e(t) represents the difference between the actual and desired position of joints. The proportional gain, KP, operates on the position error. The integral gain, KI, operates on the accumulated position error, and the derivative gain, KD, operates on the velocity error [249]. While model-free control leads to simplicity in its implementation, a disadvantage of using this method is that tuning the gains to the current setup can be time-consuming. Another disadvantage is that since this control method is not model-based and only error-driven if the exoskeleton becomes "stuck", unwanted large torques could be commanded due to accumulated error [250]. It could potentially damage the equipment and harm the patient if safety limits are not properly implemented in the system [247].

Controllers can be created that use a subset of the PID controller, such as P, PD, or PI. For example, the upper limb robotic exoskeleton ARMin III [251] uses a PD controller, while EXO-UL7 [252] uses a PID controller. Furthermore, many researchers combine elements of the PID controller with advanced control methods (such as robust control and adaptive control) and intelligent control methods (such as neural networks and fuzzy logic). For example, [253] combines PID control with robust control and fuzzy logic–based control. Depending on the application, this type of control can lead to sufficiently acceptable system performance without having to delve into the field of advanced control methods [247].

4.9.2 IMPEDANCE AND ADMITTANCE CONTROL

Impedance control is the overall philosophy that establishes a dynamic relationship between the motion of a plant and the interactive forces between the plant and its environment. It can be implemented in two ways: impedance control and admittance control.

Systems with flow (angular position) as input and effort (torque) as output are impedance. Systems with effort (torque) as inputs and flow (angular position) as outputs are called admittance. The system in these could be a controller, the plant (robot), the environment, or a human. Using these definitions for impedance control, the controller is an impedance system, while the controlled plant (robotic manipulator) is an admittance system. Conversely, admittance control features a controller that is an admittance system with the controlled plant (robotic manipulator) as an impedance system. It is important to note that for both impedance control and admittance control, the control objective is the same: determine the control torque that provides the desired relationship between the measured external torque and the deviation from the equilibrium angular joint trajectory [247].

Whereas PID controllers aim to minimize position and velocity tracking errors, impedance control is an expansion of position control [254]. This method has been proven to produce stable interactions and is efficient for lightweight, back-drivable exoskeletons [255]. However, it has been shown to not be very good at compensating for gravity, friction in the system [247], and other unmodeled dynamics in free space (where the user is allowed to move the exoskeleton without resistance). As a result, in these scenarios, accuracy and precision are compromised [256]. Using low-friction joints, direct drives, and back-drivability [255] can improve performance [247]; however, researchers have found that impedance control can become unstable when the impedance is high [257]. Impedance control strategies perform well in stiff environments and enable the robotic exoskeleton-human assembly to move compliantly with deviations from a set trajectory [258]. Impedance control has been implemented in several developments of upper limb exoskeletons, including the L-Exos [259] and SUEFUL-7 [260].

Admittance control is useful with stiff robots since forces need to be sensed at the interface between the robot and the human limb. One of the disadvantages of this method is that high admittance (low impedance) can destabilize the system [261]. This method requires high transmission ratios, such as those provided by harmonic drives to achieve precise motion control with very little backlash [247]. An advantage of using a system without backlash is smooth movement [249]. One commercial rehabilitation system that uses admittance control is the HapticMaster from Tyromotion. Two other systems that can also be controlled using admittance controllers are MGA [36] and ARMin III [251].

4.9.3 ADAPTIVE CONTROL

One of the disadvantages of impedance and admittance control systems is that they do not incorporate time-varying adjustments to the desired parameters [247] and may intervene incorrectly if participants regain some of their strength and require less assistance. It is in these kinds of situations that adaptive control methods can help. A type of adaptive controller called model reference adaptive controller (MRAC) adjusts for unknown variances of system parameters online based on ongoing operations. The controller parameter values are updated based on the difference between the measured sensor values from the system and those from the reference model.

Another advantage of adaptive controllers is that they can compensate for modeling uncertainties. Additionally, adaptive controllers do not require a priori information about the limits of the uncertain or changing parameters, as robust methods do. Adaptive methods, however, can handle neither fast-changing parameters nor systems that are exposed to external disturbances. Researchers have addressed the latter problem by combining adaptive controllers with other types of controllers, including robust control methods to handle bounded external disturbances. An example of an upper limb rehabilitation robotic exoskeleton system that uses adaptive control is ARMin V [262]. Adaptive robust control is demonstrated in [263] and [264].

4.9.4 SLIDING MODE CONTROL

Sliding mode control (SMC) is a robust nonlinear method that handles bounded external disturbances [250] and parametric uncertainties. First, a switching controller is designed, which forces the system state trajectories to converge onto a sliding surface in the state space in a finite amount of time. Then, the nominal controller is computed. One of the disadvantages of SMC is that the high-frequency switching action could cause chattering in the commanded output, resulting in wear or damage to the mechanical system and energy loss in the electrical system. However, many mathematical smoothing methods could be implemented, which may negate or mitigate this problem [247].

4.9.5 Other Control Methods

Numerous other control approaches combine the previously mentioned methods as well as others that also integrate intelligent control methods, such as neural networks [265], fuzzy logic [266], and machine learning methods [267]. Some approaches use time-delay estimation [268] and iterative learning control for repetitive tasks [269]. Other controllers integrate the use of biosignals such as EMG [270, 271] and EEG [272].

4.9.6 Control Methods for Telerobotic Systems with Time Delays

The methods discussed in the previous section can be used to control single upper limb rehabilitation robotic exoskeletons. This section presents a control method that allows humans to operate the robotic system remotely during time delays. Typically, a human operator moves the master robot to the local site to accomplish a task using the slave robot at the remote site. As the human operator interacts with the master robot, its motion information is conveyed over a communication channel to the remote side as a command signal so that the slave robot imitates the master robot while interacting with the environment [273] or another human.

Additionally, if the teleoperation is bilateral, the interaction force between the slave robot and its environment (or the human) is measured and transmitted to the human operator at the local site. As a result, the master robot not only measures motions but also displays forces to the user, simultaneously affecting the remote environment (or human) at the remote site while also perceiving the resected force from that interaction [247]. The goal is for the interaction to be so immersive and natural that the human operator is fooled into forgetting about the medium itself [247]. However, when the communication channel has issues such as time delays, the stability of the system can be compromised, resulting in undesirable and, even more critically, unsafe consequences for the humans in the loop.

There has been a lot of research over the years on telerobotics to develop control methods that compensate for time delays with the following three main objectives: stability, in that the closed-loop system is stable regardless of the behavior of the operator or the remote environment [274]; tracking performance, or how well the slave side follows the master side; and transparency (human–computer interaction) [275], or how well the operator feels that she or he is directly interacting with the remote environment [276]. Having a human operator in the control loop is desirable and advantageous in applications where the remote site interaction has unknown and unstructured characteristics. Over the last 60 years, there have been increasingly more telerobotics applications in various fields such as space [273], underwater control [277], hazardous environments [278], military [247], mobile robots [279], teledriving [280], telemedicine such as telesurgery [281], and telerehabilitation [274].

If delays exist, they cause a phase shift in the position and force signals if not addressed. Due to the delays across the communication channel, the operator acts on old data and thus keeps moving the robot forward, believing it has not yet reached the desired location. As a result, increasingly excessive forces are being applied on the slave side until the signal indicating that the robot went too far reaches the human operator. The operator tries to adjust but is also exposed to enormous forces in terms of obsolete large displacement commands. This lack of synchronization of the motion and forces between the master and the slave side leads to instability and transparency degradation. The physical consequences can include injury to the humans in the loop and damage to equipment, such as force sensors, which are sensitive and expensive [282].

Besides issues due to the communication medium, such as Internet latency, other challenges for bilateral control systems are modeling complexities and modeling uncertainties, parameter variations [283], and uncertain disturbances such as friction or payload variations [284]. Furthermore, safety and reliability are of paramount concern in telerobotics with human operators in the loop, and even more so when dealing with humans on the slave side. For example, in telesurgery, the slave robots perform a task inside the human's body, while in telerehabilitation when using exoskeletons, the robotic device encapsulates part of the human body [247].

4.9.7 Passivity-Based Control Methods

Passivity is based on energy transfer and power flow in a system. For stability, the net system power should be passive, meaning that the energy entering the system should be greater than the energy leaving the system as expected, considering that in real systems, there is always some energy dissipated internally due to friction and other damping mechanisms [285, 286].

When active elements exist in the system (time delay across the communication channel or a human at the slave side moving the robot), the control system can become unstable. However, passivity could be ensured by limiting the system energy, introducing boundedness for all the system variables, or applying damping agents [287] to remove the excess energy. However, it is important to note that if a damping agent is too conservative, the system's performance could be degraded [288].

A major advantage of using passivity-based methods is that the dynamic models of both the master and the slave systems are not required to be known [289]. As a result, passivity-based methods are ideal for systems with large uncertainties or multidegrees of freedom systems that contain nonlinearities and complexities that are hard to model. These scenarios are typical of real physical environments [285]. Although passivity-based methods cannot guarantee the achievement of desired performance, stability can always be ensured. Five popular passivity-based methods and three non-passivity-based methods are described as follows.

4.9.8 Wave Transformation

Anderson and Song [290] were the first to combine the concepts of electrical network theory, scattering transformation, and passivity for telerobotic systems to ensure stability regardless of the size of the constant time delays. They did so by treating the connection between the two robots like the equivalent of a virtual passive transmission line [291] and modeling the robots. Years later, Niemeyer and Slotine [292] improved this method while making it simpler for mechanically minded roboticists to understand. The wave impedance variable should be tuned according to the delay size. Furthermore, the wave impedance variable can be used to adjust the tradeoff between inertia and stiffness [292]. The advantage of using the wave transformation method is that neither the size of the time delay nor the model parameters need to be known to guarantee stable performance; however, the wave method has several disadvantages. Position drift, an intrinsic disadvantage, can occur when using only the velocity and force values [293]. One solution to compensate for position drift is to use a wave integral instead, which includes the position, velocity, and force in the single quantity of the wave variable [294]. Another intrinsic disadvantage of the wave transformation method is that a larger delay size can cause a wave reaction. Wave reaction is information rebounded across the communication channel between the master and slave side, leading to oscillatory behavior, like an underdamped resonance of the wave communication at its natural frequency [285]. This manifestation produces an undesirable and significant settling time for the teleoperator. Impedance matching can eliminate this issue and provide optimal tuning capabilities for the local and remote controllers [285]. An additional disadvantage of the variable wave method is that spurious dynamics may interfere with normal operation [285].

These dynamics may be problematic if this telerehabilitation method uses robotic exoskeleton control with stroke patients, as sometimes their affected arm can exhibit spurious behavior due to muscle spasticity. Additionally, this method cannot ensure stability for time-varying delays, such as those that occur over the Internet. However, extensions to the wave variable can be used to guarantee passivity, using energy-conserving dynamic filters to shape the wave responses [294].

4.9.9 WAVE PREDICTOR

A wave predictor is a wave-based control method that predicts the incoming wave variable from the slave side to compensate for constant and variable delays [295] in the communication channel on the master side and minimizes their effect. It incorporates a modified Smith predictor, an energy regulator, and a Kalman filter. This method is stable even with significant modeling uncertainties of the remote system used in the predictor. Furthermore, a wave predictor uses a position-correcting input to minimize position errors. This method enforces passivity independent of constant and possibly even time-varying delays, provided that the slave robot dissipates sufficient energy [296].

4.9.10 TIME DOMAIN PASSIVITY CONTROL (TDPC)

TDPC is one of the most popular telerobotics control methods [247]. The main advantage of using TDPC for position-force architecture is that it is model-free and works with time-varying and unknown time delays. Since its performance only relies on measurements, it can be applied to many different systems. First introduced in [247], TDPC monitors the energy input and output into a system node in real-time. The method uses passivity observers (POs) and dissipates the excess energy using passivity controllers (PCs) when the system shows a dynamic behavior.

One of the disadvantages of TDPC is that it can exhibit a jarring effect when the PC engages [247]. As a result, researchers have been expanding on this method by monitoring the power transfer between nodes instead of using a reference energy value. Improved stability and simplicity were observed in the new implementation [297]. Additionally, TDPC can suffer from the accumulation of energy dissipation. One solution is to reset the PO when the absolute value of the rendered force is less than a specified threshold for a set amount of time, meaning when the slave robot is not interacting with the environment [298]. Another disadvantage of this method can occur when the velocity or force variables are close to zero or are zero since control failure can occur due to zero division behavior [299]. Consequently, researchers have devised estimations for the conventional TDPC method to overcome these issues.

4.9.11 Passivity-Based Adaptive Control

Adaptive controllers that specifically compensate for communication delays are summarized in [300]. They can be applied to either linear or nonlinear systems. One method works by estimating an accurate environment model that gets updated in real-time. Another method suppresses uncertainties existing both in the master and the slave robot models.

Chopra et al. [301] utilized a state-feedback control law that ensures the passivity for any constant time delays, initial offsets, and parametric uncertainties. This process uses wave variables containing position, velocity, and force information [300]. Nuño et al. [302] devised a passivity-based adaptive control method that can work with variable and asymmetric time delays in both channels. During free motion, this method ensures that all signals are bounded and that the position errors and velocities diminish asymptotically and converge to zero [247].

4.9.12 Proportional-Derivative-Like Control

This method was introduced by Lee and Spong [303] and is a damping injection scheme. It treats the master and slave sides of the teleoperator as virtually connected via a spring and damper mechanism over the delayed communication channels, with an added dissipative term at each side of the teleoperator. This method, which is sometimes expressed as PDCd, guarantees the passivity of the system with constant delays and parametric uncertainties. Although it requires a known upper bound of the round-trip delay, the delays can be asymmetric, and their exact estimates are unnecessary. The advantage of this method is that the position is transmitted explicitly and passes the communication and the control blocks altogether. Nuño et al. [304] showed that this strategy provides position tracking for teleoperators with variable time-delays.

4.9.13 Non-Passivity-Based Methods

4.9.13.1 Four-Channel Architecture

This four-channel architecture requires the velocity and the force to be sent from the master to the slave and vice versa [247]. Although the four-channel method achieves perfect transparency with no time delays, it loses passivity and robustness to delays

[247]. Aziminejad et al. addressed this shortcoming by combining the four-channel method with the wave transformation. Another disadvantage of this method is that a very accurate model of the master and slave robots is required to achieve perfect transparency [305].

4.9.13.2 Sliding Mode Control

SMC requires the design of a sliding surface based on position and velocity errors. When applied to a single upper limb robotic exoskeleton, the error is between the desired and the actual positions and velocities. For teleoperated robots, however, the position and velocity errors are between the master and the slave robots. SMC has succeeded in telerobotics, as it ensures robustness against uncertainties and time delays. In [306], Park and Cho used an SMC controller on the slave side to track the master robot, which utilizes an impedance controller. One of the main disadvantages of SMC is the switching controller component's chattering effect, but numerous smoothing methods can be explored to improve performance [247].

4.9.13.3 Adaptive Robust Control

This kind of control is devoted to nonlinear systems, which do not admit the application of the superposition principle. Adaptive control is generally used in exoskeletons that contain parametric uncertainty (the structure of the model is known, but the ranges of variation of the parameters are unknown). Robust control is generally employed in exoskeletons containing non-parametric uncertainty, where the objective is to reduce the effects of unmodeled uncertainties and perturbations acting on the exoskeleton [307].

An adaptive control is robust if it guarantees signal limits in the presence of the effects of reasonable classes of unmodeled dynamics and disturbances. In the presence of disturbances and unmodeled dynamics, adaptive control schemes can be unstable, so conditions are applied that guarantee robust stability. To this end, robust, direct and indirect adaptive control schemes are applied in the design of adaptive control schemes. Some of the applications are focused on robust adaptive tracking controls, to solve problems such as dynamic uncertainties, external perturbations and interaction between humans and exoskeletons [247].

4.9.14 CONTROL METHODS FOR UPPER LIMB BILATERAL TELEREHABILITATION WITH EXOSKELETONS

An upper limb robotic exoskeleton-based telerehabilitation system consists of a therapist interacting with a robotic exoskeleton at the master side and a patient's arm fastened to a robotic exoskeleton arm at the slave side. In unidirectional teleoperation, kinematic information such as position and/or velocity is sent from the master side across a communication network to the slave side for the motion to be mimicked. In bilateral teleoperation, kinetic information, such as the force sensed on the slave side, is usually sent to the master side across the communication channel [247]. In passive-control telerehabilitation, the therapist controls the motion of the master exoskeleton, which is relayed to and mimicked by the slave robotic exoskeleton to move the patient's affected arm. The interaction during this passive control stage can include the therapist assessing and improving the patient's muscle strength, range of motion, and quality of the specific joints. The primary objectives for passive mode telerehabilitation are neural and muscular plasticity, improvement of range, and reduction of muscle tone (spasticity) in the patient at remote locations [247].

4.10 ENERGY AND METABOLIC COST

Exoskeletons are wearable robotic devices that have the potential to support employees during physical work operations. The impact of exoskeletons concerning productivity and health within sectors is characterized by a high proportion of manual work, a high average age, a shortage of skilled workers, and increasing complexity. For this reason, it is fundamental in the design of exoskeletons to consider the energy efficiency and metabolic cost of the users of the exoskeletons [306].

4.10.1 METABOLIC COST

Two goals are relevant to considering the implementation of industrial exoskeletons in operational logistics processes: improvement of productivity and optimization of ergonomics [307]. Because logistics processes are still affected by a large amount of physical work, rising requirements, cost, performance pressure, and a lack of labor, strategies to reduce back pain issues affected by repetitive lifting and moving of goods are needed to cover rising needs and requirements in this industrial sector. Exoskeletons have the potential to reduce back pain and support workers in lifting and moving processes [308], especially in areas where layouts and working conditions cannot be easily changed [309]. Exoskeletons can enhance strength, endurance, and capacity and can help cover volatile demand peaks [306].

Butler executed a field test in a welding company. He expected that the welders would feel less fatigue and would increase productivity. In a test scenario, he demonstrated an improvement in productivity of 27–86% due to the better blood supply to the workers' muscles. The workers worked more efficiently, more accurately, and longer, and muscle pain was reduced [310]. He found that exoskeletons can prevent fatigue by slowing muscle activities and reducing the risk of work-related injuries [310].

Ford tested passive exoskeletons in 2015–2016 and reported an up to 83% reduction in injuries on assembly lines [311]; Iowa State University analyzed fatigue reduction in shoulders and biceps [311, 312].

Exoskeletons can increase the range of motion, and liftable weight can be increased up to 50–70% [310, 313]. De Looze et al. reviewed 40 papers and 26 industrial exoskeletons in 2015, analyzing potential impacts on wearers [314]. Thirteen exoskeletons were evaluated regarding the effect on physical loading, holding, lifting, and bending. Reductions in muscle activities between 10% and 70% were evaluated [314]. For active exoskeletons, muscle activity reduction between 20% and 70% (dynamic lifting, holding above head) was documented [314].

Studies with arm exoskeletons showed a reduction of muscle activity in arms and shoulders (42–62%) and an extension of working endurance in realistic work activities [315]. Reduction of the physical load was measured to compare ability with and without exoskeletons. Mixed findings and mixed results were documented in the studies [315]. In another example, muscle activity reduction of between 32% and 64% was demonstrated for logisticians' bending, turning, and squatting tasks in a bank [316]. Searching for documents with an exoskeleton was faster than without, showing a connection between relaxed muscles and concentration due to less fatigue and muscle activity [316]. Reduction of muscle activity and the enhancement of weight handled during an upper-arm and upper-head task were registered in manufacturing. Muscle activities were reduced with the exoskeleton working with and without load [317]. Koopman et al. evaluated a passive back exoskeleton. They measured a reduction of compression of 21% while bending and 14% while lifting [306].

Lee and Cha did a statistical analysis of walking tasks with and without loads and exoskeleton, taking lap time as a measurement of effectiveness [318]. They demonstrated that the exoskeleton reduced the fatigue of workers while carrying loads. At the same time, their lap times increased, using an exoskeleton compared to walking without one. This means a decrease in productivity [318].

Li et al. analyzed a logistics operator who lifted 20-kg loads with motion-capture software, sensors, and a dynamometer treadmill. The oxygen level was reduced by 9.45% [318]. Poliero et al. tested exoskeletons in lifting, carrying, replacing, and walking with 1.2- to 16.2-kg loads, with and without exoskeletons. Lifting activities were supported well, but a negative impact on activities like carrying was found. Lumbar muscle activity reduction of up to 12% was measured, but no clear evidence for exoskeleton efficiency was found [319]. Schröter et al. 2020 analyzed the influence of support systems on human cognitive function in construction. The exoskeleton reduced fatigue, improved concentration, and lowered concentration errors [320].

They tested exoskeletons in static and repetitive manual tasks. A 30% performance increase due to decreased fatigue was observed, and stamina in holding was increased. Time reduction was reported in two-thirds of the cases and time extension in one-third, but three times more volunteers fulfilled the task with an exoskeleton than without [321].

Toxiri et al. compared the effects of exoskeletons while moving weights between two positions. In all cases, muscle activity with an exoskeleton was less than without one. The active one especially showed efficiency [322]. An analysis of lifting tasks based on muscle activity was conducted by Yong et al. They demonstrated a reduction of muscle activity by 24—39% [323]. Only one example of exoskeletons in logistics was found. Picking, lifting, and carrying parcels from pallets in a warehouse were evaluated with acceleration sensors, motion recording, and electromyography measurements (EMG). Moderate relief effects of 5–10%, no difference in efficiency while lifting, and decreased walking productivity were identified [324].

Roveda et al. presented a design methodology for an active exoskeleton to support the lower back by redistributing the spinal load and relieving the operator [325]. Rogge et al. present the Stuttgart Exo-jacket and describe how functions could be designed and the impact of the exoskeleton can be analyzed. However, they mention that there are no standardized test procedures for exoskeletons [326]. Designing an exoskeleton is seen as complicated, as criteria include weight, performance, and comfort [327]. Descriptions of the Robo-Mate project were summarized by O'Sullivan et al., and a qualitative study and interviews with farmers were conducted in

2020 [328]. Schnieders, Stone, Stadler, and Scherly summarized designs and exoskeleton types [329].

Due to a lack of conversion methods to identify the ergonomic impact, the most available ergonomic investigation is based on virtual simulations [307]. Computer analysis for lifting examined a reduction of muscle activity of 58% with an active exoskeleton. In addition, tests with finger exoskeletons proved the extension of movements of injured fingers [309]. Koopman et al. evaluated compression forces, muscle activity, and kinematics, emphasizing that the exoskeleton might reduce the risk of low back pain during static bending and lifting activities [306]. The compression force was reduced by 13–21% for static bending and by an average of 14% for lifting, thus indicating a reduction of strain [306].

Heart rate measurements for ship-builder analysis demonstrated a much lower heart rate working above the head with an exoskeleton than without [330]. Sylla et al. evaluated the ergonomics of an exoskeleton that hit a target 2 meters above ground with a screw gun. They used reflection markers, floor scales, and motion-capture technologies. The exoskeleton reduced the mechanical energy by up to 16.72% and decreased the process cycle time, which means a productivity increase [306].

Suitable methodologies for calculating the operational impact of exoskeletons based on key performance indicators (KPIs) are needed [331]. Methods-time measurement (MTM; or analysis according to Verband für Arbeitsgestaltung, Betriebsorganisation und Unternehmensentwicklung [REFA]) is an option for the evaluation of these KPIs [318]. Optimization of time, cost, and quality can be used to evaluate the return-on-investment potential of exoskeletons [331].

The primary analysis methods used to evaluate ergonomics are measuring muscle activity and heart rate. Alternatively, computer simulation is used. New technologies that evaluate the impact of exoskeletons are needed. Virtual simulation might be helpful, but concrete data is still missing. One option to collect data could be the transformation of exoskeletons into intelligent wearables connected to the Internet of Things (IoT). This could create feasible real-time data and the option to document productivity increases and cost savings through data analytics and machine learning [332]. Exoskeletons need sensors to analyze the impact on the human body depending on the individual attributes of the wearer [333].

4.10.2 Optimization of Soft Exosuits to Improve the Efficiency of Human Walking

Researchers have strived to develop lower-limb wearable devices to improve the efficiency of human walking. However, significant device inertia, kinematic constraints, and the lack of optimal control strategies have limited performance when testing with human subjects. To alleviate these challenges, we developed the soft exosuit, a textile-based wearable device that provides a conformal, unobtrusive, and compliant means for interfacing with the human body.

Unlike most rigid exoskeletons, the components of the soft exosuit on the lower extremity can be worn like light clothing. A soft exosuit can provide forces that are parallel to the lower limb muscles to improve the efficiency of walking.

The working principle of the soft exosuits and the development of multijoint actuation platforms that can provide real-time controlled assistance are presented. Two types of exosuit controllers, including iterative force-based position control and switching admittance-position control, are designed and evaluated. The iterative force-based position control can accurately detect the hip extension onset timing and track peak timing and peak magnitude of the assistive profile within 1% of error. The switching admittance-position controller can track the whole shape of the assistive profile with a root-mean-square error of 3.4% [334].

Human-subject studies evaluating the effects of multijoint assistance and timing of hip extension assistance are conducted to explore human-robot interaction. In the multijoint assistance study with subjects carrying a 23.8-kg backpack on a treadmill, the single-joint condition assisting hip extension with a peak force of 95 N achieves a metabolic reduction of 4.6%. In contrast, the multijoint condition assisting both hip extension and ankle plantarflexion with peak forces of 95 N and 196 N achieves a metabolic reduction of 14.6% compared to the unpowered condition. The result suggests that metabolic benefits can be added by assisting multiple joints simultaneously. Regarding the timing of the hip extension study, four different assistive profiles with two sets of onset and peak timings are evaluated with subjects carrying a 23-kg backpack on a treadmill of 1.5 ms-1. The result demonstrates that actuation timing can affect the delivered mechanical power, joint biological power, and metabolic performance. The assistive profile with an early onset and late peak timing delivers the most mechanical power and achieves the highest metabolic reduction of 8.5% compared to the unpowered condition [334].

The optimization method is first evaluated by finding the subject's optimal step frequency. It is found that the single-parameter optimization converges to the optimal step frequency in half the time of the established gradient descent method and significantly reduces the required total energy expenditure for the overall experiment protocol. Then, the multi-parameter Bayesian optimization is evaluated by optimizing the peak and offset timing of hip extension assistance with a soft exosuit. In this study, optimal timings are found over an average of 21.4 min and achieved 17.4% metabolic reduction compared to no-suit condition, representing an improvement of more than 60% on metabolic reduction compared with state-of-the-art devices that only assist hip extension. The result provides evidence for participant-specific metabolic distributions concerning peak and offset timing and metabolic landscapes, supporting the hypothesis that individualized control strategies can offer substantial benefits over fixed control strategies [334].

For the optimization running on an autonomous system, the optimization should focus on the wearer's performance and consider system efficiency. In optimizing human and system performances, it may be possible to use minimum battery power while providing maximum metabolic benefits [334].

A better understanding of this human-robot interaction allows us further to customize the actuator working range to simplify the system's design and can also guide the design of the control strategy that maximizes metabolic benefits. The definition of "apparent efficiency" is the ratio between the delivered positive mechanical power with a net metabolic reduction [335]. It might be possible that lower-limb joints have different apparent efficiencies even with optimized joint assistance. Thus, investigation of the apparent efficiency with the optimal assistance may guide the design of multijoint exosuit systems that maximize the efficiency of the overall human-robot system [334].

Adaptations have been shown to be a critical factor in reducing muscle activations in studies involving wearable devices on ankle joints [335]. Understanding how we adapt to walking with wearable devices can significantly impact more effective and intuitive uses of these devices. Thus, adaptation studies with soft exosuits for short-term and long-term use are meant for future research, especially when considering commercializing autonomous devices. Essentially, the device instructs the wearer to adjust their walking pattern during assisted walking since step frequency affects the metabolic cost of walking. Correct instructions during assisted walking may also shorten training time for a naive wearer while achieving enhanced metabolic performance [334].

4.10.3 Exoskeleton for Lifting Moderate Weights with Reduced Exhaustion

A bare-bones exoskeleton was for assistance in lifting weights up to 30 kg with reduced exhaustion. The study focused on improving productivity in small-scale industries such as refractories and packaging industries [336]. With the assistance of pneumatic power, moderately heavy materials can be handled in a limited working space, where it is impossible or feasible to utilize heavy or expensive machinery. The device also seeks to reduce workplace injuries and disorders caused by strenuous lifting or repetitive work. Lifting actions include squatting, bending, grasping, rising, and walking. By analyzing the kinematic and static characteristics of lifting, we can get an abstract idea for the design of the exostructure and control system [337]. With the object of designing an exoskeleton, the human body structure needs to be studied along with the force distribution during lifting loads within the human body [338].

Static task: In step 1, the participant lifts the weight of 20 kg without an exoskeleton and holds it in a static position until they start feeling discomfort. The time elapsed is recorded. In step 2, the participant lifts the same weight with an exoskeleton and holds it in a static position until they start feeling discomfort. In step 3, the aforementioned steps are repeated three times for all participants consecutively; in step 4, the values for each participant are plotted in the table and the effect of the exoskeleton is calculated [336].

Dynamic task: In step 1, the participant lifts and lowers the weight in reps, mirroring the movement of the exoskeleton arm joint. Reps are performed until the participant feels discomfort. In step 2, the participant lifts and similarly lowers the same weight, only this time, wearing the exoskeleton; in step 3, the aforementioned steps are repeated for all participants consecutively; in step 4, values for each participant are plotted in the table, and the effect of the exoskeleton is calculated [336].

Precision task: step 1: The participant carries the given weight and walks the predesigned path carrying the weight. A point is deducted for each digression from the path. In step 2, the participant carries a given weight and walks the predesigned path carrying the weight, this time using an exoskeleton. In step 3, the participant is asked to rate their comfort on a scale of 1–10, with 1 being the least comfortable and

10 being the most comfortable. In step 4, the aforementioned steps are repeated for all participants; and in step 5, values for each participant are noted in the observation table and the effect of the exoskeleton is estimated [336].

The test results show that the exoskeleton improved the mean time of lift for the three participants significantly in both static, dynamic, and precision tasks. The participants positively judged the exoskeleton and agreed that the exoskeleton helped them carry out heavier tasks with less physical effort. However, the downside of the exoskeleton is that sometimes the movements are not always entirely consistent with natural movement and the range of lifting is limited. The main limitation reported by participants is that although the overall experience for the user when lifting the weights was less strenuous than when they were wearing the exoskeleton, some discomfort was reported when wearing the exoskeleton for more extended periods [336].

4.10.4 REDUCING THE ENERGY COST OF HUMAN WALKING USING AN UNPOWERED EXOSKELETON

As one of the most important examples of a human-oriented system, the exoskeleton can improve the strength and endurance of the wearer. With recent technological advancements, wearable devices or exoskeletons have witnessed intense development. Passive unpowered exoskeletons are starting to emerge with advantages compared to powered solutions, such as more straightforward design, lower weight, no complex electronics, and lower price. Such an exoskeleton has a higher chance of end-user acceptance. Metabolic energy used during walking can be partly replaced by power input from an exoskeleton. We built a lightweight elastic device that acts in parallel with the user's calf muscles, off-loading muscle force and thereby reducing the metabolic energy consumed in contractions. Results show that by choosing a proper spring, the metabolic cost reduction of walking can be achieved. Improving upon walking economy in this way is analogous to altering the structure of the body such that it is more energy-effective at walking. While intense natural pressures have already shaped human locomotion, efficiency improvements are still possible [339].

With efficiencies derived from evolution, growth, and learning, humans are very well-tuned for locomotion. Metabolic energy used during walking can be partly replaced by power input from an exoskeleton. This would require an improvement in the efficiency of the human-machine system as a whole and would be remarkable given the apparent optimality of human gait. Shrinivas et al. show that an unpowered ankle exoskeleton can reduce the metabolic rate of human walking. They built a lightweight elastic device that acts in parallel with the user's calf muscles, off-loading muscle force and thereby reducing the metabolic energy consumed in contractions. The device uses a mechanical clutch to hold a spring as it is stretched and relaxed by ankle movements when the foot is on the ground, helping to fulfill one function of the calf muscles and Achilles tendon. Unlike muscles, however, the clutch sustains force passively. The exoskeleton consumes no chemical or electrical energy and delivers no net positive mechanical work yet reduces the metabolic cost of walking by $7.2 \pm 2.6\%$ for healthy human users under natural conditions, comparable to savings with powered devices. Improving upon walking economy in this way is analogous to altering the structure of the body such that it is more energy-effective at walking. While intense natural pressures have already shaped human locomotion, efficiency improvements are still possible [339].

4.11 CLOSING REMARKS AND PERSPECTIVES

The new technological trends in modeling tools are focused on the exchange of files, with which it is possible to compare files, refine the design, and apply software based on deep learning. The application of deep learning introduces predictive behavior in design software. Today, CAD software includes generative design and topology optimization tools, so it is possible to identify the best shapes according to the design requirements.

Simulation tools have evolved, focusing on concurrent engineering. This collaboration representing concurrent engineering is used to find the correlation between two simulation solvers and thus find the measured error with high precision. Multibody tools facilitate collaborative work to interact in CAD, CAE, Matlab, LabVIEW, and MSC Adams and thus obtain system performance results from several validation tools that share resources. Many software programs functioning as browser-based modelers on the cloud incorporate deep learning to predict steps in the modeling process.

Another technological leap is happening because hardware improves in harnessing the processing power of graphics processing units (GPUs); CAD users' expectations also change. The latest generation of GPUs allows working with Ray tracing (a method of graphics rendering that simulates the physical behavior of light) in real-time, thanks to the reduction in computing cost in such a way that today the rendering result is so fast. The goal of adding artificial intelligence (AI) to CAD and CAE is to ease the workflow based on deep learning to do generative design, design of experiments, CAD-CAE automation, transfer learning, visualization, and analysis. Using AI-CAD, it is possible to evaluate many 3D CAD models, estimate results, and find conceptual design candidates for the simulation stage. Also, it is convenient to evaluate shapes to optimize the design using AI-CAE.

If you're interested in learning more about exoskeletons and seeing them in action, I would like to invite you to visit our YouTube channel, "Designing Exoskeletons".

Evaluation activity. Please answer the next quiz.

https://forms.office.com/r/SQLAfSPLWB

1. A CAD model is a physical tangible representation carried out in CAD software.
   A. True
   B. False

2. What are the main types of models?
   A. Scanned and created models
   B. Part and assembly
   C. NURBs, polygon mesh, and surface
   D. Wireframe, surface, and solid

3. The animation software has a better rendering capability than CAD and incorporates better textures, illumination, and materials.
   A. True
   B. False

4. Tolerance is the acceptable error between maximum and minimum dimensions, which is searched to avoid the cumulative tolerances using tools for tolerance stack-up analysis.
   A. True
   B. False

5. According to the following list of tolerance accumulation methods, which is missing:
   RSS, Monte Carlo, worst-case, what-ifs + statistical variation, and goal seek.
   A. Adjusted RSS
   B. 3D tolerances
   C. 1D worst-case
   D. 3D worst-case

6. Setting close tolerances decreases the manufacturing cost.
   A. True
   B. False

7. Which simulation technique comprises an extensive collection of methods and applications whose objective is to reproduce the actual behavior?
   A. CAE simulations
   B. CAD simulations
   C. Animations
   D. Interference detection

8. Which item has the main objective structural lightening while maintaining the mechanical functionalities of the target component?
   A. CAD
   B. FEA
   C. Interference detection
   D. Topology optimization

9. Which study describes the mechanism of movements due to forces relative to forward and reverse dynamics?
   A. Flow CFD
   B. CAE multibody dynamics
   C. CAE motion
   D. CAE analysis by FEA

10. A CAD report shows the results of interference, sustainability, or geometric comparison reports, while a CAE report describes the simulation results.
    A. True
    B. False

REFERENCES

1. Carson, J.S., Introduction to modeling and simulation. Proceedings of the 2005 Winter Simulation Conference. IEEE, 2005.
2. Faruque, M., et al., Interfacing issues in multi-domain simulation tools. IEEE Transactions on Power Delivery, 2011.27(1): p. 439–448.
3. Zuñiga Aviles, L.A., Methodology for modeling and simulation of mobile manipulators applied in the mechatronic design of an EOD robot (in Spanish). PhD thesis, Center for Engineering and Industrial Development, CIDESI: Mexico, 2011. p. 116.
4. Stroud, I. and H. Nagy, Solid Modelling and CAD Systems: How to Survive a CAD System. Springer Science & Business Media, 2011.
5. Eiríksson, E.R., et al., Precision and accuracy parameters in structured light 3-D scanning. International Archives of the Photogrammetry, Remote Sensing and Spatial Information Sciences, 2016.5: p. 10.
6. Fischer, B., Mechanical Tolerance Stackup and Analysis. Mechanical Engineering, ed. L.L. Faulkner. 2nd ed. CRC Press Taylor & Francis Group, 2011. p. 486.
7. Dawei, T. and K. Zakrisson, Non-rigid FE-Based Variation Simulation for Furniture. Chalmers University of Technology, 2016.
8. Lee, H.-H., Finite Element Simulations with ANSYS Workbench 2021: Theory, Applications, Case Studies. SDC Publications, 2021.
9. Dos Santos, F.L., et al., Multiphysics NVH modeling: Simulation of a switched reluctance motor for an electric vehicle. IEEE Transactions on Industrial Electronics, 2013.61(1): p. 469–476.
10. Buhl, J., R. Israr, and M. Bambach, Modeling and convergence analysis of directed energy deposition simulations with hybrid implicit/explicit and implicit solutions. Journal of Machine Engineering, 2019.19.
11. García, M., et al., Computational steering of CFD simulations using a grid computing environment. International Journal on Interactive Design and Manufacturing (IJIDeM), 2015.9(3): p. 235–245.
12. Stolzenburg, M.R. and P.H. McMurry, Equations governing single and tandem DMA configurations and a new lognormal approximation to the transfer function. Aerosol Science and Technology, 2008.42(6): p. 421–432.
13. Peng, J.-S., et al., Nonlinear electro-dynamic analysis of micro-actuators: Effect of material nonlinearity. Applied Mathematical Modelling, 2014.38(11–12): p. 2781–2790.
14. Hivet, G. and P. Boisse, Consistent 3D geometrical model of fabric elementary cell. Application to a meshing preprocessor for 3D finite element analysis. Finite Elements in Analysis and Design, 2005.42(1): p. 25–49.
15. Boundary Conditions, August 31, 2021; Available from: www.simscale.com/docs/simulation-setup/boundary-conditions/.
16. Singh, R., H. Garg, and V. Guleria, Haar wavelet collocation method for Lane–Emden equations with Dirichlet, Neumann and Neumann–Robin boundary conditions. Journal of Computational and Applied Mathematics, 2019.346: p. 150–161.
17. Cuillière, J.-C. and V. Francois, Integration of CAD, FEA and topology optimization through a unified topological model. Computer-Aided Design and Applications, 2014.11(5): p. 493–508.
18. Marcé Nogué, J., et al., Coupling finite element analysis and multibody system dynamics for biological research. Palaeontologia Electronica, 2015(18.2.5T): p. 1–14.
19. Nedelcu, D., et al., The kinematic and kinetostatic study of the shaker mechanism with SolidWorks motion. In Journal of Physics: Conference Series. IOP Publishing, 2020.
20. Lange, C., et al., Impact of HPC and automated CFD simulation processes on virtual product development—a case study. Applied Sciences, 2021.11(14): p. 6552.

21. Sherman, M.A., A. Seth, and S.L. Delp, Simbody: Multibody dynamics for biomedical research. Procedia Iutam, 2011.2: p. 241–261.
22. Gomes, C., et al., Co-simulation: A survey. ACM Computing Surveys (CSUR), 2018.51(3): p. 1–33.
23. Gomes, C., et al., Co-simulation: State of the art. arXiv preprint arXiv:1702.00686, 2017.
24. Liu, Z.L., Multiphysics in porous materials. In Multiphysics in Porous Materials. Springer, 2018. p. 29–34.
25. Multiphysics Solutions Features. October 21, 2021; Available from: www.ozeninc.com/ansys-multiphysics/multiphysics-solutions-features/.
26. Multiphysics Simulation. August 31, 2021; Available from: www.plm.automation.siemens.com/global/en/products/simulation-test/multiphysics-simulation.html.
27. Bernhardt, R., H. Schafstall, and I. Hwang, Simulate reality-deliver certainty through the virtual weld. Journal of Welding and Joining, 2016.34(5): p. 41–46.
28. Rodda, J. and H. Graham, Classification of gait patterns in spastic hemiplegia and spastic diplegia: A basis for a management algorithm. European Journal of Neurology, 2001.8: p. 98–108.
29. Durkin, M.S., et al., Prevalence of cerebral palsy among 8-year-old children in 2010 and preliminary evidence of trends in its relationship to low birthweight. Paediatric and Perinatal Epidemiology, 2016.30(5): p. 496–510.
30. Armand, S., G. Decoulon, and A. Bonnefoy-Mazure, Gait analysis in children with cerebral palsy. EFORT Open Reviews, 2016.1(12): p. 448.
31. Cifuentes, C., F. Martínez, and E. Romero, Theoretical and computational analysis of normal and pathological gait: A review (in Spanish). Medical Journal, 2010.18(2): p. 182–196.
32. Standford University, Neuromuscular Biomechanics Laboratory, 2023; Available from: https://nmbl.stanford.edu/.
33. Horsman, M.K., et al., Morphological muscle and joint parameters for musculoskeletal modelling of the lower extremity. Clinical Biomechanics, 2007.22(2): p. 239–247.
34. Rose, J., and J.G. Gamble, Human Walking. 3rd ed. Lippincott Williams & Wilkins, 2005: p. 234.
35. Zajac, F.E., R.R. Neptune, and S.A. Kautz, Biomechanics and muscle coordination of human walking: Part II: Lessons from dynamical simulations and clinical implications. Gait & Posture, 2003.17(1): p. 1–17.
36. Zajac, F.E., R.R. Neptune, and S.A. Kautz, Biomechanics and muscle coordination of human walking: Part I: Introduction to concepts, power transfer, dynamics and simulations. Gait & Posture, 2002.16(3): p. 215–232.
37. Ivanenko, Y.P., R.E. Poppele, and F. Lacquaniti, Five basic muscle activation patterns account for muscle activity during human locomotion. The Journal of Physiology, 2004.556(1): p. 267–282.
38. Lara Romero, M.F., M.T. Angulo Carrere, and L.F. Llanos Alcazar, Normal electromyographic activity in human walking (in Spanish). Biomecanica, 1996.IV(7): p. 110–116.
39. Komura, T., et al., Simulating pathological gait using the enhanced linear inverted pendulum model. IEEE Transactions on Biomedical Engineering, 2005.52(9): p. 1502–1513.
40. Delp, S.L. and J.P. Loan, A graphics-based software system to develop and analyze models of musculoskeletal structures. Computers in Biology and Medicine, 1995.25(1): p. 21–34.
41. Baker, R., Gait analysis methods in rehabilitation. Journal of Neuroengineering and Rehabilitation, 2006.3: p. 1–10.
42. Ackermann, M., Dynamics and Energetics of Walking with Prostheses. Institute of Engineering and Computational Mechanics, University of Stuttgart, 2007: p. 192.

43. Inaba, H., S.-Y. Miyazaki, and J.-I. Hasegawa, Muscle-driven motion simulation based on deformable human model constructed from real anatomical slice data. In Articulated Motion and Deformable Objects: Second International Workshop, AMDO 2002 Palma de Mallorca, Spain, November 21–23, 2002 Proceedings 2.2002. Springer.

44. Barrett, R.S., T.F. Besier, and D.G. Lloyd, Individual muscle contributions to the swing phase of gait: An EMG-based forward dynamics modelling approach. Simulation Modelling Practice and Theory, 2007.15(9): p. 1146–1155.

45. Naruse, K., Biped walking pattern by virtual muscle oscillation in growing physical parameter of robot model. In 2009 ICCAS-SICE. IEEE, 2009.

46. Hill, A.V., The heat of shortening and the dynamic constants of muscle. Proceedings of the Royal Society of London. Series B-Biological Sciences, 1938.126(843): p. 136–195.

47. Nielsen, D.H., et al., Comparison of energy cost and gait efficiency during ambulation in below-knee amputees using different prosthetic feet—a preliminary report. JPO: Journal of Prosthetics and Orthotics, 1988.1(1): p. 24–31.

48. Pandy, M.G., Computer modeling and simulation of human movement. Annual Review of Biomedical Engineering, 2001.3(1): p. 245–273.

49. Dong, F., et al., An anatomy-based approach to human muscle modeling and deformation. IEEE Transactions on Visualization and Computer Graphics, 2002.8(2): p. 154–170.

50. Goujon, H., et al., A functional evaluation of prosthetic foot kinematics during lower limb amputee gait. Prosthetics and Orthotics International, 2006.30(2): p. 213–223.

51. Kuruvilla, A., et al., Characterization of gait parameters in patients with Charcot-Marie-Tooth disease. Neurology India, 2000.48(1): p. 49.

52. Buchli, J. and A.J. Ijspeert, Distributed central pattern generator model for robotics application based on phase sensitivity analysis. In Biologically Inspired Approaches to Advanced Information Technology: First International Workshop, BioADIT 2004, Lausanne, Switzerland, January 29–30, 2004, Revised Selected Papers 1.2004. Springer.

53. Taga, G., A model of the neuro-musculo-skeletal system for human locomotion: I. Emergence of basic gait. Biological Cybernetics, 1995.73(2): p. 97–111.

54. Abbas, J.J. and R.J. Full, Neuromechanical interaction in cyclic movements. Biomechanics and Neural Control of Posture and Movement, 2000: p. 177–191.

55. Taga, G., A model of the neuro-musculo-skeletal system for anticipatory adjustment of human locomotion during obstacle avoidance. Biological Cybernetics, 1998.78(1): p. 9–17.

56. Cruz Martínez, G.M., Generation of trajectories of an exoskeleton for rehabilitation of upper limbs (in Spanish). In Faculty of Engineering. UAEMex, 2018. p. 101.

57. Secco, E.L. and A.M. Tadesse, A wearable exoskeleton for hand kinesthetic feedback in virtual reality. In Wireless Mobile Communication and Healthcare: 8th EAI International Conference, MobiHealth 2019, Dublin, Ireland, November 14–15, 2019, Proceedings 8.2020. Springer.

58. Norkin, C.C. and P.K. Levangie, Joint Structure & Function: A Comprehensive Analysis. FA Davis Company, 1983.

59. Dickmann, T., et al., An adaptive mechatronic exoskeleton for force-controlled finger rehabilitation. Frontiers in Robotics and AI, 2021.8: p. 716451.

60. Gordon, B.L., A.L. Wolff, and A. Daluiski, Elbow kinematics during gait improve with age in children with hemiplegic cerebral palsy. Journal of Pediatric Orthopaedics, 2018.38(8): p. 436–439.

61. Porciuncula, F., et al., Wearable movement sensors for rehabilitation: A focused review of technological and clinical advances. Pm&r, 2018.10(9): p. S220–S232.

62. Tong, K. and M.H. Granat, A practical gait analysis system using gyroscopes. Medical Engineering & Physics, 1999.21(2): p. 87–94.

63. Williamson, R. and B.J. Andrews, Gait event detection for FES using accelerometers and supervised machine learning. IEEE Transactions on Rehabilitation Engineering, 2000.8(3): p. 312–319.

64. Mayagoitia, R.E., A.V. Nene, and P.H. Veltink, Accelerometer and rate gyroscope measurement of kinematics: An inexpensive alternative to optical motion analysis systems. Journal of Biomechanics, 2002.35(4): p. 537–542.

65. Kavanagh, J.J. and H.B. Menz, Accelerometry: A technique for quantifying movement patterns during walking. Gait & Posture, 2008.28(1): p. 1–15.

66. Chen, K.Y. and J. David R. Bassett, The technology of accelerometry-based activity monitors: Current and future. Medicine & Science in Sports & Exercise, 2005.37(11): p. S490–S500.

67. Rueterbories, J., et al., Methods for gait event detection and analysis in ambulatory systems. Medical Engineering & Physics, 2010.32(6): p. 545–552.

68. Haji Ghassemi, N., et al., Segmentation of gait sequences in sensor-based movement analysis: A comparison of methods in Parkinson's disease. Sensors, 2018.18(1): p. 145.

69. Wüest, S., et al., Reliability and validity of the inertial sensor-based Timed" Up and Go" test in individuals affected by stroke. Journal of Rehabilitation Research & Development, 2016.53(5).

70. Heldman, D.A., et al., Clinician versus machine: Reliability and responsiveness of motor endpoints in Parkinson's disease. Parkinsonism & Related Disorders, 2014.20(6): p. 590–595.

71. Kegelmeyer, D.A., et al., Quantitative biomechanical assessment of trunk control in Huntington's disease reveals more impairment in static than dynamic tasks. Journal of the Neurological Sciences, 2017.376: p. 29–34.

72. Mancini, M., et al., Continuous monitoring of turning in Parkinson's disease: Rehabilitation potential. NeuroRehabilitation, 2015.37(1): p. 3.

73. Isho, T., H. Tashiro, and S. Usuda, Accelerometry-based gait characteristics evaluated using a smartphone and their association with fall risk in people with chronic stroke. Journal of Stroke and Cerebrovascular Diseases, 2015.24(6): p. 1305–1311.

74. Bergamini, E., et al., Multi-sensor assessment of dynamic balance during gait in patients with subacute stroke. Journal of Biomechanics, 2017.61: p. 208–215.

75. Byl, N., et al., Clinical impact of gait training enhanced with visual kinematic biofeedback: Patients with Parkinson's disease and patients stable post stroke. Neuropsychologia, 2015.79: p. 332–343.

76. Carpinella, I., et al., Wearable sensor-based biofeedback training for balance and gait in Parkinson disease: A pilot randomized controlled trial. Archives of Physical Medicine and Rehabilitation, 2017.98(4): p. 622–630. e3.

77. Dowling, A.V., D.S. Fisher, and T.P. Andriacchi, Gait modification via verbal instruction and an active feedback system to reduce peak knee adduction moment. Journal of Biomechanical Engineering ASME, 2010.132(071007): p. 1–5.

78. Massé, F., et al., Improving activity recognition using a wearable barometric pressure sensor in mobility-impaired stroke patients. Journal of Neuroengineering and Rehabilitation, 2015.12(1): p. 1–15.

79. Fulk, G.D., et al., Predicting home and community walking activity poststroke. Stroke, 2017.48(2): p. 406–411.

80. French, M.A., et al., Self-efficacy mediates the relationship between balance/walking performance, activity, and participation after stroke. Topics in Stroke Rehabilitation, 2016.23(2): p. 77–83.

81. Danks, K.A., et al., A step activity monitoring program improves real world walking activity post stroke. Disability and Rehabilitation, 2014.36(26): p. 2233–2236.

82. Capela, N., et al., Evaluation of a smartphone human activity recognition application with able-bodied and stroke participants. Journal of Neuroengineering and Rehabilitation, 2016.13(1): p. 1–10.

83. Rodríguez-Molinero, A., et al., Validation of a portable device for mapping motor and gait disturbances in Parkinson's disease. JMIR mHealth and uHealth, 2015.3(1): p. e3321.

84. Delrobaei, M., et al., Towards remote monitoring of Parkinson's disease tremor using wearable motion capture systems. Journal of the Neurological Sciences, 2018.384: p. 38–45.

85. Cavanaugh, J.T., et al., Toward understanding ambulatory activity decline in Parkinson disease. Physical Therapy, 2015.95(8): p. 1142–1150.

86. Schlachetzki, J.C., et al., Wearable sensors objectively measure gait parameters in Parkinson's disease. PLoS One, 2017.12(10): p. e0183989.

87. Dunlop, D.D., et al., Objective physical activity measurement in the osteoarthritis initiative: Are guidelines being met? Arthritis & Rheumatism, 2011.63(11): p. 3372–3382.

88. Lee, J., et al., Sedentary behavior and physical function: Objective evidence from the Osteoarthritis Initiative. Arthritis Care & Research, 2015.67(3): p. 366–373.

89. Semanik, P.A., et al., Accelerometer-monitored sedentary behavior and observed physical function loss. American Journal of Public Health, 2015.105(3): p. 560–566.

90. White, D.K., et al., Do radiographic disease and pain account for why people with or at high risk of knee osteoarthritis do not meet physical activity guidelines? Arthritis & Rheumatism, 2013.65(1): p. 139–147.

91. White, D.K., et al., Walking to meet physical activity guidelines in knee osteoarthritis: Is 10,000 steps enough? Archives of Physical Medicine and Rehabilitation, 2013.94(4): p. 711–717.

92. Kumar, D., K.T. Manal, and K.S. Rudolph, Knee joint loading during gait in healthy controls and individuals with knee osteoarthritis. Osteoarthritis and Cartilage, 2013.21(2): p. 298–305.

93. Bennell, K.L., et al., Higher dynamic medial knee load predicts greater cartilage loss over 12 months in medial knee osteoarthritis. Annals of the Rheumatic Diseases, 2011.70(10): p. 1770–1774.

94. Van Gent, R., et al., Incidence and determinants of lower extremity running injuries in long distance runners: A systematic review. British Journal of Sports Medicine, 2007.41(8): p. 469–480.

95. Zadpoor, A.A. and A.A. Nikooyan, The relationship between lower-extremity stress fractures and the ground reaction force: A systematic review. Clinical Biomechanics, 2011.26(1): p. 23–28.

96. Davis, I.S., B.J. Bowser, and D.R. Mullineaux, Greater vertical impact loading in female runners with medically diagnosed injuries: A prospective investigation. British Journal of Sports Medicine, 2016.50(14): p. 887–892.

97. Hennig, E.M. and M.A. Lafortune, Relationships between ground reaction force and tibial bone acceleration parameters. Journal of Applied Biomechanics, 1991.7(3): p. 303–309.

98. Daniels, J., Daniels' Running Formula. Human Kinetics, 2013.

99. Heiderscheit, B.C., et al., Effects of step rate manipulation on joint mechanics during running. Medicine and Science in Sports and Exercise, 2011.43(2): p. 296.

100. Lenhart, R.L., et al., Increasing running step rate reduces patellofemoral joint forces. Medicine and Science in Sports and Exercise, 2014.46(3): p. 557.

101. Willy, R., et al., In-field gait retraining and mobile monitoring to address running biomechanics associated with tibial stress fracture. Scandinavian Journal of Medicine & Science in Sports, 2016.26(2): p. 197–205.

102. Rice, H.M., S.T. Jamison, and I.S. Davis, Footwear matters: Influence of footwear and foot strike on load rates during running. Medicine & Science in Sports & Exercise, 2016.48(12): p. 2462–2468.

103. Cheung, R.T. and I.S. Davis, Landing pattern modification to improve patellofemoral pain in runners: A case series. Journal of Orthopaedic & Sports Physical Therapy, 2011.41(12): p. 914–919.

104. Diebal, A.R., et al., Forefoot running improves pain and disability associated with chronic exertional compartment syndrome. The American Journal of Sports Medicine, 2012.40(5): p. 1060–1067.

105. Godinho, C., et al., A systematic review of the characteristics and validity of monitoring technologies to assess Parkinson's disease. Journal of Neuroengineering and Rehabilitation, 2016.13(1): p. 1–10.

106. Johansson, D., K. Malmgren, and M. Alt Murphy, Wearable sensors for clinical applications in epilepsy, Parkinson's disease, and stroke: A mixed-methods systematic review. Journal of Neurology, 2018.265: p. 1740–1752.

107. Provot, T., et al., Validation of a high sampling rate inertial measurement unit for acceleration during running. Sensors, 2017.17(9): p. 1958.

108. Group, B.D.W., et al., Biomarkers and surrogate endpoints: Preferred definitions and conceptual framework. Clinical Pharmacology & Therapeutics, 2001.69(3): p. 89–95.

109. Kumari, U. and E. Tan, LRRK2 in Parkinson's disease: Genetic and clinical studies from patients. The FEBS Journal, 2009.276(22): p. 6455–6463.

110. Mirelman, A., et al., Gait alterations in healthy carriers of the LRRK2 G2019S mutation. Annals of Neurology, 2011.69(1): p. 193–197.

111. Mirelman, A., et al., Arm swing as a potential new prodromal marker of Parkinson's disease. Movement Disorders, 2016.31(10): p. 1527–1534.

112. Berardelli, A., et al., Pathophysiology of chorea and bradykinesia in Huntington's disease. Movement Disorders: Official Journal of the Movement Disorder Society, 1999.14(3): p. 398–403.

113. Tabrizi, S.J., et al., Predictors of phenotypic progression and disease onset in premanifest and early-stage Huntington's disease in the TRACK-HD study: Analysis of 36-month observational data. The Lancet Neurology, 2013.12(7): p. 637–649.

114. Porciuncula, F., et al., Sensory modulation of postural control in Huntington's disease. In Movement Disorders. Wiley 111 River ST, Hoboken 07030–5774, NJ USA, 2017.

115. Esser, P., et al., Insights into gait disorders: Walking variability using phase plot analysis, Parkinson's disease. Gait & Posture, 2013.38(4): p. 648–652.

116. Reinkensmeyer, D.J., et al., Computational neurorehabilitation: Modeling plasticity and learning to predict recovery. Journal of Neuroengineering and Rehabilitation, 2016.13(1): p. 1–25.

117. Clark, D.J., et al., Merging of healthy motor modules predicts reduced locomotor performance and muscle coordination complexity post-stroke. Journal of Neurophysiology, 2010.103(2): p. 844–857.

118. Veerbeek, J.M., et al., Effects of augmented exercise therapy on outcome of gait and gait-related activities in the first 6 months after stroke: A meta-analysis. Stroke, 2011.42(11): p. 3311–3315.

119. Ferrante, S., et al., A personalized multi-channel FES controller based on muscle synergies to support gait rehabilitation after stroke. Frontiers in Neuroscience, 2016.10: p. 425.

120. Jacobs, D.A., et al., Motor modules during adaptation to walking in a powered ankle exoskeleton. Journal of Neuroengineering and Rehabilitation, 2018.15(1): p. 1–15.

121. Winters, J.M., Telerehabilitation research: Emerging opportunities. Annual Review of Biomedical Engineering, 2002.4(1): p. 287–320.

122. Polisena, J., et al., Home telehealth for chronic disease management: A systematic review and an analysis of economic evaluations. International Journal of Technology Assessment in Health Care, 2009.25(3): p. 339–349.

123. Chen, J., et al., Telerehabilitation approaches for stroke patients: Systematic review and meta-analysis of randomized controlled trials. Journal of Stroke and Cerebrovascular Diseases, 2015.24(12): p. 2660–2668.

124. Hall, J.L. and D. McGraw, For telehealth to succeed, privacy and security risks must be identified and addressed. Health Affairs, 2014.33(2): p. 216–221.

125. Rezaeibagha, F. and Y. Mu, Practical and secure telemedicine systems for user mobility. Journal of Biomedical Informatics, 2018.78: p. 24–32.

126. Esquenazi, A., et al., The ReWalk powered exoskeleton to restore ambulatory function to individuals with thoracic-level motor-complete spinal cord injury. American Journal of Physical Medicine & Rehabilitation, 2012.91(11): p. 911–921.

127. Veale, A.J. and S.Q. Xie, Towards compliant and wearable robotic orthoses: A review of current and emerging actuator technologies. Medical Engineering & Physics, 2016.38(4): p. 317–325.

128. Panizzolo, F.A., et al., A biologically-inspired multi-joint soft exosuit that can reduce the energy cost of loaded walking. Journal of Neuroengineering and Rehabilitation, 2016.13(1): p. 1–14.

129. Lee, G., et al., Reducing the metabolic cost of running with a tethered soft exosuit. Science Robotics, 2017.2(6): p. eaan6708.

130. Awad, L.N., et al., A soft robotic exosuit improves walking in patients after stroke. Science Translational Medicine, 2017.9(400): p. eaai9084.

131. Bae, J., et al., A lightweight and efficient portable soft exosuit for paretic ankle assistance in walking after stroke. In 2018 IEEE International Conference on Robotics and Automation (ICRA). IEEE, 2018.

132. Chou, L.-W., et al., Motor unit rate coding is severely impaired during forceful and fast muscular contractions in individuals post stroke. Journal of Neurophysiology, 2013.109(12): p. 2947–2954.

133. Li, X., et al., Motor unit number reductions in paretic muscles of stroke survivors. IEEE Transactions on Information Technology in Biomedicine, 2011.15(4): p. 505–512.

134. Kallenberg, L.A. and H.J. Hermens, Motor unit action potential rate and motor unit action potential shape properties in subjects with work-related chronic pain. European Journal of Applied Physiology, 2006.96: p. 203–208.

135. Falla, D., et al., Effect of pain on the modulation in discharge rate of sternocleidomastoid motor units with force direction. Clinical Neurophysiology, 2010.121(5): p. 744–753.

136. De Luca, C.J., et al., Decomposition of surface EMG signals. Journal of Neurophysiology, 2006.96(3): p. 1646–1657.

137. De Luca, C.J., et al., Decomposition of surface EMG signals from cyclic dynamic contractions. Journal of Neurophysiology, 2015.113(6): p. 1941–1951.

138. Pope, Z.K., et al., Action potential amplitude as a noninvasive indicator of motor unit-specific hypertrophy. Journal of Neurophysiology, 2016.115(5): p. 2608–2614.

139. Roy, S.H., et al., High-resolution tracking of motor disorders in Parkinson's disease during unconstrained activity. Movement Disorders, 2013.28(8): p. 1080–1087.

140. Roy, S., et al., Autonomous tracking of body bradykinesia during unconstrained activities in Parkinson's disease. In Movement Disorders. Wiley 111 River ST, Hoboken 07030–5774, NJ USA, 2017.

141. Roy, S.H., et al., A combined sEMG and accelerometer system for monitoring functional activity in stroke. IEEE Transactions on Neural Systems and Rehabilitation Engineering, 2009.17(6): p. 585–594.

142. Lonini, L., et al., Automatic detection of spasticity from flexible wearable sensors. In Proceedings of the 2017 ACM International Joint Conference on Pervasive and Ubiquitous Computing and Proceedings of the 2017 ACM International Symposium on Wearable Computers, 2017.

143. Van Meulen, F.B., et al., Objective evaluation of the quality of movement in daily life after stroke. Frontiers in Bioengineering and Biotechnology, 2016.3: p. 210.

144. Gilgien, M., et al., Mechanics of turning and jumping and skier speed are associated with injury risk in men's world cup alpine skiing: A comparison between the competition disciplines. British Journal of Sports Medicine, 2014.48(9): p. 742–747.

145. Cheung, R., et al., Intrinsic foot muscle volume in experienced runners with and without chronic plantar fasciitis. Journal of Science and Medicine in Sport, 2016.19(9): p. 713–715.

146. Willemsen, A.T.M., J.A. van Alste, and H. Boom, Real-time gait assessment utilizing a new way of accelerometry. Journal of Biomechanics, 1990.23(8): p. 859–863.

147. Constantinescu, G., et al., Epidermal electronics for electromyography: An application to swallowing therapy. Medical Engineering & Physics, 2016.38(8): p. 807–812.

148. Mengüç, Y., et al., Wearable soft sensing suit for human gait measurement. The International Journal of Robotics Research, 2014.33(14): p. 1748–1764.

149. Atalay, A., et al., Batch fabrication of customizable silicone-textile composite capacitive strain sensors for human motion tracking. Advanced Materials Technologies, 2017.2(9): p. 1700136.

150. Atalay, O., et al., A highly sensitive capacitive-based soft pressure sensor based on a conductive fabric and a microporous dielectric layer. Advanced Materials Technologies, 2018.3(1): p. 1700237.

151. Araromi, O.A., C.J. Walsh, and R.J. Wood, Hybrid carbon fiber-textile compliant force sensors for high-load sensing in soft exosuits. In 2017 IEEE/RSJ International Conference on Intelligent Robots and Systems (IROS). IEEE, 2017.

152. Araromi, O.A., C.J. Walsh, and R.J. Wood, Fabrication of stretchable composites with anisotropic electrical conductivity for compliant pressure transducers. In 2016 IEEE SENSORS. IEEE, 2016.

153. Association, A.P.T. Physical therapist practice and the movement system. 2015; Available from: https://www.apta.org/patient-care/interventions/movement-system-management/movement-system-white-paper. August 22, 2022.

154. Qiu, S., et al., Systematic review on wearable lower extremity robotic exoskeletons for assisted locomotion. Journal of Bionic Engineering, 2022: p. 1–34.

155. Liu, D., et al., A brain-controlled lower-limb exoskeleton for human gait training. Review of Scientific Instruments, 2017.88(10): p. 104302.

156. Lyu, M., et al., Development of an EMG-controlled knee exoskeleton to assist home rehabilitation in a game context. Frontiers in Neurorobotics, 2019.13: p. 67.

157. Deng, L.Y., et al., EOG-based human–computer interface system development. Expert Systems with Applications, 2010.37(4): p. 3337–3343.

158. Sarajchi, M., M.K. Al-Hares, and K. Sirlantzis, Wearable lower-limb exoskeleton for children with cerebral palsy: A systematic review of mechanical design, actuation type, control strategy, and clinical evaluation. IEEE Transactions on Neural Systems and Rehabilitation Engineering, 2021.29: p. 2695–2720.

159. Vantilt, J., et al., Model-based control for exoskeletons with series elastic actuators evaluated on sit-to-stand movements. Journal of Neuroengineering and Rehabilitation, 2019.16(1): p. 1–21.

160. Al-Shuka, H.F., et al., Biomechanics, actuation, and multi-level control strategies of power-augmentation lower extremity exoskeletons: An overview. International Journal of Dynamics and Control, 2019.7: p. 1462–1488.

161. Anam, K. and A.A. Al-Jumaily, Active exoskeleton control systems: State of the art. Procedia Engineering, 2012.41: p. 988–994.

162. Young, A.J. and D.P. Ferris, State of the art and future directions for lower limb robotic exoskeletons. IEEE Transactions on Neural Systems and Rehabilitation Engineering, 2016.25(2): p. 171–182.

163. Eguren, D., et al., Design of a customizable, modular pediatric exoskeleton for rehabilitation and mobility. In 2019 IEEE International Conference on Systems, Man and Cybernetics (SMC). IEEE, 2019.

164. Bayon, C., et al., Development and evaluation of a novel robotic platform for gait rehabilitation in patients with Cerebral Palsy: CPWalker. Robotics and Autonomous Systems, 2017.91: p. 101–114.

165. Bayon, C., et al., CPWalker: Robotic platform for gait rehabilitation in patients with Cerebral Palsy. In 2016 IEEE International Conference on Robotics and Automation (ICRA). IEEE, 2016.

166. Baud, R., et al., Review of control strategies for lower-limb exoskeletons to assist gait. Journal of Neuroengineering and Rehabilitation, 2021.18(1): p. 1–34.

167. Hussain, S., S.Q. Xie, and G. Liu, Robot assisted treadmill training: Mechanisms and training strategies. Medical Engineering & Physics, 2011.33(5): p. 527–533.

168. Bortole, M., et al., The H2 robotic exoskeleton for gait rehabilitation after stroke: Early findings from a clinical study. Journal of Neuroengineering and Rehabilitation, 2015.12: p. 1–14.

169. Campeau-Lecours, A., et al., Kinova modular robot arms for service robotics applications. In Rapid Automation: Concepts, Methodologies, Tools, and Applications. IGI Global, 2019. p. 693–719.

170. Xu, D., X. Liu, and Q. Wang, Knee exoskeleton assistive torque control based on real-time gait event detection. IEEE Transactions on Medical Robotics and Bionics, 2019.1(3): p. 158–168.

171. Shepherd, M.K. and E.J. Rouse, Design and validation of a torque-controllable knee exoskeleton for sit-to-stand assistance. IEEE/ASME Transactions on Mechatronics, 2017.22(4): p. 1695 1704.

172. Zhang, J., C.C. Cheah, and S.H. Collins, Torque control in legged locomotion. In Bioinspired Legged Locomotion. Elsevier, 2017. p. 347–400.

173. Del Prete, A., et al., Implementing torque control with high-ratio gear boxes and without joint-torque sensors. International Journal of Humanoid Robotics, 2016.13(01): p. 1550044.

174. Li, W.-Z., G.-Z. Cao, and A.-B. Zhu, Review on control strategies for lower limb rehabilitation exoskeletons. IEEE Access, 2021.9: p. 123040–123060.

175. Quintero, H.A., et al., Preliminary assessment of the efficacy of supplementing knee extension capability in a lower limb exoskeleton with FES. In 2012 Annual International Conference of the IEEE Engineering in Medicine and Biology Society. IEEE, 2012.

176. Winter, D.A., Biomechanics and motor control of human gait: normal, elderly and pathological. 2nd ed., Vol. 1. Waterloo Biomechanics, 1991: p. 143.

177. Harib, O., et al., Feedback control of an exoskeleton for paraplegics: Toward robustly stable, hands-free dynamic walking. IEEE Control Systems Magazine, 2018.38(6): p. 61–87.

178. Li, Y., et al., Design and preliminary validation of a lower limb exoskeleton with compact and modular actuation. IEEE Access, 2020.8: p. 66338–66352.

179. Esquenazi, A., et al., The ReWalk powered exoskeleton to restore ambulatory function to individuals with thoracic-level motor-complete spinal cord injury. American Journal of Physical Medicine & Rehabilitation, 2012.91(11): p. 911–921.

180. Bach Baunsgaard, C., et al., Gait training after spinal cord injury: Safety, feasibility and gait function following 8 weeks of training with the exoskeletons from Ekso Bionics. Spinal Cord, 2018.56(2): p. 106–116.

181. Riener, R., The Cybathlon promotes the development of assistive technology for people with physical disabilities. Journal of Neuroengineering and Rehabilitation, 2016.13: p. 1–4.

182. Hogan, N., Impedance control: An approach to manipulation: Part II—Implementation. Journal of Dynamic Systems, Measurement, and Control, ASME, 1985.107: p. 8–16.

183. Ott, C., R. Mukherjee, and Y. Nakamura, A hybrid system framework for unified impedance and admittance control. Journal of Intelligent & Robotic Systems, 2015.78: p. 359–375.

184. Veneman, J.F., et al., Design and evaluation of the LOPES exoskeleton robot for interactive gait rehabilitation. IEEE Transactions on Neural Systems and Rehabilitation Engineering, 2007.15(3): p. 379–386.

185. Farris, R.J., H.A. Quintero, and M. Goldfarb, Preliminary evaluation of a powered lower limb orthosis to aid walking in paraplegic individuals. IEEE Transactions on Neural Systems and Rehabilitation Engineering, 2011.19(6): p. 652–659.

186. Wang, J., et al., Comfort-centered design of a lightweight and backdrivable knee exoskeleton. IEEE Robotics and Automation Letters, 2018.3(4): p. 4265–4272.

187. Zhu, H., et al., Design and validation of a torque dense, highly backdrivable powered knee-ankle orthosis. In 2017 IEEE International Conference on Robotics and Automation (ICRA). IEEE, 2017.

188. Murray, S.A., et al., An assistive control approach for a lower-limb exoskeleton to facilitate recovery of walking following stroke. IEEE Transactions on Neural Systems and Rehabilitation Engineering, 2014.23(3): p. 441–449.

189. Martínez, A., C. Durrough, and M. Goldfarb, A single-joint implementation of flow control: Knee joint walking assistance for individuals with mobility impairment. IEEE Transactions on Neural Systems and Rehabilitation Engineering, 2020.28(4): p. 934–942.

190. Martinez, A., et al., A velocity-field-based controller for assisting leg movement during walking with a bilateral hip and knee lower limb exoskeleton. IEEE Transactions on Robotics, 2018.35(2): p. 307–316.

191. Holm, J.K. and M.W. Spong, Kinetic energy shaping for gait regulation of underactuated bipeds. In 2008 IEEE International Conference on Control Applications. IEEE, 2008.

192. Lv, G. and R.D. Gregg, Orthotic body-weight support through underactuated potential energy shaping with contact constraints. In 2015 54th IEEE Conference on Decision and Control (CDC). IEEE, 2015.

193. Lin, J., G. Lv, and R.D. Gregg, Contact-invariant total energy shaping control for powered exoskeletons. In 2019 American Control Conference (ACC). IEEE, 2019.

193 Byrnes, C.I. and A. Isidori, A frequency domain philosophy for nonlinear systems, with applications to stabilization and to adaptive control. In the 23rd IEEE Conference on Decision and Control. IEEE, 1984.

194. Chevallereau, C., et al., Rabbit: A testbed for advanced control theory. IEEE Control Systems Magazine, 2003.23(5): p. 57–79.

195. Gregg, R.D., et al., Virtual constraint control of a powered prosthetic leg: From simulation to experiments with transfemoral amputees. IEEE Transactions on Robotics, 2014.30(6): p. 1455–1471.

196. Righetti, L., J. Buchli, and A.J. Ijspeert, Dynamic hebbian learning in adaptive frequency oscillators. Physica D: Nonlinear Phenomena, 2006.216(2): p. 269–281.

197. Ronsse, R., et al., Oscillator-based assistance of cyclical movements: Model-based and model-free approaches. Medical & Biological Engineering & Computing, 2011.49: p. 1173–1185.

198. Yan, T., et al., Review of assistive strategies in powered lower-limb orthoses and exoskeletons. Robotics and Autonomous Systems, 2015.64: p. 120–136.

199. Gams, A., et al., Effects of robotic knee exoskeleton on human energy expenditure. IEEE Transactions on Biomedical Engineering, 2013.60(6): p. 1636–1644.

200. Zhang, Y., K.J. Nolan, and D. Zanotto, Oscillator-based transparent control of an active/semiactive ankle-foot orthosis. IEEE Robotics and Automation Letters, 2018.4(2): p. 247–253.

201. Seo, K., et al., Adaptive oscillator-based control for active lower-limb exoskeleton and its metabolic impact. In 2018 IEEE International Conference on Robotics and Automation (ICRA). IEEE, 2018.

202. Ijspeert, A.J., Central pattern generators for locomotion control in animals and robots: A review. Neural Networks, 2008.21(4): p. 642–653.

203. Yu, J., et al., A survey on CPG-inspired control models and system implementation. IEEE Transactions on Neural Networks and Learning Systems, 2013.25(3): p. 441–456.

204. Gams, A., et al., On-line learning and modulation of periodic movements with nonlinear dynamical systems. Autonomous Robots, 2009.27: p. 3–23.

205. Cavanagh, P.R. and P.V. Komi, Electromechanical delay in human skeletal muscle under concentric and eccentric contractions. European Journal of Applied Physiology and Occupational Physiology, 1979.42: p. 159–163.

206. Sitaram, R., et al., Closed-loop brain training: The science of neurofeedback. Nature Reviews Neuroscience, 2017.18(2): p. 86–100.

207. Johansson, B.B., Brain plasticity and stroke rehabilitation: The Willis lecture. Stroke, 2000.31(1): p. 223–230.

208. Campbell, E., A. Phinyomark, and E. Scheme, Current trends and confounding factors in myoelectric control: Limb position and contraction intensity. Sensors, 2020.20(6): p. 1613.

209. Hogan, N., A review of the methods of processing EMG for use as a proportional control signal. Biomedical Engineering, 1976.11(3): p. 81–86.

210. Graupe, D. and W.K. Cline, Functional separation of EMG signals via ARMA identification methods for prosthesis control purposes. IEEE Transactions on Systems, Man, and Cybernetics, 1975(2): p. 252–259.

211. Farry, K.A., I.D. Walker, and R.G. Baraniuk, Myoelectric teleoperation of a complex robotic hand. IEEE Transactions on Robotics and Automation, 1996.12(5): p. 775–788.

212. Fukuda, O., et al., EMG-based human-robot interface for rehabilitation aid. In Proceedings. 1998 IEEE International Conference on Robotics and Automation (Cat. No. 98CH36146). IEEE, 1998.

213. Song, J., et al., Human body mixed motion pattern recognition method based on multi-source feature parameter fusion. Sensors, 2020.20(2): p. 537.

214. Durandau, G., et al., Voluntary control of wearable robotic exoskeletons by patients with paresis via neuromechanical modeling. Journal of Neuroengineering and Rehabilitation, 2019.16: p. 1–18.

215. Hill, A.V., The heat of shortening and the dynamic constants of muscle. Proceedings of the Royal Society of London. Series B-Biological Sciences, 1938.126(843): p. 136–195.

216. Sartori, M., D.G. Lloyd, and D. Farina, Corrections to "neural data-driven musculoskeletal modeling for personalized neurorehabilitation technologies" [May 16 879–893]. IEEE Transactions on Biomedical Engineering, 2016.63(6): p. 1341–1341.

217. Karavas, N., et al., Tele-impedance based assistive control for a compliant knee exoskeleton. Robotics and Autonomous Systems, 2015.73: p. 78–90.

218. Horn, J.C., et al., Hybrid zero dynamics of bipedal robots under nonholonomic virtual constraints. IEEE Control Systems Letters, 2018.3(2): p. 386–391.

219. Furukawa, J.-I., et al., An EMG-driven weight support system with pneumatic artificial muscles. IEEE Systems Journal, 2014.10(3): p. 1026–1034.

220. Grazi, L., et al., Gastrocnemius myoelectric control of a robotic hip exoskeleton can reduce the user's lower-limb muscle activities at push off. Frontiers in Neuroscience, 2018.12: p. 71.

221. Benabid, A.L., et al., An exoskeleton controlled by an epidural wireless brain–machine interface in a tetraplegic patient: A proof-of-concept demonstration. The Lancet Neurology, 2019.18(12): p. 1112–1122.

222. Del-Ama, A.J., et al., Review of hybrid exoskeletons to restore gait following spinal cord injury. Journal of Rehabilitation Research & Development, 2012.49(4).

223. Anaya, F., P. Thangavel, and H. Yu, Hybrid FES–robotic gait rehabilitation technologies: A review on mechanical design, actuation, and control strategies. International Journal of Intelligent Robotics and Applications, 2018.2: p. 1–28.

224. Del-Ama, A.J., et al., Hybrid FES-robot cooperative control of ambulatory gait rehabilitation exoskeleton. Journal of Neuroengineering and Rehabilitation, 2014.11(1): p. 1–15.

225. To, C.S., et al., Design of a variable constraint hip mechanism for a hybrid neuroprosthesis to restore gait after spinal cord injury. IEEE/ASME Transactions on Mechatronics, 2008.13(2): p. 197–205.

226. Bao, X., et al., Using person-specific muscle fatigue characteristics to optimally allocate control in a hybrid exoskeleton—preliminary results. IEEE Transactions on Medical Robotics and Bionics, 2020.2(2): p. 226–235.

227. Nandor, M., et al., A muscle-first, electromechanical hybrid gait restoration system in people with spinal cord injury. Frontiers in Robotics and AI, 2021.8: p. 645588.

228. Molazadeh, V., et al., An iterative learning controller for a switched cooperative allocation strategy during sit-to-stand tasks with a hybrid exoskeleton. IEEE Transactions on Control Systems Technology, 2021.30(3): p. 1021–1036.

229. Alibeji, N.A., et al., A muscle synergy-inspired control design to coordinate functional electrical stimulation and a powered exoskeleton: Artificial generation of synergies to reduce input dimensionality. IEEE Control Systems Magazine, 2018.38(6): p. 35–60.

230. d'Avella, A., P. Saltiel, and E. Bizzi, Combinations of muscle synergies in the construction of a natural motor behavior. Nature Neuroscience, 2003.6(3): p. 300–308.

231. Singh, R.E., et al., A systematic review on muscle synergies: From building blocks of motor behavior to a neurorehabilitation tool. Applied Bionics and Biomechanics, 2018.2018.

232. Alibeji, N.A., N.A. Kirsch, and N. Sharma, A muscle synergy-inspired adaptive control scheme for a hybrid walking neuroprosthesis. Frontiers in Bioengineering and Biotechnology, 2015.3: p. 203.

233. Griffin, R., et al., Stepping forward with exoskeletons: Team IHMC? s design and approach in the 2016 CYBATHLON. IEEE Robotics & Automation Magazine, 2017.24(4): p. 66–74.

234. Choi, J., et al., Walkon suit: A medalist in the powered exoskeleton race of cybathlon 2016. IEEE Robotics & Automation Magazine, 2017.24(4): p. 75–86.

235. Zhang, T., M. Tran, and H. Huang, Admittance shaping-based assistive control of SEA-driven robotic hip exoskeleton. IEEE/ASME Transactions on Mechatronics, 2019.24(4): p. 1508–1519.

236. Martinez, A., B. Lawson, and M. Goldfarb, A controller for guiding leg movement during overground walking with a lower limb exoskeleton. IEEE Transactions on Robotics, 2017.34(1): p. 183–193.

237. Nagarajan, U., G. Aguirre-Ollinger, and A. Goswami, Integral admittance shaping: A unified framework for active exoskeleton control. Robotics and Autonomous Systems, 2016.75: p. 310–324.

238. Aguirre-Ollinger, G. and H. Yu, Omnidirectional platforms for gait training: Admittance-shaping control for enhanced mobility. Journal of Intelligent & Robotic Systems, 2021.101: p. 1–17.

239. Lv, G. and R.D. Gregg, Towards total energy shaping control of lower-limb exoskeletons. In 2017 American Control Conference (ACC). IEEE, 2017.

240. Cardona, M., et al., ALICE: Conceptual development of a lower limb exoskeleton robot driven by an on-board musculoskeletal simulator. Sensors, 2020.20(3): p. 789.

241. Alibeji, N.A., N.A. Kirsch, and N. Sharma, A muscle synergy-inspired adaptive control scheme for a hybrid walking neuroprosthesis. Frontiers in Bioengineering and Biotechnology, 2015.3: p. 203.

242. Lv, G., et al., A task-invariant learning framework of lower-limb exoskeletons for assisting human locomotion. In 2020 American Control Conference (ACC). IEEE, 2020.

243. Song, S. and S.H. Collins, Optimizing exoskeleton assistance for faster self-selected walking. IEEE Transactions on Neural Systems and Rehabilitation Engineering, 2021.29: p. 786–795.

244. Khan, S.G., et al., Reinforcement learning based compliance control of a robotic walk assist device. Advanced Robotics, 2019.33(24): p. 1281–1292.

245. Kelly, M., An introduction to trajectory optimization: How to do your own direct collocation. SIAM Review, 2017.59(4): p. 849–904.

246. Duburcq, A., et al., Online trajectory planning through combined trajectory optimization and function approximation: Application to the exoskeleton atalante. In 2020 IEEE International Conference on Robotics and Automation (ICRA). IEEE, 2020.

247. Bauer, G. and Y.-J. Pan, Review of control methods for upper limb telerehabilitation with robotic exoskeletons. IEEE Access, 2020.8: p. 203382–203397.

248. Khairuddin, I.M., et al., Assistive-as-needed strategy for upper-limb robotic systems: An initial survey. In IOP Conference Series: Materials Science and Engineering. IOP Publishing, 2017.

249. Proietti, T., et al., Upper-limb robotic exoskeletons for neurorehabilitation: A review on control strategies. IEEE Reviews in Biomedical Engineering, 2016.9: p. 4–14.

250. Islam, M.R., et al., A brief review on robotic exoskeletons for upper extremity rehabilitation to find the gap between research porotype and commercial type. Advances in Robotics & Automation, 2017.6(3): p. 2.

251. Nef, T., M. Mihelj, and R. Riener, ARMin: A robot for patient-cooperative arm therapy. Medical & Biological Engineering & Computing, 2007.45: p. 887–900.

252. Yu, W., X. Li, and R. Carmona, A novel PID tuning method for robot control. Industrial Robot: An International Journal, 2013.40(6): p. 574–582.

253. Wu, Q., et al., Fuzzy sliding mode control of an upper limb exoskeleton for robot-assisted rehabilitation. In 2015 IEEE International Symposium on Medical Measurements and Applications (MeMeA) Proceedings. IEEE, 2015.

254. Anam, K. and A.A. Al-Jumaily, Active exoskeleton control systems: State of the art. Procedia Engineering, 2012.41: p. 988–994.

255. Ott, C., R. Mukherjee, and Y. Nakamura, Unified impedance and admittance control. In 2010 IEEE International Conference on Robotics and Automation. IEEE, 2010.

256. MacLean, K.E. and V. Hayward, Do it yourself haptics: Part ii [tutorial]. IEEE Robotics & Automation Magazine, 2008.15(1): p. 104–119.

257. Riener, R., et al., Patient-cooperative strategies for robot-aided treadmill training: First experimental results. IEEE Transactions on Neural Systems and Rehabilitation Engineering, 2005.13(3): p. 380–394.

258. Riener, R., L. Lünenburger, and G. Colombo, Human-centered robotics applied to gait training and assessment. Journal of Rehabilitation Research & Development, 2006.43(5).

259. Frisoli, A., et al., A force-feedback exoskeleton for upper-limb rehabilitation in virtual reality. Applied Bionics and Biomechanics, 2009.6(2): p. 115–126.

260. Kiguchi, K. and Y. Hayashi, An EMG-based control for an upper-limb power-assist exoskeleton robot. IEEE Transactions on Systems, Man, and Cybernetics, Part B (Cybernetics), 2012.42(4): p. 1064–1071.

261. Carignan, C., et al., A configuration-space approach to controlling a rehabilitation arm exoskeleton. In 2007 IEEE 10th International Conference on Rehabilitation Robotics. IEEE, 2007.

262. Just, F., et al., Online adaptive compensation of the ARMin Rehabilitation Robot. In 2016 6th IEEE International Conference on Biomedical Robotics and Biomechatronics (BioRob). IEEE, 2016.

263. Kang, H.-B. and J.-H. Wang, Adaptive robust control of 5 DOF upper-limb exoskeleton robot. International Journal of Control, Automation and Systems, 2015.13: p. 733–741.

264. Brahmi, B., et al., Robust adaptive tracking control of uncertain rehabilitation exoskeleton robot. Journal of Dynamic Systems, Measurement, and Control, 2019.141(12).

265. Yang, C., et al., Neural control of bimanual robots with guaranteed global stability and motion precision. IEEE Transactions on Industrial Informatics, 2016.13(3): p. 1162–1171.

266. Xu, L.-J., C.-Y. Dong, and Y. Chen, An adaptive fuzzy sliding mode control for networked control systems. In 2007 International Conference on Mechatronics and Automation. IEEE, 2007.

267. Wu, Q., et al., Development of an RBFN-based neural-fuzzy adaptive control strategy for an upper limb rehabilitation exoskeleton. Mechatronics, 2018.53: p. 85–94.

268. Brahmi, B., et al., Adaptive tracking control of an exoskeleton robot with uncertain dynamics based on estimated time-delay control. IEEE/ASME Transactions on Mechatronics, 2018.23(2): p. 575–585.

269. Shokri-Ghaleh, H. and A. Alfi, Bilateral control of uncertain telerobotic systems using iterative learning control: Design and stability analysis. Acta Astronautica, 2019.156: p. 58–69.

270. Ugurlu, B., et al., Proof of concept for robot-aided upper limb rehabilitation using disturbance observers. IEEE Transactions on Human-Machine Systems, 2014.45(1): p. 110–118.

271. Pang, M., S. Guo, and Z. Song, Study on the sEMG driven upper limb exoskeleton rehabilitation device in bilateral rehabilitation. Journal of Robotics and Mechatronics, 2012.24(4): p. 585.

272. Simonetti, D., et al., Multimodal adaptive interfaces for 3D robot-mediated upper limb neuro-rehabilitation: An overview of bio-cooperative systems. Robotics and Autonomous Systems, 2016.85: p. 62–72.

273. Zhong, X. and Y. ShiQiang, A review of on-orbit servicing robot teleoperation control system. International Journal of Signal Processing, Image Processing and Pattern Recognition, 2016.9(11): p. 83–92.

274. Buongiorno, D., et al., Multi-dofs exoskeleton-based bilateral teleoperation with the time-domain passivity approach. Robotica, 2019.37(9): p. 1641–1662.

275. Nisky, I., F.A. Mussa-Ivaldi, and A. Karniel, Analytical study of perceptual and motor transparency in bilateral teleoperation. IEEE Transactions on Human-Machine Systems, 2013.43(6): p. 570–582.

276. Muradore, R. and P. Fiorini, A review of bilateral teleoperation algorithms. Acta Polytechnica Hungarica, 2016.13(1): p. 191–208.

277. Serna, M., et al., Bilateral teleoperation of a commercial small-sized underwater vehicle for academic purposes. In OCEANS 2015-MTS/IEEE Washington. IEEE, 2015.

278. Wei, W. and Y. Kui, Teleoperated manipulator for leak detection of sealed radioactive sources. In IEEE International Conference on Robotics and Automation, 2004. Proceedings. ICRA'04.2004. IEEE, 2004.

279. Slawiñski, E., et al., Force and position–velocity coordination for delayed bilateral teleoperation of a mobile robot. Robotica, 2019.37(10): p. 1768–1784.

280. Dong, Y. and N. Chopra, Passivity-based bilateral tele-driving system with parametric uncertainty and communication delays. IEEE Control Systems Letters, 2018.3(2): p. 350–355.

281. Hokayem, P.F. and M.W. Spong, Bilateral teleoperation: An historical survey. Automatica, 2006.42(12): p. 2035–2057.

282. Richert, D., C.J. Macnab, and J.K. Pieper, Adaptive haptic control for telerobotics transitioning between free, soft, and hard environments. IEEE Transactions on Systems, Man, and Cybernetics-Part A: Systems and Humans, 2011.42(3): p. 558–570.

283. Chen, Z., Y.J. Pan, and J. Gu, Integrated adaptive robust control for multilateral teleoperation systems under arbitrary time delays. International Journal of Robust and Nonlinear Control, 2016.26(12): p. 2708–2728.

284. Tzafestas, S.G. and A.-I. Mantelos, Time delay and uncertainty compensation in bilateral telerobotic systems: State-of-art with case studies. In Engineering Creative Design in Robotics and Mechatronics. IGI Global, 2013. p. 208–238.

285. Niemeyer, G. and J.-J.E. Slotine, Telemanipulation with time delays. The International Journal of Robotics Research, 2004.23(9): p. 873–890.

286. Hannaford, B. and J.-H. Ryu, Time-domain passivity control of haptic interfaces. IEEE transactions on Robotics and Automation, 2002.18(1): p. 1–10.

287. Duong, M.D., K. Terashima, and T. Miyoshi, A novel stable teleoperation with haptic feedback by means of impedance adjustment via arbitrary time delay environment for rehabilitation. In 2009 IEEE Control Applications, (CCA) & Intelligent Control, (ISIC). IEEE, 2009.

288. Ware, J.R., Power based time domain passivity control and its application to bilateral teleoperated robotic vehicles. Mechanical Engineering, Dalhousie University, 2010: p. 110.

289. Ware, J. and Y.-J. Pan, Realisation of a bilaterally teleoperated robotic vehicle platform with passivity control. IET Control Theory & Applications, 2011.5(8): p. 952–962.

290. Anderson, R.J. and M.W. Spong, Bilateral control of teleoperators with time delay. In Proceedings of the 1988 IEEE International Conference on Systems, Man, and Cybernetics. IEEE, 1988.

291. Carignan, C.R. and H.I. Krebs, Telerehabilitation robotics: Bright lights, big future? Journal of Rehabilitation Research and Development, 2006.43(5): p. 695.

292. Niemeyer, G. and J.-J. Slotine, Stable adaptive teleoperation. IEEE Journal of Oceanic Engineering, 1991.16(1): p. 152–162.

293. Sun, D., F. Naghdy, and H. Du, Application of wave-variable control to bilateral teleoperation systems: A survey. Annual Reviews in Control, 2014.38(1): p. 12–31.

294. Niemeyer, G. and J.-J. Slotine, Towards force-reflecting teleoperation over the internet. In Proceedings. 1998 IEEE International Conference on Robotics and Automation (Cat. No. 98CH36146). IEEE, 1998.

295. Munir, S. and W.J. Book, Internet-based teleoperation using wave variables with prediction. In 2001 IEEE/ASME International Conference on Advanced Intelligent Mechatronics. Proceedings (Cat. No. 01TH8556). IEEE, 2001.

296. Rodriguez-Seda, E.J., D. Lee, and M.W. Spong, Experimental comparison study of control architectures for bilateral teleoperators. IEEE Transactions on Robotics, 2009.25(6): p. 1304–1318.

297. Ye, Y., Y. Pan, and Y. Gupta, A simplified time domain passivity control of haptic interfaces. In Proceedings of the 11th IASTED International Conference, Intelligent Systems and Control (ISC 2008), 2008.

298. Kim, Y.S. and B. Hannaford, Some practical issues in time domain passivity control of haptic interfaces. In Proceedings 2001 IEEE/RSJ International Conference on Intelligent Robots and Systems. Expanding the Societal Role of Robotics in the Next Millennium (Cat. No. 01CH37180). IEEE, 2001.

299. Sheng, L., et al., A time domain passivity control scheme for bilateral teleoperation. Electronics, 2019.8(3): p. 325.

300. Chan, L., F. Naghdy, and D. Stirling, Application of adaptive controllers in teleoperation systems: A survey. IEEE Transactions on Human-Machine Systems, 2014.44(3): p. 337–352.

301. Chopra, N. and M.W. Spong, Adaptive coordination control of bilateral teleoperators with time delay. In 2004 43rd IEEE Conference on Decision and Control (CDC) (IEEE Cat. No. 04CH37601). IEEE, 2004.

302. Nuno, E., I. Sarras, and L. Basanez, An adaptive controller for bilateral teleoperators: Variable time-delays case. IFAC Proceedings Volumes, 2014.47(3): p. 9341–9346.

303. Lee, D. and M.W. Spong, Passive bilateral teleoperation with constant time delay. IEEE Transactions on Robotics, 2006.22(2): p. 269–281.

304. Nuño, E., L. Basañez, and R. Ortega, Passivity-based control for bilateral teleoperation: A tutorial. Automatica, 2011.47(3): p. 485–495.

305. Aziminejad, A., et al., Transparent time-delayed bilateral teleoperation using wave variables. IEEE Transactions on Control Systems Technology, 2008.16(3): p. 548–555.

306. Kaupe, V., C. Feldmann, and H. Wagner, Exoskeletons: Productivity and ergonomics in logistics: A systematic review. In Hamburg International Conference of Logistics (HICL) 2021. Epubli, 2021.

307. Dahmen, C. and C. Constantinescu, Methodology of employing exoskeleton technology in manufacturing by considering time-related and ergonomics influences. Applied Sciences, 2020.10(5): p. 1591.

308. Constantinescu, C., et al., Exoskeleton-centered process optimization in advanced factory environments. Procedia CIRP, 2016.41: p. 740–745.

309. Ippolito, D., C. Constantinescu, and C.A. Rusu, Enhancement of human-centered workplace design and optimization with Exoskeleton technology. Procedia CIRP, 2020.91: p. 243–248.

310. Butler, T. and D. Wisner, Exoskeleton technology: Making workers safer and more productive. In ASSE Professional Development Conference and Exposition. OnePetro, 2017.

311. Bances, E., et al., Exoskeletons towards industrie 4.0: Benefits and challenges of the IoT communication architecture. Procedia Manufacturing, 2020.42: p. 49–56.

312. Burton, S.D., Responsible use of exoskeletons and exosuits: Ensuring domestic security in a European context. Paladyn, Journal of Behavioral Robotics, 2020.11(1): p. 370–378.

313. Brown, M., N. Tsagarakis, and D.G. Caldwell, Exoskeletons for human force augmentation. Industrial Robot: An International Journal, 2003.30(6): p. 592–602.

314. De Looze, M.P., et al., Exoskeletons for industrial application and their potential effects on physical workload. Ergonomics, 2016.59(5): p. 671–681.

315. De Vries, A. and M. De Looze, The effect of arm support exoskeletons in realistic work activities: A review study. Journal Ergonomic, 2019.9(4): p. 1–9.

316. Geregei, A., et al., Up-to-date techniques for examining safety and physiological efficiency of industrial exoskeletons. Health Risk Analysis, 2020(3): p. 147–158.

317. Hyun, D.J., et al., A light-weight passive upper arm assistive exoskeleton based on multi-linkage spring-energy dissipation mechanism for overhead tasks. Robotics and Autonomous Systems, 2019.122: p. 103309.

318. Lee, G. and D. Cha, Statistical analysis of the effectiveness of wearable robot. Electronics, 2021.10(9): p. 1006.

319. Poliero, T., et al., Applicability of an active back-support exoskeleton to carrying activities. Frontiers in Robotics and AI, 2020.7: p. 579963.

320. Schroeter, F., et al., Cognitive effects of physical support systems: A study of resulting effects for tasks at and above head level using exoskeletons. In Annals of Scientific Society for Assembly, Handling and Industrial Robotics. Springer, 2020.

321. Spada, S., et al., Investigation into the applicability of a passive upper-limb exoskeleton in automotive industry. Procedia Manufacturing, 2017.11: p. 1255–1262.

322. Toxiri, S., et al., Rationale, implementation and evaluation of assistive strategies for an active back-support exoskeleton. Frontiers in Robotics and AI, 2018.5: p. 53.

323. Yong, X., et al., Ergonomic mechanical design and assessment of a waist assist exoskeleton for reducing lumbar loads during lifting task. Micromachines, 2019.10(7): p. 463.

324. Winter, G., C. Felt a en, and J. Hedtmann, Testing of exoskeletons in the context of logistics-application and limits of use. In HCI International 2019-Posters: 21st International Conference, HCII 2019, Orlando, FL, USA, July 26–31, 2019, Proceedings, Part II 21.2019. Springer.

325. Roveda, L., et al., Design methodology of an active back-support exoskeleton with adaptable backbone-based kinematics. International Journal of Industrial Ergonomics, 2020.79: p. 102991.

326. Rogge, T., U. Daub, and A. Ebrahimi, Status demonstration of the interdisciplinary development regarding the upper limb exoskeleton. Stuttgart Exo-Jacket. In 17. Internationales Stuttgarter Symposium: Automobil-und Motorentechnik. Springer, 2017.

327. Lanotte, F., et al., Design and characterization of a multi-joint underactuated low-back exoskeleton for lifting tasks. In 2020 8th IEEE RAS/EMBS International Conference for Biomedical Robotics and Biomechatronics (BioRob). IEEE, 2020.

328. Omoniyi, A., et al., Farmers' perceptions of exoskeleton use on farms: Finding the right tool for the work (er). International Journal of Industrial Ergonomics, 2020.80: p. 103036.

329. Schnieders, T.M. and R.T. Stone, Current work in the human-machine interface for ergonomic intervention with exoskeletons. International Journal of Robotics Applications and Technologies (IJRAT), 2017.5(1): p. 1–19.

330. Moyon, A., E. Poirson, and J.-F. Petiot, Experimental study of the physical impact of a passive exoskeleton on manual sanding operations. Procedia CIRP, 2018.70: p. 284–289.

331. Dahmen, C., et al., Approach of optimized planning process for exoskeleton centered workplace design. Procedia CIRP, 2018.72: p. 1277–1282.

332. Constantinescu, C., P.-C. Muresan, and G.-M. Simon, JackEx: The new digital manufacturing resource for optimization of exoskeleton-based factory environments. Procedia CIRP, 2016.50: p. 508–511.

333. Bances, E., et al., Exoskeletons towards industrie 4.0: Benefits and challenges of the IoT communication architecture. Procedia Manufacturing, 2020.42: p. 49–56.

334. Sawicki, G.S. and D.P. Ferris, Mechanics and energetics of level walking with powered ankle exoskeletons. Journal of Experimental Biology, 2008.211(9): p. 1402–1413.

335. Gordon, K.E., C.R. Kinnaird, and D.P. Ferris, Locomotor adaptation to a soleus EMG-controlled antagonistic exoskeleton. Journal of Neurophysiology, 2013.109(7): p. 1804–1814.

336. De Bock, S., et al., An occupational shoulder exoskeleton reduces muscle activity and fatigue during overhead work. IEEE Transactions on Biomedical Engineering, 2022.69(10): p. 3008–3020.

337. Simon, A.A., M.M. Alemi, and A.T. Asbeck, Kinematic effects of a passive lift assistive exoskeleton. Journal of Biomechanics, 2021.120: p. 110317.

338. Durante, F., M.G. Antonelli, and P.B. Zobel, Development of an active exoskeleton for assisting back movements in lifting weights. International Journal of Mechanical Engineering and Robotics Research, 2018.7(4): p. 353–360.

339. Shrinivas G. Nagekar, S.K.P., Mohammed Yaseen, reducing the energy cost of human walking using an unpowered exoskeleton. IOSR Journal of Mechanical and Civil Engineering (IOSR-JMCE), 2020: p. 26–31.

5 Technology Readiness Level in Exoskeleton Development

5.1 INTRODUCTION

While CAD handles the design of a workpiece and CAE performs analysis tasks, CAM focuses on how to manufacture the workpiece. CAM prepares a CAD model for machining, checking for any geometry errors, creating a machining path, setting machine parameters, and setting up nesting to maximize machining efficiency. These are CAD-CAM-CAE software tools that are fundamental during the design cycle, helping to reach the nine levels of technological maturity (TRL), the nine levels of maturity for manufacturing (MRL), and the nine levels of maturity for investment (IRL). This chapter addresses the considerations for generating a work plan that allows reaching a certain level of technological maturity, as well as evaluating whether the prototype of an exoskeleton meets a certain level of technological maturity. In this context, the gathering of user requirements, the generation of the design concept, the operating principle, the experimental physical model, the prototypes for laboratory evaluation, prototypes for demonstration, the released products, certified products, and products in production are of essential relevance. This chapter covers the topics of requirements of the user, requirements to reach TRL, functional requirements, design parameters, critical design parameters, process variables, manufacturing tools, and prototyping.

5.2 REQUIREMENTS

The success of an exoskeleton is the acceptance of the product in the market, which can be an incremental or radical innovation when the users recognize the product. Incremental innovation is when users assimilate the technology quickly due to known operating paradigms. Radical innovation has slower assimilation due to the change in operating paradigms. Once users assimilate and adopt it, this innovation forms a new operating paradigm; an example of radical innovation is replacing motors with soft actuators.

The acceptance of new products is related to establishing appropriate requirements, which allows an understanding of user needs through an exhaustive analysis of requirements. Various tools are used to establish requirements, such as the Kano model, storytelling, mapping journey, and an affinity diagram.

With the advancement of technology, the classification of requirements depends on the design area. In the case of exoskeleton design, the requirements are determined

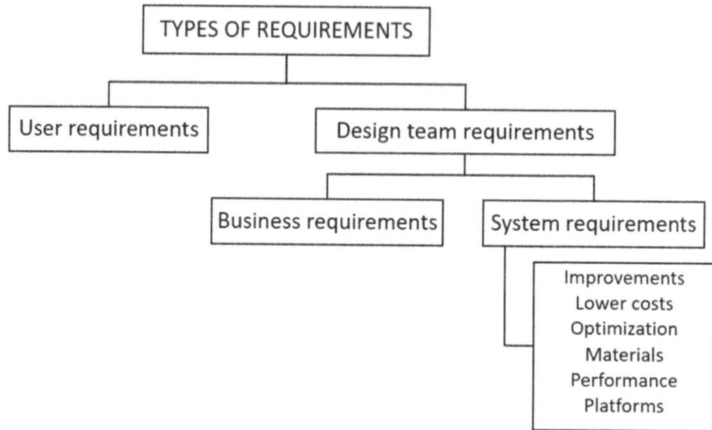

FIGURE 5.1 Types of requirements for exoskeleton design.

based on the type of use of the exoskeleton. In general, requirements are established based on the user's needs and the required performance of the exoskeleton. For this, the design team proposes improvements in various areas, such as weight reduction, material selection, coatings, manufacturing processes, manufacturing costs reduction, ease of manufacture, interchangeability, refurbishment, maintenance, compatibility between accessories, customization, styling, security, parameters (position, velocity, force, dimensions), and part control.

The satisfaction of user requirements is fundamental; for this reason, understanding the technology tendency according to the requirements of every market segment allows the product to be accepted, assimilated, and adopted. Overall, the types of requirements are divided into user and design team requirements; the latter are divided into business and system requirements. The business requirements are dedicated to linking the market opportunity with the exoskeleton design [1]. The system requirements are divided into improvements, lower costs, optimization, materials, performance, and platforms, as shown in Figure 5.1.

5.3 REQUIREMENTS TO REACH READINESS OF A SYSTEM

There are several requirements by phase of readiness during exoskeleton development, such as the TRL, MRL, and IRL [2]. Figure 5.2 shows the requirements to reach the readiness of technology, manufacturing, and investment levels as well as how they are related to each other according to the research, development, and deployment stages.

The research stage has three sections. The first and second sections include requirements to reach TRL1 and TRL2, and the third section includes requirements to reach TRL3, which is at the laboratory level. At this level, the operating evaluation is done on a test bench using controlled parameters [3]. The laboratory level includes requirements for TRL3 and MRL1 of the research stage, as well as requirements for TRL4, MRL2, and IRL1 of the development stage.

	REQUIREMENTS TO REACH TRL/MRL/IRL	TRL/MRL/IRL	LEVEL
RESEARCH	❑ User Requirements, References of Principles from Basic Research, Benchmarking, and Potential Market Segments. External Constraints and Ideation.	TRL1	
	❑ Internal Constraints, Formulation of Solution, Design Concept, Value Offer, and Capacity from Design Team.	TRL2	
	❑ Operating Principle, Experimental Physical Model and Feasibility Evaluation. ➢ Initial Materials and Manufacturing Implications.	TRL3 MRL1	
DEVELOPMENT	❑ Experimental Physical Model Pilot and its Effectiveness Evaluation. Usability Testing and Risk Management Plan. ➢ Manufacturing Strategies for Users' Needs. ❖ Business Model.	TRL4 MRL2 IRL1	LABORATORY
	❑ Prototype with Components of High Reliability and Experimental Lot. ➢ New Manufacturing Process Developed with Limited Functionality. ❖ Market Analysis, Market Size and Competitive Analysis.	TRL5 MRL3 IRL2	DEMONSTRATION Conditions that Emulate Real Environment
	❑ Prototype by Complete Exoskeleton Testing. ➢ Manufacturing Technologies, Producibility Assessments, Facilities and Skills. ❖ Problem-Solution Validation.	TRL6 MRL4 IRL3	INDUSTRIAL DEMONSTRATION Real Environment
DEPLOYMENT	❑ Prototype by Complete System Validation in Hospital and Clinical Tasks. ➢ Manufacturing Refined and Integrated with Risk Management Plan; Processes in Development. Materials and Tooling defined to Produce Prototype Components. ❖ MVP Low Fidelity and Testing with Users and Potential Clients.	TRL7 MRL5 IRL4	
	➢ Capability to Produce the Prototype Following the Process Sheet Using Tooling and Materials, Refining the Process.	MRL6	PRODUCTION BY SYSTEM
	❖ Validate Product and Market Fit.	IRL5	
	❖ Validate Revenue Model.	IRL6	
	❑ Certified Product with User Manual, Technical Support and Maintenance. ➢ Pilot Line and Final Materials, Production Improvements, and Risk Assessments. ❖ MVP High Fidelity.	TRL8 MRL7 IRL7	FDA AND COMMERCIAL CLEARANCES
	❑ Released Product. Outlining New Versions and Scaling.	TRL9	
	➢ Initial Production and Minimal System Changes. Optimization of Manufacturing Process.	MRL8	
	➢ Continuous Production and Process Statistical Control.	MRL9	
	➢ Manufacturing Process Required based on Quality and Costs.	MRL10	FULL-RATE PRODUCTION
	❖ Validate Value Delivery.	IRL8	
	❖ Metrics to Growth.	IRL9	MARKET EXPANSION

FIGURE 5.2 Requirements to reach TRL, MRL, and IRL by stage and level.

The demonstration level is where the conditions that emulate the real operating environment are implemented. The prototype describes the system; this level includes TRL5, MRL3, and IRL2, corresponding to the development stage.

The industrial demonstration is where the exoskeleton requires operating in a real environment. This level includes the requirement to reach the TRL6, MRL4, and IRL3 of the development stage and the requirements to reach the TRL7 and MRL5. In addition, IRL4 corresponds to the deployment stage.

The deployment stage includes 11 sections. The first section was described earlier. The second section includes the MRL6 level, which in turn corresponds to the level of production by the system. The third and fourth sections include the IRL5 and IRL6 levels, respectively. The fifth section includes TRL8, MRL7, and IRL7, which correspond to FDA and commercial clearance levels. The sixth, seventh, eighth, and tenth sections include TRL9, MRL8, MRL9, and IRL8, respectively. The ninth section includes MRL10, which corresponds to the level of full-rate production. Finally, the eleventh section includes IRL9, which corresponds to the level of market expansion.

5.4 REQUIREMENT IDENTIFICATION

The design gives solutions to opportunities, needs, or problems, depending on the design team's approach. The necessity requires fast solutions; a problem is solved over a long time due to the planning of the research project, so the identification of market opportunity is the main motivation to define the requirements. Figure 5.3 shows the interaction of tools to get the user requirements as a job mapping framework, customer journey mapping, and job to be done, as well as the requirements to project as business model in CANVAS, FODA, and GANTT.

The job mapping framework is a visual representation that describes the job of customers; for instance, in the vigilance job are depicted the specific steps which allow the design team to capture the customer requirements throughout the process [4]. The customer journey mapping (CJM) is a group of several schemes describing the interaction of the client to purchase flow; in some stores, there are steps to achieve the client to purchase their first exoskeleton. This CJM helps to identify the expectation of customers in the acquisition of an exoskeleton, and the team design considers these requirements for new designs [5]. The job to be done is a framework for customer requirements; the perspective of this methodology is to understand the customer motivations to use a product [6]. The client buys a product for the task it solves, but not for the product itself. So, a client thinks an exoskeleton can help them to perform better in their job, sport, or training. Maybe the clients are looking for esteem, status, comfort, and values that an exoskeleton represents. Clayton Christensen spread the concept of jobs to be done (JTBD) in his book *The Innovator's Dilemma* [7]. The steps to implement JTBD are as follows: 1. define the market segments in the function of the job, 2. list customer expectations, 3. quantify the attention of competency (analyze the actual competitors) to the job, 4. list hidden opportunities, and 5. list requirements for the new exoskeleton.

The functional architecture focuses specifically on operating exoskeletons. For this, the interaction of different aspects is taken into account (Figure 5.4). The

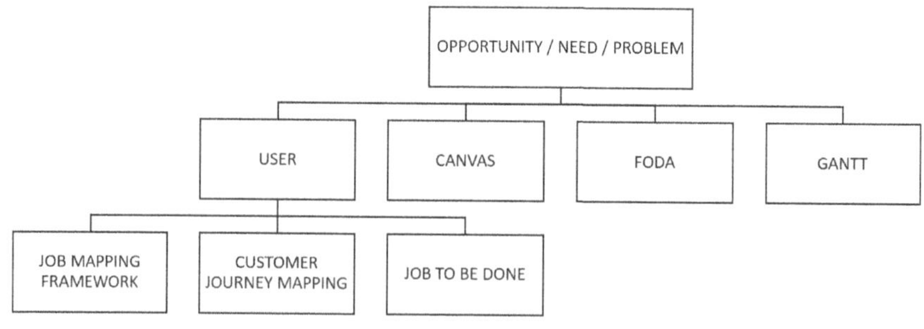

FIGURE 5.3 Interaction of tools to get the user and project requirements.

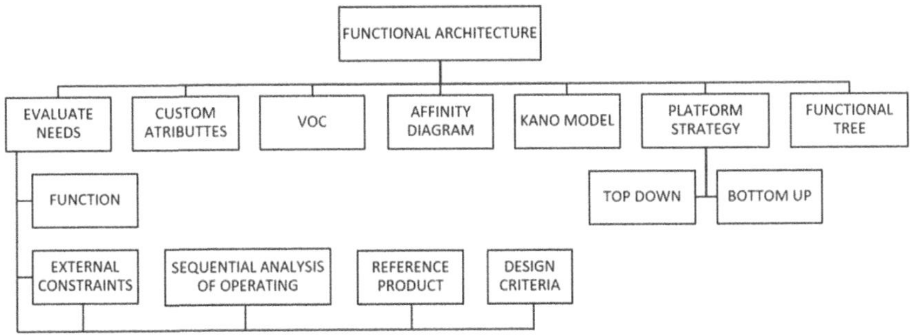

FIGURE 5.4   Interaction of topics to planning the functional architecture.

evaluation of needs includes the function of an exoskeleton, which refers to the operating modes and security aspects. The external constraints refer to the conditions of use, anthropometric aspects, and accessories. The sequential analysis of operating indicates the diagrams of moving parts in the motion phases and the times for every function phase. The reference product is distinguished based on the market segment, which defines the competence and identifies the attributes of our product.

The custom attributes are the dimensional parameters and usability issues. The VOC corresponds to the responses by questionnaires realized to focal groups [7]. The affinity diagram is the list of custom preferences by market segment. The Kano model is an approach to prioritizing five types of requirements: performance, basic, excitement, indifferent, and reverse [8]. Platform strategy is the business strategy with multiple products based on a modular architecture; a platform is designed either top-down, from a platform to several products, or bottom-up, from a product by scaling to the platform [9].

A functional tree is a hierarchical structure; it considers FR and DP. FR is a function with a required level of performance. Usually, the user requirements are continuously increasing and then the technical evolution occurs. When the FR is satisfied and it does not change, the increasing technical property becomes slow. DP is referred to as the design component (DC), which is the method to accomplish a given FR. Thus, DP is a certain parameter of a specific component. The function tree includes the following nine steps: extract functions from existing engineering systems, categorize functions (function module), change functions to function requirements, arrange the FR, expand the function tree, analyze function performance, select a scenario for the function tree, build a new function tree, and evaluate the new design [10].

5.5   DETERMINATION OF FR AND ASSESSMENT OF ITS DIFFICULTY

The QFD usually includes four houses of quality (HOQ), which concern the client, product design, process planning, and control [11]. In this chapter five HOQs are developed, namely HOQ1, HOQ2, HOQ3, HOQ4, and HOQ5.

Aspects		Symbol / Values
Relationships	Strong	● = 5
	Medium	○ = 3
	Weak	▽ = 1
Improvement direction	To maximize	▲
	Target	◇
	To minimize	▼
Priority		From 1 to 9 (9 = more priority)
Difficulty		From 1 to 9 (9 = more difficulty)

FIGURE 5.5   Aspects, symbols, and values of HOQ.

The QFD is a diagram comprising several sections and elements organized to visualize requirements and solutions compared to competitors. Figure 5.5 shows aspects, symbols, and/or values of HOQ. The aspects include relationships, improvement direction, priority, and difficulty. The relationship is divided into three categories: strong, medium, and weak. Improvement considers if it maximizes, targets, or minimizes the goal. The values are multiplied to calculate the technical importance rating (TIR).

The House of Quality 1 (HOQ1) is where the determination of FR is done from the VOC, which is a list of requirements. Figure 5.6 shows an example of HOQ1 designing an exoskeleton platform that includes two products. A list of eight items numbering the VOC includes its priority. The list from 1 to 3 is a group to product 1, the list from 6 to 8 is a group to product 2, and items 4 and 5 are requirements shared by both products.

Consequently, for instance, the lightweight requirement is solved by an FR of material property; then, five FRs solve eight requirements. Every FR is conditioned to improving the direction, being necessary to diminish any material property such as density to lighten the exoskeleton and reach the improvement target by essential parts, modular architecture, and force regulator. The most useful life is indicated with the improvement direction. Once the relationship between VOC and FR is analyzed, the TIR is obtained. According to the priority and relationship, the most TIR is a material property and the least is useful life. The target of function in the FR must be numerically expressed. This HOQ1 considers the difficulty (D), which is analyzed by the design team according to its installed capacity; so, the new priority (NP) is obtained by dividing the TIR between D; NP is an index that includes the difficulty value and helps to outline the design strategy.

HOQ1 does not show the competitive customer and technical assessments because benchmarking graphics would not allow an in-depth appreciation of these aspects.

The House of Quality 2 (HOQ2) assesses the FR difficulty. It could result in two ways: 1. where the greater difficulty level makes it necessary to feedback on the HOQ1 and 2. where the difficulty is solved with an action planned by the design team.

Improvement		▼	◇	◇	◇	▲	Customer competitive assessment
Priority	VOC \\ FR	Material property	Essential parts	Modular architecture	Force regulator	Useful life	
1	8	Lightweight	●	○	▽	○	▽	
2	9	1 million of units by year	▽	●	○	▽	▽	
3	5	Model for women	▽	▽	●	○	▽	
4	6	Adjustable force	▽	▽	▽	●	▽	
5	4	Engraving name	▽	▽	●	▽	▽	
6	7	Cheap magazine	●	▽	▽	▽	▽	
7	9	2 million of units by year	▽	●	○	○	▽	
8	8	Durable parts	●	▽	▽	▽	●	
		Target	70% of the components are made of polymeric material	DFA > 60%	C > 60%	Force from 20 and 40 N	Acceptable operating conditions > 12,000 cycles	
		Technical Importance Rating (TIR)	148	144	128	124	88	
		Difficulty (D)	9	6	4	8	5	
		New priority (NP)= TIR/D	16.4	24	32	15.5	16.4	
Technical competitive assessment								

FIGURE 5.6 HOQ1 to obtain FR from VOC.

The latter is the case presented in Figure 5.7. The NP has multiplied per relationship values. Infrastructure, training, technology transfer, collaboration agreement, and test bench are the actions to solve the difficulties analyzed by the design team. The importance of each column is the result of the sum of multiplications between NP and every action. In the target section, it is possible to observe in detail the action to do by the design team. The action is related to improvement direction, so the action is reading as more infrastructure, more training, technology transfer, collaboration agreement, and test bench.

5.6 DETERMINATION OF DPS USING AXIOMATIC DESIGN

Once the FRs and difficulty analysis are obtained, the DPs are attained from FRs; the axiomatic design is used. An axiom is a fundamental truth for which there are no counterexamples or exceptions and cannot be derived from other laws of nature or principles [12]. It is important to mention that the implementation of axiomatic design is done before the House of Quality 3 (HOQ3) because it is here where the DPs regarding FRs are proposed and refined.

The axiomatic design includes two axioms: the independence axiom and the information axiom. The independence axiom analyzes the effects in the relationships FR among DP. During the relationships, collateral effects appear which result in three types of design matrix. The first matrix is referred to as coupled design when the design matrix is completely filled with collateral effects. The second matrix is referred to as decoupled design when the design matrix is semi-filled with collateral effects. The third matrix is the ideal matrix, which is referred to as uncoupled design, meaning that the collateral effects are null or almost null and each DP accomplishes every FR. It should be noted that although the uncoupled design is ideal, most designs in a real environment reach the decoupled design after refining the design. Usually, the first DPs results in a coupled design and, once the design parameters are refined or replanned, the design matrix represents a decoupled or uncoupled design. In summary, the design of an exoskeleton in relation to its independence matrix is interpreted as the coupled design being a poor design and the decoupled design being the best design [13]. Figure 5.8 shows the kinds of design matrices according to collateral effects.

	NP	Improvement / Action / Difficulty	▲ Infrastructure	▲ Training	◇ Technology transfer	◇ Collaboration agreement	◇ Test bench
1	16.4	70% of the components are made of polymeric material	●	○	▽	▽	▽
2	24	DFA >60%	▽	●	▽	▽	▽
3	32	C >60%	▽	●	▽	○	▽
4	15.5	Force from 20 to 40 N	○	○	●	●	●
5	16.4	Acceptable operational conditions >12,000 cycles	▽	▽	●	▽	●
		Target	To instrument the dynamic laboratory	Specialists in sintering process	Agreement with patent owner	Agreement with factories and universities	Testing of components' lifetime
		Importance	200.9	392.1	231.9	230.3	231.9

FIGURE 5.7   HOQ2 to assess FR difficulty.

Coupled design

$$\begin{bmatrix} X & X & X & X & X \\ X & X & X & X & X \\ X & X & X & X & X \\ X & X & X & X & X \\ X & X & X & X & X \end{bmatrix}$$

Decoupled design

$$\begin{bmatrix} X & X & X & X & X \\ 0 & X & X & X & X \\ 0 & 0 & X & X & X \\ 0 & 0 & 0 & X & X \\ 0 & 0 & 0 & 0 & X \end{bmatrix}$$

Uncoupled design

$$\begin{bmatrix} X & 0 & 0 & 0 & 0 \\ 0 & X & 0 & 0 & 0 \\ 0 & 0 & X & 0 & 0 \\ 0 & 0 & 0 & X & 0 \\ 0 & 0 & 0 & 0 & X \end{bmatrix}$$

FIGURE 5.8   Types of design from the design matrix.

The FRs are taken to propose the corresponding DPs, which have been refined to reach an uncoupled design. Figure 5.9 shows the independence axiom equation and the relationships between FR and DP. As you can see, insert molding is related to components made of polymers and 10% more essential parts. DFA >60% is related to insert molding, 10% to more essential parts, and 15% to more common parts. C >60% is only related to the spring-elastomer mechanism. A force of 20–40 N is only related to the spring elastomer mechanism. Acceptable operation >12,000 cycles is related to the spring-elastomer mechanism.

The information axiom aims to minimize the information content of the design; this is recommended to simplify the design. Information content, I, is defined as the probability of satisfying a given FR, which is expressed in Equation 5.1 [13].

$$I = log_2 \frac{1}{P} = \frac{System\ range}{Common\ range} \tag{5.1}$$

where I is the information expressed in bits and P is the probability of success. The system range is the range of values of FR, DP, or PV according to the application of the information axiomatic equation; the common range is the common area (intersection) between the system range and the common range. The design range is the range of DP values that will satisfy the FR.

Among DPs that satisfy FR, the DP with the minimum information content has the highest probability of success; this axiom provides a quantitative way to reach the optimum from DP. Figure 5.10 shows the graph realized with the data obtained

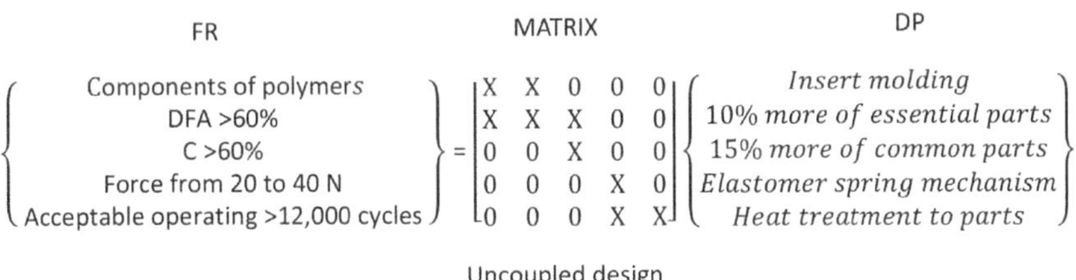

FIGURE 5.9   Design matrix of the independence axiom for an exoskeleton.

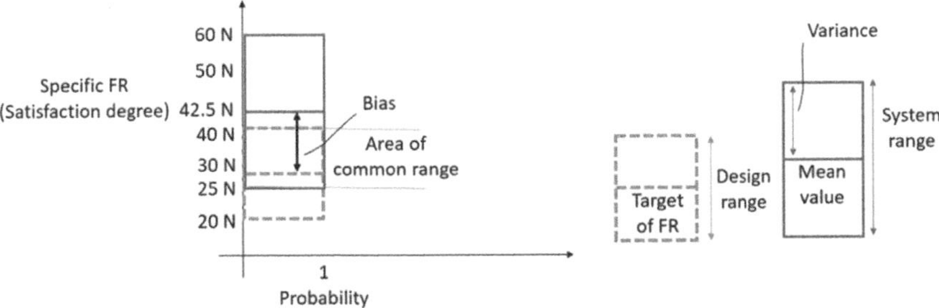

FIGURE 5.10   Graph of the information axiom for an exoskeleton.

from FR for exoskeleton design. The elements shown in the graph are the design range from 20 N to 40 N and the system range from 25 N to 60 N, which are the measures in competitive exoskeletons. Bias is a measure of the "exactitude" of the measurement and representation system to the systematic error of the system. It is the contribution to the total error due to the combined effects of all sources of variation, known or unknown [14]; bias, in this case, is the value among the target of FR (30 N) and the mean value of the system range (42.5 N). Using Equation 5.1, the information content is calculated as:

$$I = log_2 \frac{(60-25)}{(40-25)}$$

$$I = log_2 \frac{35}{15}$$

$$I = 1.222 \; bits$$

5.7 RELATIONSHIP OF DP TO FR

The HOQ3 is where the FRs are related to DPs, adjusting the priority after having analyzed the difficulty and refining the DPs using the axiomatic design.

The result of most importance is the mechanism and that of the minor importance is the insert molding. The insert molding is related to the use of polyamide in components of moving parts and encasements and the use of Makrolon in the magazine. In addition, the target design in the physical domain indicates 10% more essential parts, 15% more common parts, spring-elastomer mechanism, and hard chrome plating. The target DPs are the components necessary to solve the FRs.

The DPs are related to improvement direction. The DP is the solution to reach insert molding to at least 70% of exoskeleton components, 10% more essential parts, and 15% more common parts. In addition to reaching the mechanism with regulated force from 20 N to 40 N, applying a covering using heat treatment on components to improve the performance is desired. Figure 5.11 shows that the priority is multiplied per relationship values: relationship essential parts, common parts, mechanism, and cover.

5.8 RELATIONSHIP OF CRITICAL DESIGN PARAMETER (CDP) TO TEST BENCH FEATURE (TBF)

A critical design parameter is a requirement that must be driven with high accuracy and evaluated on its behavior repeatedly to verify the permanence of performance in an operating range. TBFs are conditions to satisfy each CDP, which are implemented in the instrumentation of the test bench, experimental protocol, and certification of the event. Figure 5.12 shows the analysis of relationships between CDPs and TBFs.

	Priority	FR \ DP	Insert molding	Essential parts	Common parts	Mechanism	Internal hole covering
		Improvement	◇	▲	▲	◇	◇
1	7	70% of components made of polymer	●	○	○	○	▽
2	6	DFA >60%	▽	●	○	○	▽
3	6	CI >60%	▽	○	●	○	▽
4	8	Force from 20 to 40 N	▽	▽	▽	●	▽
5	9	Acceptable operating conditions >12,000 cycles	▽	▽	▽	●	●
		Target	Insert molding using polyamide and Makrolon	10% more of essential parts	15% more of common parts	Spring-elastomer mechanism	Hard chrome plating of critical component
		Importance	64	86	86	142	72

FIGURE 5.11 HOQ3 of design parameters from functional requirements.

	Priority	CDP \ TBF	Devices to avoid deformation of plastic parts	Clinical test	Ultrahigh-speed sensors	Force verification	Data acquisition
		Improvement	▲	◇	◇	◇	◇
1	5	70% of components made of polymer material	●	○	▽	▽	▽
2	8	Prevent component fractures	▽	●	○	▽	○
3	9	Operating exoskeleton	▽	○	●	○	○
4	7	Force from 20 to 40 N	▽	○	▽	●	○
5	6	Acceptable operational conditions >12,000 cycles	▽	○	○	○	●
		Target	Interchangeability	Conditions of usability	Repeatability of operating sequence	Reliability range	Durability range
		Importance	55	121	99	93	107

FIGURE 5.12 HOQ4 of test bench features from critical design parameters.

The House of Quality 4 (HOQ4) related each CDP to every TBF, considering the priority of CDP defined by the design team. The priority is multiplied per relationship value. Devices to avoid the deformation of plastic parts guarantee the dimensional parameters to correct exoskeleton operating, allowing interchangeability among components and groups. Ultra-high-speed sensors and transparent covers allow verifying the operating of the exoskeleton, reaching the repeatability of the operating sequence. Pull-force verification satisfies a force from 20 N to 40 N, reaching the reliability range. Data acquisition satisfies the acceptable operating conditions >12,000 cycles, reaching the expected durability range.

The multiplication result is the importance of setting up the elements in the test bench or several test benches and planning a schedule to converge the times to testing with a test bench supplier or the same design team.

5.9 RELATIONSHIP OF PROCESS VARIABLE (PV) TO DP

PV is a process value or parameter measured in a particular part of the manufacturing or testing process in the development stage. This PV is monitored and controlled; for instance, the manufacturing is monitored and controlled to reach the desired tolerance [15].

In the House of Quality 5 (HOQ5), the PVs are established in a general way, which includes specific process variables according to each DP requirement. Figure 5.13 shows the analysis of relationships among DPs and PVs. The HOQ5 related each DP to every PV, considering the priority of DP defined by the design and manufacturing teams. The priority is multiplied per relationship value. The injection parameters to make the moving parts and covers of polyamide and magazine of Makrolon must be defined, specifying in the target the materials to satisfy the insert molding. Using the DFA algorithm to define the essential parts, the required 10% more is satisfied, reaching the classification in the BOM of the commercial and manufacturing parts.

	Priority	Improvement / PV \ DP	◇ Moving parts and covers	◇ Algorithm to essential parts	◇ Market segments	◇ Material to spring and elastomer	◇ Manufacturing process and heat treatment
1	9	Insert molding using polyamide and Makrolon	●	○	▽	▽	●
2	6	10% more of essential parts	▽	●	○	▽	○
3	4	15% more of common parts	▽	○	●	○	○
4	8	Spring-elastomer mechanism	●	▽	▽	●	●
5	5	High durability	▽	▽	▽	▽	●
		Target	Vestamid (PA 66) and Astamid, Makrolon (3107)	Commercial parts and manufacturing parts	2 product families, 3 products	Material to spring and elastomer	Process sheet to parts durability
		Importance	100	82	60	72	140

FIGURE 5.13 HOQ5 of process variables from design parameters.

Market segments satisfy the 15% more required for modular architecture according to the product platform. Material to spring and elastomer satisfy the mechanism to regulate the pull-force. The manufacturing process satisfies the hard chrome plating, reaching the durability required.

The multiplication result is the importance of setting up the PVs in the manufacturing process and planning a schedule to converge the times to manufacture the parts and acquire the commercial parts. The improvement of this HOQ5 has no direction because the PVs are aiming for a specific measure.

5.10 DETERMINATION OF INSTRUMENTS TO TECHNOLOGY TRANSFER

Technology transfer is the transmission of rights implemented by intellectual property and author rights or copyrights. As mentioned, the requirements for designing an exoskeleton are distinct depending on the design team's approach. For this, some designers focus on the design, starting with intellectual property. The intellectual property registers documents to certify the idea owner in the invention, design, and utility patents; names change according to the country. These patents are the instruments to carry out the technology transfer based on a strategy to reach expected revenues.

Figure 5.14 shows the analysis of relationships between technology transfer and patent valuation. In the House of Quality 6 (HOQ6), the patent valuation is established in a general way, which includes specific patents according to each requirement of

	Priority	Technology transfer / Patent valuation	Trademark	Invention patent	Design patent	Distributor	Manufacturing license
		Improvement	◇	◇	◇	▲	◇
1	6	Product portfolio	●	○	○	○	○
2	3	Operating principle	▽	●	▽	▽	○
3	7	Styling and customization	▽	▽	●	○	▽
4	8	Sell	○	○	○	●	▽
5	9	Manufacturing	○	○	○	▽	●
		Target	Platform and product family	Radical innovation	Incremental innovation	Exoskeleton license	Exoskeleton license
		Importance	91	91	107	91	87

FIGURE 5.14 HOQ6 to technology transfer of the exoskeleton.

technology transfer. HOQ6 is related to each patent valuation to every technology transfer, considering the priority of technology transfer defined by design, manufacturing, and commercial teams. The priority is multiplied per relationship value. Trademarks for model and product family satisfy the transferable product portfolio [16]. Invention patent by each design in the exoskeleton, utility, and invention allows transferring the operating principle and the requirements of styling and customization [17]. Distributor and manufacturing licensing allows the planning of business models and guiding design requirements for current and future product generations [17].

5.11   EXOSKELETON PROTOTYPING

In the literature, there is information on rapid prototyping for the manufacture of exoskeletons. This information requires certain clarifications since it is information of disclosure of manufacturing processes that lacks scientific rigor and details of implementation. Some methodologies show the immediate manufacture of prototypes until their perfection, making the exoskeleton development process more expensive.

Design and manufacturing are activities that must be balanced according to the infrastructure and technical capacity of the design team and manufacturing team. Suppose the designers do not have enough skill and knowledge. In that case, the manufacturing team is expected to compensate for this disadvantage with infrastructure and technical capacity to deduce design aspects and consider good manufacturing practices to achieve the design of the exoskeleton components, reaching the required tolerances and the principle of operation of the exoskeleton when assembled. Now suppose the manufacturing team does not have sufficient skills. In that case, the designers compensate for this disadvantage by performing more specialized computing work, from modeling, interference detection, tolerance analysis, motion, FEA, CFD, and MBD simulations until an acceptable correlation is achieved comparing the solutions of each solver.

As described in Chapters 3 and 4, models or dummies are used during CAD modeling, which are tangible physical models that assist in formulating the solution. In addition, during CAE simulation, experimental physical models (EPMs) are used to validate the operating principle. For these activities, which correspond from TRL1 to TRL3 and later to TRL4 as described in Section 5.12, a CAM assessment is carried out to determine the materials and manufacturing process of rapid prototypes: models, dummies, experimental physical models, and prototypes controlled in a laboratory setting. Then, rapid prototypes refer to tangible physical models that formulate the solution and validate the operating principle. The solution formulation and the operating principle are developed from TRL1 to TRL 4. They do not refer to a prototype as the first type to be replicated in a TRL5, TRL6, or TRL7. The former is used for experimental lots, and the last two are used in a real environment (Figure 5.3).

5.12   CAM ASSESSMENT

The manufacturing assessment is performed to obtain the rapid prototypes required in low-volume and high-volume manufacturing [18]. The CAM assessment for low-volume manufacturing is performed based on the following considerations (Figure 5.15):

- Clamping devices include rapid holding systems and flexible positioning clamping [19].
- CAD drawings to be used as a template for laser cutting or dimensioning in optical comparators and approbation of rapid prototypes.
- Required parts to the experimental process.
- Difficulty degree, considering the quick modification and assembly conditions for solution formulation, as well as controllable error in critical tolerances and verification of mechanical properties for functional testing.
- Dimensional requirements according to styling process, interaction, simplification, and assembly.
- Manufacturing processes, where polymer and metal 3D printing, computer numerical control (CNC) machining, laser cutting, and rapid tooling are taken into account.

The CAM assessment for high-volume manufacturing is accomplished based on the following aspects (Figure 5.16):

- Accessories, which include clamping devices and gauges
- Process sheets to be used as a guide to fabrication and approbation of the product

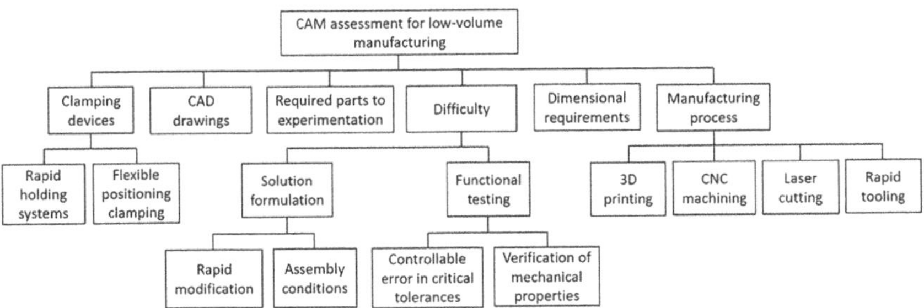

FIGURE 5.15   Consideration of CAM assessment for exoskeleton prototyping.

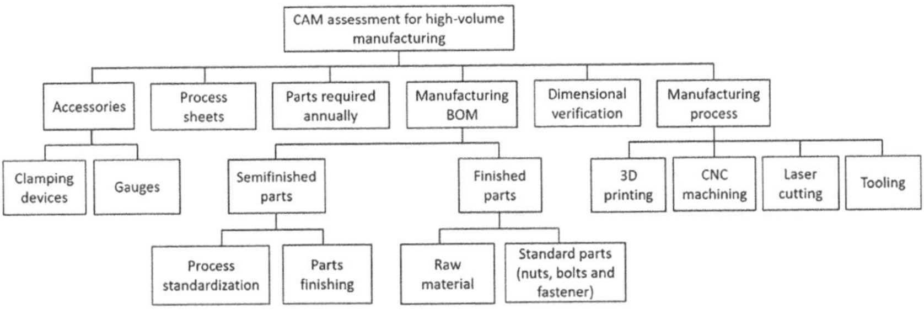

FIGURE 5.16   Consideration of CAM assessment for high-volume manufacturing.

- Parts are required annually at the beginning of the pilot lot and later for sale
- Manufacturing BOM, considering the process standardization and part finishing for semi-finished parts, as well as raw material and standard parts for finished parts
- Dimensional verification in each component and permissible gaps in assembly using scanning sensors (vision systems) on a coordinate measuring machine (CMM)
- The manufacturing process to high-volume manufacturing, considering polymer and metal 3D printing, CNC machining, laser cutting, and tooling

Figure 5.17 shows the workflow to manufacture a rapid prototype (RP) of an exoskeleton by CNC machining, laser cutting, or 3D printing, which considers the variation among each type of process used for this purpose. For the case of CNC machining, it is possible to obtain a model in an exclusive extension depending on CAD software: *.sldprt from SolidWorks or generic extension as Parasolid *.x_t. The CAD file is converted to *.step or *.iges formats, which are valid input data as CAM files and are opened in CAM software such as Mastercam, Edgecam, SURFCAM, or Cimatron, where the manufacturing parameters as toolpaths are analyzed [20]. In the case of CAM software, the CAM file is converted to a cutter location (CL) file or CL-data and later from the postprocessing phase to G-code, which includes the (axis movements) G-code and M-code (auxiliary code) [21]. The G-code, also known as ISO 6983, or with the most modern version as STEP-NC, is used by CNC machines, laser cutters, and 3D printers to operate [22]. Today, the drive control can operate up to ten axes driving the spindle to work RPs in composite, aluminum, and steel. The CNC control panel is the human-machine interface (HMI) for movement programming, backup, and file upload and download. The drive control operates the X, Y, Z, A, and B axes according to the number of CNC machine axes [23].

For the case of laser cutting, it is also possible to obtain a model in an exclusive extension depending on CAD software: *.sldprt from SolidWorks or generic extension as Parasolid *.x_t. Depending on vectorizing requirements, CorelDRAW with the *.cdr format can be used. The CAD file is converted to *.dxf format, which is

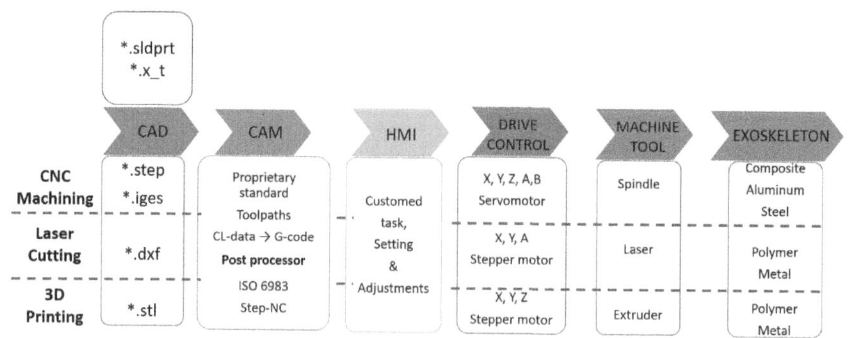

FIGURE 5.17 Scheme of workflow to get RPs.

valid input data as a CAM file and is opened in CAM software such as SmartCarve, DraftSight, or SketchUp, where the manufacturing parameters as toolpaths are analyzed. CAM software converts the CAM file to CL-data and, later, from the post-processing phase to G-code, including the G and M codes [24]. The HMI assists in uploading files, turning on the laser, and visualizing the cutting progress. The drive control operates the X and Y axes and the rotational movement A to move the laser during the cutting of an RP part in polymer or metal [23].

For the case of 3D printing, it is also possible to obtain a model in an exclusive extension depending on CAD software: *.sldprt from SolidWorks or generic extension as Parasolid *.x_t. The CAD file is converted to *.stl format and transferred to a 3D printer where Slicer software is used. The Slicer file is opened in Slicer software as Slic3r, Cura, Simplify3D, 3DXpert, or 3D Sprint, where the manufacturing parameters are analyzed and the slice errors are verified and corrected. The Slicer file is converted to CL-data in the Slicer software and later from the postprocessing phase to G-code [25]. The drive control operates X, Y, and Z axes in cartesian or delta types to position the extruder when printing an RP part in thermoplastic and metal materials.

5.13   CNC MACHINING

One of the ways to manufacture RPs is using CNC machinery, which includes milling, turning, grinding, drilling, router, and the machining center (MC). Numerical control (NC) is a system of movement programming on the HMI of the machine tool by an operator [26]. When this action is made through CAM software, it is called CNC, and when this action is carried out by means of a network to allow simultaneous upload and download instructions of multiple CNC machines, it is called direct numerical control (DNC) [27]. In the manufacture of exoskeletons, the evolution of the machinery began using the DNC; the creation of multi-operation machines (MMs) emerged later. An MM can perform up to 150 operations, from component machining to exoskeleton manufacturing. A disadvantage of MMs is that they are designed with an integral and custom design approach, making it difficult to repair, scale, and upgrade. Currently, this approach has changed to using a modular design approach. These modules work as MCs with multifunction programming, automatic tool changer, and tool storage. An MC comprises a control cabinet, tool magazine, head, HMI with programs backup, uninterruptible power supply (UPS), worktable, machine bed, servomotors to the axis, drives, and automatic tool changer [28]. The DC servomotors were used formerly in the MCs; today, the features of the MCs have changed to supply AC 3x400 V using, for instance, Siemens technology such as SINUMERIK 840D, conveyor, feeder, security network, and coolant system [29].

CNC machines are classified based on the following characteristics: motion control, point to point (PTP), and continuous path; control loops such as open and closed loops; power drives, such as hydraulic, electric, and pneumatic; and positioning, such as absolute and incremental [30]. The assessment of the process allows considering some techniques to optimize the RPs, such as reducing the machining time of the workpiece, dividing a small linear toolpath to curve or spline, and using perform blocks. Some advantages of this process are greater accuracy, repeatability, and obtaining complex part geometries [31].

CNC programming is classified into three types (Figure 5.18): the G-code (includes M-code) RS-274, Open Architecture Control (OAC), and STEP-NC, the most modern code [32]. G-code is classified into the following versions: Binary Cutter Language (BCL); Deutsches Institut für Normung (German Institute for Standardization—DIN) 66025; PN-73M-55256 and PN-93M-55251; International Organization for Standardization (ISO) 6983; Electronic Industries Alliance (EIA) RS274D and the version EIA RS274X, which is used for the fabrication of printed circuit boards (PCBs); and conversational programming, which is a wizard-like mode that hides G-code, for instance, the IPS from Haas, MAZATROL from Yamazaki Mazak Corporation, UltiMax from Hurco Companies, ProtoTRAK from Southwestern Industries, and CAPS from DMG Mori Seiki [33]. OAC is growing due to the tendency to create open-source machine designs. OAC is not as suitable for high-volume manufacturing due to a lack of compatibility, scalability, and technical support. However, OAC is an excellent option for RPs, as it is possible to use open source by combining rapid manufacturing processes to low cost and with sufficient characteristics for the fabrication and testing of exoskeletons. STEP-NC is classified into the following types: indirect, interpreted, and adaptive; the latter is organized into geometric adaptive and technological adaptive [32]. Adaptive control constraint and adaptive control optimization are control modes of the technological adaptive type.

STEP-NC-based exchange of product data in product lifecycle management (PLM) software helps in faster information processing and reduces errors owing to human intervention. A new format of STEP-NC, called STEP-NC AP238, was recently implemented and included geometric dimension and tolerance, as well as product data management (PDM) [34]. STEP-NC AP238 allows adaptive manufacturing with bidirectional information. These data include continuous feedback verifying the geometric dimensioning and tolerancing (GD&T), minimizing the errors, estimating process data, and converting to machine-specific code for the case of sending manufacturing data to CNC machines and 3D printers [34].

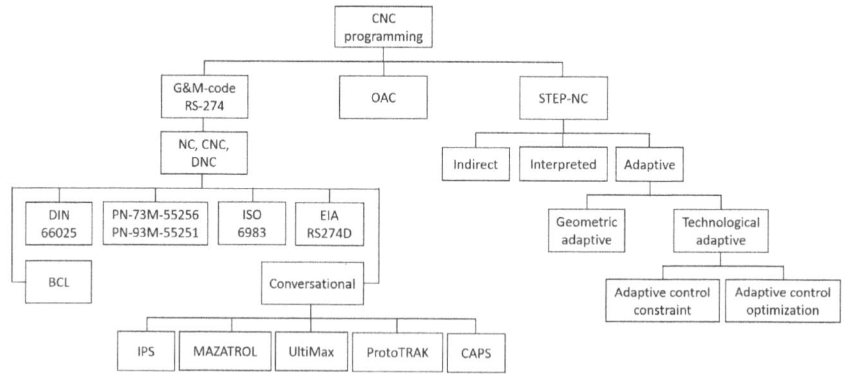

FIGURE 5.18 Types of CNC programming.

5.14 LASER CUTTING

Laser cutting is another beneficial manufacturing technology for exoskeleton RPs, especially for the evaluation of design concepts in mechanisms such as the firing mechanism and recoil system. Its versatility makes its applications very convenient since the time to obtain components is faster than in a 3D printer; in addition, tolerances of ± 0.03 mm for 10-mm thickness can be attained [35]. Also, considering the reduced dimensions of small exoskeleton components, laser cutting is better for getting RPs than water jet cutting and plasma cutting due to the average speed of 300 mm/s, cut finish, tolerance, and kerf thickness [36]. Figure 5.19 shows a schema of a component produced by laser cutting, where the features of the process are indicated. It is required to consider that the thicker the component to be cut, the larger the bevel angle, and it should be oversized in the critical dimension to fit it later, thereby removing the dross buildup and the kerf thickness.

There are several kinds of laser cutting machines, but the most used for exoskeleton RPs are CO_2 machines for cutting polymers and doped silica fiber machines for cutting metals [37]. For instance, depending on metal thickness, it can be used at 750 W with the fiber laser generator Raycus [38] or at 10 kW, considered the best quality of an IPG fiber laser [39].

Advances in adaptive manufacturing and the advantages of STEP-NC have improved the versatility and performance of laser cutting, thus compensating for errors and improving the characteristics of the obtained component. The stepper motors drive the movements of the laser tool in the X and Y axes and the A rotary axis within the workspace for both CO_2 and fiber machines [40].

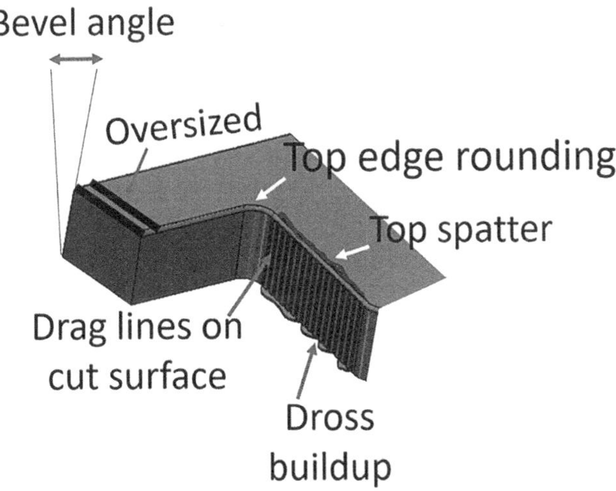

FIGURE 5.19 Exoskeleton component features manufactured by laser cutting.

5.15 3D PRINTING

It is common to refer to additive manufacturing as a synonym for 3D printing. However, it is important to highlight its appropriate use according to the capabilities of this manufacturing process for RPs. 3D printing is suitable for evaluating the design concept, solution formulations, and the principle of operation, but not suitable for patient testing. As mentioned before, important advances have been made in implementing adaptive manufacturing, which is why 3D printing has increased its uses and scope. The design of exoskeletons depends to a large extent on the speed of proofs-of-concept validation and principles of operation of their mechanisms. In this sense, 3D printing is fundamental, starting from the design concept tests with the manufacture of powders to verify appearance and with the fused deposition modeling (FDM) process to evaluate the interaction of mechanisms. These evaluations are compared with those carried out in the simulation, allowing the refinement of the design concept until meeting the design requirements. For instance, an exoskeleton design begins with the 3D printing by the stereolithography (SLA) process for evaluating its appearance and cosmetic aspects; later, the design concept is evaluated with an RP printed by FDM, considering a tolerance of ± 0.1 mm [19]. The evaluations of RPs, for instance, are focused on the interaction of the mechanism and bolt body. Once verified, the interaction is evaluated with refined FDM and metal inserts in the parts that operate as arm links. A transparent exoskeleton model is used to verify the mechanism's operation and acquire the testing data; Chapter 7 will focus on test bench experimentation.

As can be seen in Figure 5.20, 3D printing is classified as follows:

- Architecture is divided into polar and cartesian. The latter includes rectilinear, which can be H-bot, core XY or belt, delta, and Scara.

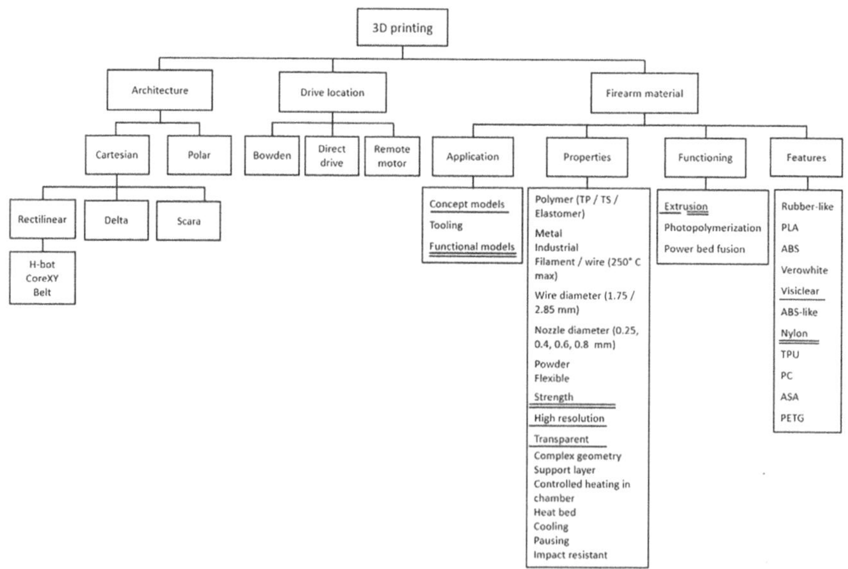

FIGURE 5.20 Considerations for 3D printing assessment.

- Drive location can be of three types: Bowden if a Bowden extruder is used, direct drive if the extruder and nozzle are in the same assembly, and small motor if the motor and extruder are separated from the nozzle [41].
- Exoskeleton material refers to the application, properties, functioning, and features of materials used for 3D printing. The application includes concept models, tooling, and functional models. Properties are classified into the polymer which can be thermoplastic (TP), thermosetting (TS) or elastomer, metal, industrial use, filament characteristics, nozzle, powder, flexible, strength, high resolution, transparent, complex geometry, support layer, controlled heating in the chamber, heat bed, cooling, pausing, and impact resistant [42]. Functioning is divided into extrusion, photopolymerization, and powder bed fusion. Features are classified into rubber-like, polylactic acid (PLA), acrylonitrile butadiene styrene (ABS), Verowhite, Visiclear, ABS-like, nylon, thermoplastic polyurethane elastomer (TPU), polycarbonate (PC), acrylic styrene acrylonitrile (ASA), and polyethylene terephthalate glycol (PETG) [43].

Different considerations to evaluate 3D printing can be taken into account. For instance, if the concept model is required with a transparent appearance and high resolution, the extrusion functioning and the Visiclear material should be selected; if the functional model is required with strength, the extrusion functioning and the nylon material should be selected. According to the material used for 3D printing, there are features that perform better with a specific material type; for instance, layer adhesion is better achieved with PLA, heat resistance with PC and ABS, impact resistance with TPU, visual quality with nylon, maximum strength with PC, and ease of printing with PLA. Although multicolor is attractive, the use of black and white is preferable for RP manufacturing [44]. Concerning the types of processes, FDM and selective laser sintering (SLS) are the most used. Further, it is important to consider acquiring a 3D machine for spare parts, support, maintenance, and standardization to obtain RPs [45].

5.16 PROTOTYPING WORKSHOP

The creation of exoskeleton RPs requires an area with suitable equipment for their efficient manufacture. A prototyping workshop for manufacturing exoskeleton RPs should at least contain the following (Figure 5.21):

- CNC machining includes CAM software, machine center, wire and sinker, electrical discharge machining (EDM), CNC spring coiling machine, and CNC grinder.
- 3D printing should comprise cartesian and delta printers and support cleaning apparatus, including soluble substances to remove the support.
- Laser cutting may consist of a fiber laser cutting machine, a CO_2 laser cutting machine, and laser cut part cleaning.
- Programmable logic controller (PLC) machines with programming software, devices to start up machines, and a design and integration area to create simple PLC machines based on input and output to movement coordination [46].

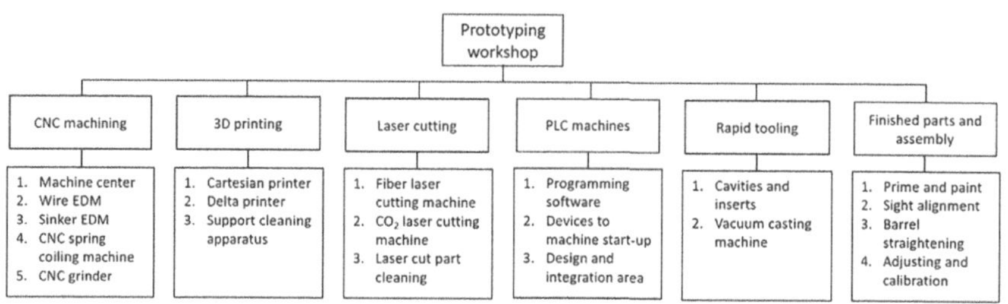

FIGURE 5.21 Prototyping workshop for exoskeleton RPs.

- Rapid tooling (RT) includes cavities and inserts and vacuum casting machines.
- Area of finished parts and assembly, provided with prime and paint, adjusting, and calibration.
- Further, the prototyping workshop must be provided with 440V three-phase electric power and pneumatic and water lines.

5.17 RAPID PROTOTYPING

Rapid prototyping is a group of techniques that allow fast and flexible manufacturing. Together with rapid tooling (RT), it is part of rapid manufacturing for low-volume manufacturing from TRL1 to TRL4 (Figure 3.5). Table 5.1 shows a comparison of RPs features to describe some advantages and disadvantages of generating exoskeleton RPs.

Rapid prototyping machines must possess versatile manufacturing, modularity, compatibility, and scalability to anticipate early obsolescence and underutilization. There are two types of RPs. One type is used to get concept design, solution formulation, and test the operation principle using an experimental physical model tested under controlled laboratory parameters. The other type of RP is used to define the high-volume manufacturing process. Other companies have developed adaptive machining processes using custom CNC machines that reduce operator intervention and machining errors.

5.18 RAPID TOOLING AND MANUFACTURING DEVICES

RT refers to mold cavities that are either directly or indirectly fabricated using rapid prototyping techniques. Figure 5.22 makes a classification of manufacturing devices and rapid tooling. When an RP is being validated, material properties, accuracy, cost, and lead time are determined to design production tools. Manufacturing devices are classified into gauges and clamping devices and elements. Gauges include several measuring instruments for different exoskeleton components [47]. The group of clamping devices and elements covers different clamps and accessories [19]. Rapid tooling includes direct and indirect tools. The former is tooling obtained by a manufacturing process, while the latter uses an RP pattern to model molding, casting,

TABLE 5.1

Comparison of RP Features

Item	Advantage	Disadvantage
1	Quick solution formulation, design concepts, and EPMs	Thermal shrinkage and warping of the model
2	Multiple iterations for optimization	Model size limitation due to the printer or laser cutter workspace
3	Systematic refinement	Postprocessing time and resources are required
4	Ideation traceability	Limited mechanical properties of raw material
5	Reduced time and cost	Problems due to part surface by layering
6	Fast detection of critical dimensions	Limited control of material variability
7	Customizing	High manufacturer dependence on raw materials, upgrades, and technical support

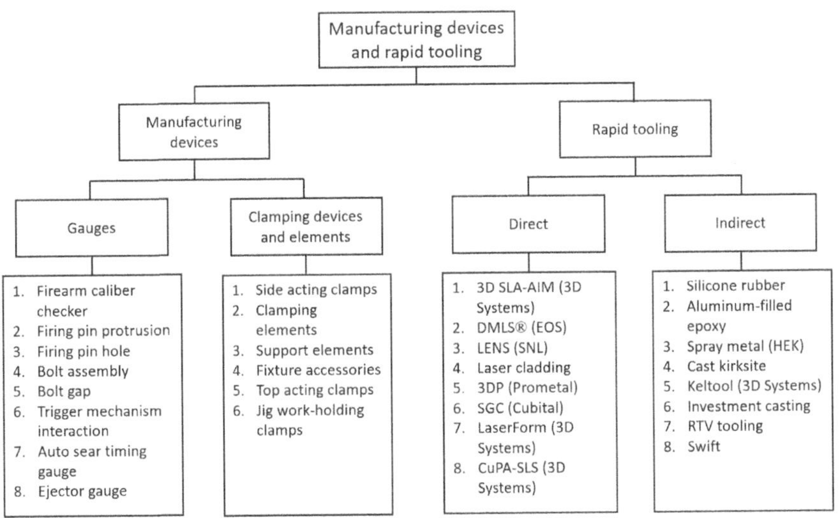

FIGURE 5.22 Manufacturing devices and rapid tooling for exoskeleton RPs.

and die-making [47]. Direct RTs are classified into 3D SLA-AIM (3D systems) [48], DMLS (EOS) [49], LENS (SNL) [50], laser cladding [51], 3DP (Prometal) [52], SGC (Cubital) [53], LaserForm (3D systems) [54], and CuPASLS (3D systems) [55]. Indirect RTs are divided into silicone rubber [56], aluminum-filled epoxy [57], spray metal (HEK) [58], cast Kirksite [59], Keltool (3D systems) [60], Investment casting [61], RTV tooling [62], and Swift [63].

5.19 INDUSTRY 4.0

As new technologies advance in the third Internet wave (IW), RP manufacturing evolves, adapting to the technological pace of Industry 4.0, which represents the fourth industrial revolution. Figure 5.23 shows the characteristics of Industry 4.0, which is considered to have started in 2006 and became broadly known in 2011 [64]. Industry 4.0 is focused on manufacturing digital transformation, Lean and Agile manufacturing, smart reconfigurable manufacturing machines, and adaptive manufacturing. The impact of Industry 4.0 is reflected in product fabrication from manufacturing technologies, supply chain monitoring, and PLM [65]. Likewise, digital twin (DT) technology is a significant characteristic of getting an RP. A digital model has manual data flow. The digital shadow occurs when there is automatic data flow from the physical exoskeleton model to the digital exoskeleton model [66]. A digital twin has automatic data flow from the physical exoskeleton model to the digital exoskeleton model and inversely [67]. A digital twin has the following features: connectivity; modularity homogenization; digital traces; reprogramming; simulation models forward with varying degrees of fidelity; updates continuously change in terms of the states, conditions, and contexts of the asset; and provides values through visualization, analysis, prediction, and optimization [68]. A digital twin receives real-time data from its real-world counterpart; therefore, a digital twin simulation is active, changing as the data is delivered [69].

Other characteristics of Industry 4.0 are related to the Industrial Internet of Things (IIoT) such as IIoT ecosystem, IIoT levels, IIoT hardware, and IIoT software [70]. The IIoT ecosystem includes sensors and devices, data processing, connectivity, and HMI. IIoT levels are classified into a device, resource, service controller, database, web service, analysis component, and application [71]. IIoT hardware includes the implementation of interfaces with the physical world, task execution, and microcontroller-run software that interprets inputs and control [72]. IIoT software is divided into execution functions, cybersecurity, services, communication, accesses, alarms, and data processing [73].

Based on the evolution of manufacturing technology, some authors pointed to the start of Industry 5.0 in 2020 [74]. Industry 5.0 focuses on the interaction of human

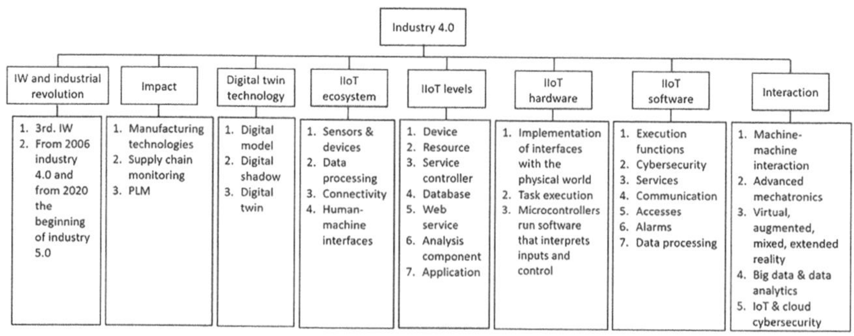

FIGURE 5.23 Characteristics of Industry 4.0.

intelligence and cognitive computing to improve machine-machine interaction in implementing advanced mechatronics technology [75]. This interaction is developed based on virtual, augmented, mixed, and extended reality, big data, and data analytics as machine and deep learning applied to manufacturing, the Internet of Things (IoT), and cloud cybersecurity [76].

5.20 CASE STUDY OF ERMIS EXOSKELETON

Many exoskeletons in scientific communications and patents only reach a technology readiness level corresponding to an experimental physical model or a low-fidelity prototype. While only operational in a laboratory environment, the increasing technology readiness level (TRL) in exoskeletons is not widely studied. For the rehabilitation process of a physical disability of the upper limb, an EPM of 7 degrees of freedom (DOF) was developed. This exoskeleton of the upper limb received the name "ERMIS" [77].

This section presents a study to reach this aim based on a methodology that includes two phases, 11 steps, and four case studies from EPM (TRL3) of ERMIS up to TRL 5 of ERMIS. The results show the increase in TRL based on the analysis of the operational parameters of the ERMIS exoskeleton. The passive rehabilitation movements were validated by characterizing the points of their trajectories assisted by an anthropomorphic mechanism used to measure the end-effector position of ERMIS by acquiring data and obtaining an error of 20 mm. The real performance parameters are detailed, explaining their causes according to the behavior of the exoskeleton in a real environment operating the four case studies. It presents the group of parameters that reach TRL 5 [78].

ERMIS development focuses on passive rehabilitation and faces specific challenges due to the patient's conditions, ensuring that the position of the arms is maintained and that the arms are within the ranges of each exercise, as well as exerting pull and push at the appropriate locations where therapists apply force during the exercises [78]. Figure 5.24 shows the CAD model of the proposed exoskeleton assembly and the ERMIS built and validated in a laboratory environment.

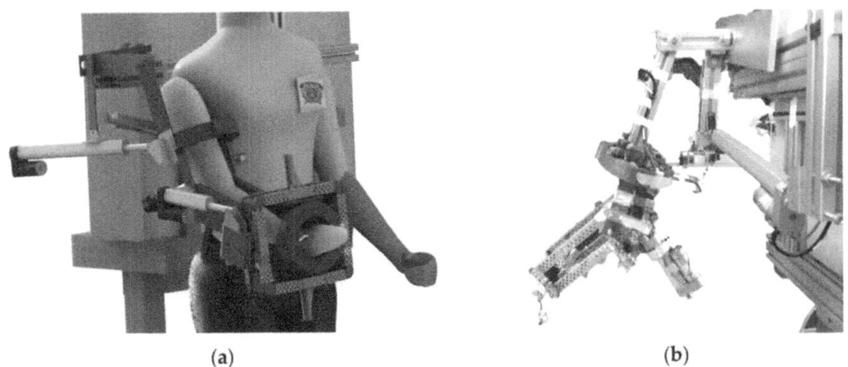

FIGURE 5.24   (a) CAD model of the ERMIS exoskeleton and (b) EPM of the ERMIS.

TABLE 5.2

Ranges of Motion of ERMIS Exoskeleton

Item	Movement	ROM (°)
1	Shoulder adduction-abduction	0 to 164
2	Shoulder flexion-extension	0 to 173
3	Internal and external shoulder rotation	−86 to 74
4	Elbow flexion-extension	0 to 140
5	Wrist flexion-extension	−53 to 74
6	Radial cubital deviation	−10 to 30
7	Pronation and supination	−80 to −90

The ERMIS exoskeleton as a rehabilitation tool presents an original configuration based on the requirements and limitations of four case studies of passive rehabilitation of the upper limb that can generate functional ranges of movement, which allow the patient to regain autonomy [79]. Their ranges of motion for each of the degrees of freedom are shown in Table 5.2.

In the design process of a medical product, its purpose, fields of application, associated risks, and user benefits must be clearly specified. The main objective of product development is to demonstrate the knowledge available or obtained by the different aspects of the project in prototypes, pilot plants, and models to validate their usefulness in satisfying a need.

It is necessary to know the level of technological development, which is understood as the application of research results, or any other type of scientific knowledge, for the manufacture of new materials or products, in the design of new processes or production systems, as well as in the provision of services [80].

TRLs are a type of measurement system used to assess the maturity level of a particular technology. The technological maturity of the designs is carried out with the improvement of the development phases of the devices, from the design concept, the experimental physical model, and, subsequently, the characteristics of the prototype concerning the maturity of the product proposed in the TRLs, are reached [81, 82]. Each development is evaluated according to the requirements of each technological level which is assigned a TRL rating [80].

5.20.1 METHODOLOGY TO INCREASE THE TRL IN EXOSKELETONS

The ergonomic aspect, the good mechanical strength of materials, and lower weight in the development of exoskeletons are fundamental topics in the design; however, such aspects should be reviewed in the experimental physical model stage. There are many challenges during the development of an upper extremity exoskeleton. From the mechanical point of view, the mobility of the mechanism is the most important part of improving its effectiveness [83].

Product development must go beyond the traditional steps of acquiring and implementing design technologies as a solution. It should focus on the end user's needs, including these requirements in the product design [77]. A methodology was developed and implemented to evaluate the mechanical design of the ERMIS exoskeleton. This methodology was divided into two phases. Phase 1 consisted of identifying the design needs, and phase 2 involved the design of a virtual, mathematical, and prototype model. It was composed of 11 steps [77], described next.

Testbench: A testbench is a platform for the experimentation of large development projects; this provides a rigorous, reliable, efficient, and repeatable form of testing [77]. It is possible to verify the performance and service life of the components, and it allows for the detection and elimination of weak points from the very beginning. Each time a new product is designed, it is necessary to verify that the actual performance meets the design specifications. For this purpose, test benches are built to analyze these products. The data derived from the test benches are conditioned, processed, dated, and recorded; using data processing techniques, these data are reprocessed and interpreted [77].

Identification of TRL3 operating parameters of ERMIS exoskeleton: Studies are conducted to establish the system attributes' product parameters, and they reflect important properties or capabilities, possible system states, and critical dimensions [84]. This step looks for the area of interest where there is an opportunity for improvement. This makes it vitally important to collect information such as identifying the operation; conducting a needs analysis, which provides support in the project strategy; basic assumptions; and limitations. Determination of design parameters: These are detailed statements, which are generally quantitative, of the expected operating values, environmental conditions in which the device must operate, space or weight limitations, or available materials and components that may be used [77].

Implementation of tasks: Once the tasks for the analysis are identified and defined, they are implemented through a precise, descriptive, and routine process that is adapted to the actual system conditions. This allows us to parameterize the requirements and processes designed in the previous phase, working with real data to be validated by the system. The proper implementation of tasks depends on the correct development of the process, which in turn conditions the results. These tasks allow the detection of errors, times, attributes, and physical aspects that will shape the product from the engineering point of view. Conceptual design: This is the design step in which the following activities are carried out: identification of needs and their expression; functional specification of the system; synthesis, analysis, and evaluation; and, finally, conceptual design.

System grouping: From the CAD conceptual model, it is possible to identify the groups that make up the system; it is important to ensure that these groups are independent in their functions to be able to work on the detailed engineering at the same time while seeking to reduce development time. The deliverable of this step is a structural diagram that identifies the assemblies, subassemblies, and parts through an identification code.

Detailed engineering: This phase takes the conceptual solutions of the different subsystems or work packages as a starting point and proceeds with the preliminary design and basic engineering of the product and manufacturing process. Parameters, processes, tolerances, and materials must be definitively established to generate mechanical analyses, simulations, CAD prototypes, and virtual and rapid prototypes. Unified architecture: The assemblies are integrated into a single CAD and migrated to specific software for the analysis of the system, where different analyses can be performed to learn its behavior. The objective of this migration is to generate the synthesis of the mathematical model. The parts are replaced with their equivalents in materials and technical design specifications that allow performance testing. The deliverable of this step is the virtual prototype with a technical design file. Emulation and simulation: Emulation is understood as the effect of performing tests with the experimental physical model of the different tasks defined in the conceptual design. The importance of an emulation system lies in being able to observe the system's behavior to subsequently make decisions, comparing the characteristics of the system [85].

A simulation is a form of design validation with an important role during research: targeting a product. With this, generating the product and performing the necessary iterations is possible. Simulation is performed using the CAD model, where it is possible to analyze the system according to the operating parameters [77]. The emulation and simulation of the system are validated by comparing the correlation of its results, taking the simulation results as ideal and the emulation results as real.

Prototype specifications: The prototype specifications are generated to allow the corresponding assembly of the parts and the functional testing. In the methodology, the steps establish the points where the analysis must be made and evaluated and the points where it is necessary to provide feedback to improve the system.

5.20.2 IMPLEMENTATION OF THE METHODOLOGY

Test bench: The test bench was selected for the experiment to provide a reliable, efficient, and repeatable way of testing the position of the ERMIS, which is an anthropomorphic mechanism [77]. This type of mechanism simulates an arm's movements, is fast, has great accessibility and maneuverability, and is a small device considering the work field it is used in. The anthropomorphic three-DOF mechanism for positioning rehabilitation devices is a structure with three rotational joints. The end-effector position is specified in angular coordinates or cartesian coordinates with a transformation of the data. The mechanism has a cardan joint as an end effector. This mechanical component allows the transmission of rotational movement between two non-collinear axes. The purpose of the cardan joints is to enable the links of the rehabilitation device and the anthropomorphic mechanism to rotate in regard to the links.

Mathematical model position: The representation of the position in the workspace of the ERMIS, by means of the anthropomorphic mechanism, is obtained through mathematical expressions from a mathematical model. The success of the model lies in the accuracy with which it can represent the object or phenomenon under study [86]. A mathematical model capable of describing the direct kinematics of the system is developed; this model is used for the location of points in the trajectories generated by the ERMIS movements. Through the analysis of direct kinematics, a set of kinematic equations helpful in calculating the position of the end-effector of the anthropomorphic mechanism, using specific values of the angles between the links, is obtained.

Critical points were taken from the different ERMIS trajectories to analyze their position in the working space. The movements were characterized using the trajectories generated with an anthropomorphic mechanism and contrasted with the ideal trajectory for each movement of the exoskeleton. The analysis in unloaded conditions covered different values of the absolute error at the selected point of its trajectories: 54.5 mm in the Y axis and as a maximum value for the external-internal rotation movement of the shoulder. The analysis under loading conditions covered different values of the absolute error at the selected point of its trajectories: 39.0 mm in the Z axis as the maximum value for the abduction-adduction movement of the shoulder. This error represented a variation according to the type of analysis and case, which could indicate different situations. This error was caused by working, component wear, construction without adequate materials, and system vibration. The error values were analyzed, obtaining a permissible error rate for each joint between 5 and 15 mm.

The trajectory point values on each axis were a guide to the repeatability and accuracy of the trajectory, which served as a guide for improving the ERMIS design. The error, repeatability, and accuracy values indicated whether the rehabilitation objectives could be met; the implementation of the tasks was set to be as complementary to the ERMIS analysis. This gave us the requirements and constraints from which the design improvement proposal was formulated. From this data, it was possible to estimate where the exoskeleton worked efficiently and the critical points where a greater error occurred. Keeping a permissible error requires paying special attention to the materials, shafts, bushings, and links [77]. So, the ERMIS exoskeleton can increase its TRL 3 to TRL 5, validating its performance according to TRL requirements defined in Figure 5.2.

5.21 CLOSING REMARKS AND PERSPECTIVES

The requirements are a group of conditions to guide the project, which depend on the approach of the design team and all teams involved, like manufacturing and commercial teams. The research, development, and deployment stages have the technology, manufacturing, and investment readiness requirements. The design methodologies like axiomatic design, QFD, TRL, MRL, and IRL help establish the requirements to reach the objectives in every phase and stage. The evolution of technology in the exoskeleton design impulses the creation of new ways to define the user requirements every time with more feedback, experimental physical models, and prototypes, and increase the proposals in the market.

Current markets demand the design of exoskeletons that include state-of-the-art technological levels to ensure efficient operation in the environment. Speed in establishing design requirements is critical and affects exoskeleton development times. Methodologies such as Lean design, Lean manufacturing, design thinking, and Agile design focus on the speed of design while maintaining quality and safety in the performance of each system.

The most used equipment for manufacturing prototypes is CNC machines and 3D printers, which have had various technological advances, from the range of printing materials and extrusion technologies to control systems. Today some parts are fabricated by 3D printing using the direct metal laser sintering (DMLS) process, whereas they were previously only obtained by subtractive manufacturing.

Currently, it is possible to have applications using 4D printing, also known as shape-morphing systems, which uses 3D deposition, but the material is deformable; this is perfect for printing assemblies that include parts within others, impossible to obtain by traditional methods. However, it is necessary to point out that with technology, there are also low-cost alternatives. In most cases, it is advisable to verify the benefits considering the spare parts and technical support. There are technology tools that are open source, such as Cura software, which is compatible with many low-cost 3D printing and control hardware that can be implemented in these printers, which means having modular and scalable systems.

Fiber-optic laser cutting technology is becoming a very useful tool for prototyping. Consolidated companies in manufacturing technologies have also focused on manufacturing modular systems with the appropriate capacity to manufacture rapid prototypes. In this way, companies such as DMG stand out for their small-size CNC machinery, from three to five axes; Chevalier, with its wire and penetration EDM machines; and 3D Systems and Stratasys with their Vantage and Fortus models, which include polycarbonate, ABS, and nylon fabrication.

Clay-based composites and aluminum are materials that allow rapid machining that can be easily adjusted according to necessary design changes based on the functioning of the exoskeleton components to be subsequently scanned, parameterized, and refined.

Evaluation activity. Please answer the next quiz.
https://forms.office.com/r/DKLZDAjdkq

1. How many levels of technological readiness exist?
   A. 7
   B. 8
   C. 9
   D. 10

2. Radical innovation is when users assimilate the technology quickly due to known operating paradigms. Incremental innovation has slower assimilation due to the change in operating paradigms.
   A. True
   B. False

3. Choose the types of requirements
   A. Business and system requirements
   B. User and design team requirements
   C. Improvements, lower costs, and optimization
   D. Materials, performance, and platforms

4. To which TRL does the released product and outlining new versions and scaling correspond?
   A. TRL 7
   B. TRL 8

   C. TRL 9
   D. TRL 10

5. What types of requirements does the Kano approach prioritize?
   A. Performance, basic, excitement, indifferent, and reverse
   B. Performance, complex, excitement, indifferent, and reverse
   C. Performance, basic, excitement, and indifferent
   D. Performance, excitement, indifferent, and reverse

6. What is the term for a diagram constituted by several sections and elements organized to visualize requirements and solutions compared to competitors?
   A. QFD
   B. FR
   C. DC
   D. TIR

7. In the axiomatic design, an axiom is a fundamental truth for which there are no counterexamples or exceptions.
   A. True
   B. False

8. What is a requirement that must be driven with high accuracy and evaluated on its repeatable behavior to verify the permanence of performance in an operating range?
   A. Technology transfer
   B. Process variable
   C. Critical design parameter
   D. Test bench feature

9. What is the transmission of rights implemented by the intellectual property and author rights or copyrights?
   A. Technology transfer
   B. Process variable
   C. Critical design parameter
   D. Test bench feature

10. Methodologies such as Lean design, Lean manufacturing, design thinking, and Agile design focus on the speed of design while maintaining quality and safety in the performance of each system.
   A. True
   B. False

REFERENCES

1. Lehtola, L., M. Kauppinen, and S. Kujala, Linking the business view to requirements engineering: Long-term product planning by roadmapping. In 13th IEEE International Conference on Requirements Engineering (RE'05). IEEE, 2005.
2. Fernandez, J.A., Contextual role of TRLs and MRLs in technology management. Sandia National Lab, California, SAND2010-7595, 2010.
3. Sauser, B., et al., From TRL to SRL: The concept of systems readiness levels. In Conference on Systems Engineering Research, Los Angeles, CA. 2006. Citeseer.

4. Bettencourt, L.A. and A.W. Ulwick, The customer-centered innovation map. Harvard Business Review, 2008.86(5): p. 109.

5. Marquez, J.J., A. Downey, and R. Clement, Walking a mile in the user's shoes: Customer journey mapping as a method to understanding the user experience. Internet Reference Services Quarterly, 2015.20(3–4): p. 135–150.

6. Christensen, C.M., et al., Finding the right job for your product. MIT Sloan Management Review, 2007.48(3): p. 38.

7. Christensen, C.M., The Innovator's Dilemma: The Revolutionary Book That Will Change the Way You Do Business. Harper Business Essentials, 2003.

8. Xu, Q., et al., An analytical Kano model for customer need analysis. Design Studies, 2009.30(1): p. 87–110.

9. Simpson, T.W., J.R. Maier, and F. Mistree, Product platform design: Method and application. Research in Engineering Design, 2001.13(1): p. 2–22.

10. Romli, F.I., A.S.M. Rafie, and S. Wiriadidjaja, Conceptual product design methodology through functional analysis. In Advanced Materials Research. Trans Tech Publications, 2014.

11. Moubachir, Y. and D. Bouami, A new approach for the transition between QFD phases. Procedia CIRP, 2015.26: p. 82–86.

12. Kulak, O., S. Cebi, and C. Kahraman, Applications of axiomatic design principles: A literature review. Expert Systems with Applications, 2010.37(9): p. 6705–6717.

13. Suh, N.P., Axiomatic design theory for systems. Research in Engineering Design, 1998.10(4): p. 189–209.

14. Helander, M.G. and L. Lin, Axiomatc design in ergonomics and an extension of the information axiom. Journal of Engineering Design, 2002.13(4): p. 321–339.

15. Hanumaiah, N., B. Ravi, and N. Mukherjee, Rapid hard tooling process selection using QFD-AHP methodology. Journal of Manufacturing Technology Management, 2006.17(3): p. 332–350.

16. Cooper, R.G., S.J. Edgett, and E.J. Kleinschmidt, New product portfolio management: Practices and performance. Journal of Product Innovation Management: An International Publication of The Product Development & Management Association, 1999.16(4): p. 333–351.

17. Liu, Y., et al., Integrating requirements analysis and design around strategy for designing around patents. In 2011 IEEE 2nd International Conference on Computing, Control and Industrial Engineering. IEEE, 2011.

18. Abdulhameed, O., et al., Additive manufacturing: Challenges, trends, and applications. Advances in Mechanical Engineering, 2019.11(2): p. 1687814018822880.

19. Clamping devices and elements. October 31, 2021; Available from: https://unitygroup. co.in/clamping-devices-and-elements/.

20. Boboulos, M.A., CAD-CAM & Rapid Prototyping Application Evaluation. Ventus Publishing ApS, 2010.

21. Integrating Advanced Computer-Aided Design, Manufacturing, and Numerical Control: Principles and Implementations: Principles and Implementations. IGI Global, 2009.

22. Hatem, Noor, Y. Yusof, Aini Zuhra A. Kadir, and M.A. Mohammed, Reviewing of STEP-NC standards related to manufacturing industries. International Journal of Scientific & Technology Research, 2020.9(4): p. 6.

23. Understanding laser automation axis controls. October 31, 2021; Available from: www. controllaser.com/blog/2018/12/11/understanding-laser-automation-axis-controls/.

24. Autodesk, Fundamentals of CNC Machining: A Practical Guide for Beginners. Autodesk inc., United States of America, 2014. p. 256.

25. 3D Printing, in Thematic Research Reports, T.R. Technology, Editor. 2019, GlobalData. p. 57.

26. Zhang, Y., X. Xu, and Y. Liu, Numerical control machining simulation: A comprehensive survey. International Journal of Computer Integrated Manufacturing, 2011.24(7): p. 593–609.
27. Yudianto, Y., An overview of direct or distributed Numerical Control in Computer Numerical Control Applications. Journal of Mechanical Science and Engineering, 2020.7(2): p. 025–029.
28. İç, Y.T. and M. Yurdakul, Development of a decision support system for machining center selection. Expert Systems with Applications, 2009.36(2): p. 3505–3513.
29. Control sinumerik. October 31, 2021; Available from: https://new.siemens.com/global/en/products/automation/systems/cnc-sinumerik/automation-systems/sinumerik-840.html.
30. Types of CNC machines. October 31, 2021; Available from: www.cnclathing.com/guide/classification-of-cnc-machine-system-what-are-the-types-of-cnc-machines-cnclathing.
31. Fitzpatrick, M., Machining and CNC technology. McGraw Hill Higher Education, 2013.
32. Latif, K., et al., A review of G code, STEP, STEP-NC, and open architecture control technologies based embedded CNC systems. The International Journal of Advanced Manufacturing Technology, 2021.114: p. 1–18.
33. Creation of G-code. October 31, 2021; Available from: www.ajpdsoft.com/modules.php?name=News&file=article&sid=664.
34. Rodriguez, E. and A. Alvares, A STEP-NC implementation approach for additive manufacturing. Procedia Manufacturing, 2019.38: p. 9–16.
35. How it Works 3D Printing with FDM. Stratasys. Israel, 2018. p. 7.
36. Types of FDM 3D Printers. October 31, 2021; Available from: https://all3dp.com/2/cartesian-3d-printer-delta-scara-belt-corexy-polar/.
37. Ligon, S.C., et al., Polymers for 3D printing and customized additive manufacturing. Chemical Reviews, 2017.117(15): p. 10212–10290.
38. How to choose the right 3D printing materials. October 31, 2021; Available from: www.emergingedtech.com/2021/02/how-to-choose-right-3d-printing-materials-for-classroom/.
39. What materials can be 3D printed. October 31, 2021; Available from: https://blogmech.com/flexible-3d-printing-materials-material-strength/.
40. Ismail, K.I., T.C. Yap, and R. Ahmed, 3D-printed fiber-reinforced polymer composites by fused deposition modelling (FDM): Fiber length and fiber implementation techniques. Polymers, 2022.14(4659): p. 1–36.
41. McGetrick, P.J., et al., Experimental testing and analysis of the axial behaviour of intermeshed steel connections. Proceedings of the Institution of Civil Engineers-Structures and Buildings, 2020: p. 1–21.
42. Olivero, M., et al., Measurement techniques for the evaluation of photodarkening in fibers for high-power lasers. Proceedings SPIE 7914, Fiber Lasers VIII: Technology, Systems, and Applications. 79142U 2011. International Society for Optics and Photonics.
43. Raycus laser. October 31, 2021; Available from: https://en.raycuslaser.com/.
44. IPG photonics. October 31, 2021; Available from: www.ipgphotonics.com/en/products/lasers/high-power-cw-fiber-lasers/1-micron-1/yls-sm-1-10-kw.
45. Dobelis, J. and V. Beresnevich, Fundamental precision dependencies of a CNC laser cutter. Transport & Engineering, 2015.36.
46. Simatic technology. October 31, 2021; Available from: https://new.siemens.com/global/en/products/automation/systems/industrial/simatic-technology.html.
47. Equbal, A., A.K. Sood, and M. Shamim, Rapid tooling: A major shift in tooling practice. Manufacturing and Industrial Engineering, 2015.14(3–4).
48. Stereolithography. October 31, 2021; Available from: www.3dsystems.com/stereolithography.

49. 3D printing metal. October 31, 2021; Available from: www.eos.info/en/additive-manu facturing/3d-printing-metal.
50. Smith, M.F., Additive Manufacturing at Sandia. Sandia National Lab. (SNL-NM), Albuquerque, NM (United States), 2015.
51. Laser cladding. October 31, 2021; Available from: www.laserline.com/en-int/laser-cladding/.
52. 3D print. October 31, 2021; Available from: https://prometal3d.com/en/content/8-3d-print.
53. Solid ground curing. October 31, 2021; Available from: https://galraz.wixsite.com/il-am-industry/solid-ground-curing-sgc-by-cubital.
54. Laserform. October 31, 2021; Available from: www.3dsystems.com/materials/laser form-ni718.
55. Selective laser sintering. October 31, 2021; Available from: www.3dsystems.com/selective-laser-sintering.
56. Methods of rapid tooling worldwide. October 31, 2021; Available from: https://wohler-sassociates.com/Oct00MMT.htm.
57. Khushairi, M.T.M., et al., Effects of metal fillers on properties of epoxy for rapid tooling inserts. International Journal on Advanced Science, Engineering and Information Technology, 2017.7: p. 1155–1161.
58. Metal sprayed moulds. October 31, 2021; Available from: www.ronald-simmonds.de/tcchnologic/mctal-spraycd-moulds/.
59. Cast Kirksite re-emerges as RT approach for molding plastics. October 31, 2021; Available from: www.armstrongrm.com/pages/kirksitearticle.html.
60. 3D Keltool. October 31, 2021; Available from: www.3dsystems.ru/products/production-tooling/3dkeltool/products_3dkel_howitworks.asp.htm.
61. Nagahanumaiah, R.B. and N. Mukherjee, Tool path planning for investment casting of functional prototypes/production molds. In National Conference on Investment Casting, 2003.
62. Silicone rubber tooling technology. October 31, 2021; Available from: www.simtec-silicone.com/silicone-rubber-tooling-technology/.
63. Levy, G.N., R. Schindel, and J.-P. Kruth, Rapid manufacturing and rapid tooling with layer manufacturing (LM) technologies, state of the art and future perspectives. CIRP Annals, 2003.52(2): p. 589–609.
64. Industry 4.0 and the fourth industrial revolution explained. October 31, 2021; Available from: www.i-scoop.eu/industry-4-0/.
65. Finance, A., Industry 4.0 Challenges and solutions for the digital transformation and use of exponential technologies. Finance, Audit Tax Consulting Corporate: Zurich, Swiss, 2015: p. 1–12.
66. Boschert, S. and R. Rosen, Digital twin—the simulation aspect. In Mechatronic Futures. Springer, 2016. p. 59–74.
67. Fuller, A., et al., Digital twin: Enabling technologies, challenges and open research. IEEE Access, 2020.8: p. 108952–108971.
68. Understanding the digital twin. October 31, 2021; Available from: www.chemengonline.com/understanding-the-digital-twin/?printmode=1.
69. Digital twins: The doppelgänger approach to digital success. October 31, 2021; Available from: www.devopsonline.co.uk/digital-twins-the-doppelganger-approach-to-digital-success/.
70. Usländer, T., et al., Smart factory web—A blueprint architecture for open marketplaces for industrial production. Applied Sciences, 2021.11(14): p. 1–28.
71. Smart sensors for industry 4.0. October 31, 2021; Available from: www.te.com/usa-en/industries/sensor-solutions/applications/iot-sensors/industry-4-0.html.
72. Industrial internet of things. October 31, 2021; Available from: https://internetofthing-sagenda.techtarget.com/definition/Industrial-Internet-of-Things-IIoT.
73. Dhirani, L.L., E. Armstrong, and T. Newe, Industrial IoT, Cyber threats, and standards landscape: Evaluation and roadmap. Sensors, 2021.21(11): p. 3901.

74. Di Nardo, M. and H. Yu, Special Issue "Industry 5.0: The Prelude to the Sixth Industrial Revolution". Multidisciplinary Digital Publishing Institute, 2021.
75. George, A.S. and A.H. George, Industrial revolution 5.0: The transformation of the modern manufacturing process to enable man and machine to work hand in hand. Journal of Seybold Report ISSN NO, 2020.1533: p. 9211.
76. Maddikunta, P.K.R., et al., Industry 5.0: A survey on enabling technologies and potential applications. Journal of Industrial Information Integration, 2021: p. 100257.
77. Cruz Martínez, G.M., Generation of trajectories of an exoskeleton for rehabilitation of upper limbs (in spanish). In Faculty of Engineering. UAEMex, 2018. p. 101.
78. Medina-Valdes, J.L., et al., Study to increase the TRL of exoskeleton ERMIS based on a methodology to the identification of real performance parameters. Applied Sciences, 2021.11(19): p. 9245.
79. Cruz-Martínez, G., et al., Diseño de exoesqueleto con base en cuatro casos de estudio de rehabilitación de miembro superior. Revista mexicana de ingeniería biomédica, 2018.39(1): p. 81–94.
80. NASA. Technology readiness level. January 31, 2023; Available from: www.nasa.gov/directorates/heo/scan/engineering/.
81. Behdinan, K., M. Fahimian, and R. Pop-Iliev, A tool for systematically accessing the level of readiness of engineering design in product development. Proceedings of the Canadian Engineering Education Association (CEEA), 2017.
82. Olechowski, A., S.D. Eppinger, and N. Joglekar, Technology readiness levels at 40: A study of state-of-the-art use, challenges, and opportunities. In 2015 Portland International Conference on Management of Engineering and Technology (PICMET). IEEE, 2015.
83. Majidi Fard Vatan, H., et al., A review: A comprehensive review of soft and rigid wearable rehabilitation and assistive devices with a focus on the shoulder joint. Journal of Intelligent & Robotic Systems, 2021.102: p. 1–24.
84. Han, X., et al., Identification of key design characteristics for complex product adaptive design. The International Journal of Advanced Manufacturing Technology, 2018.95: p. 1215–1231.
85. Gregor, M., et al., Design of a system for verification of automatic guided vehicle routes using computer emulation. Applied Sciences, 2022.12(7): p. 1–25.
86. Grinchenkov, D., V. Mokhov, and I. Spiridonova, Object-oriented approach to design of the complex mechanical system dynamics mathematical models. Procedia Engineering, 2015.129: p. 356–361.

6 Standards

6.1 INTRODUCTION

The design process follows guidelines, rules, and guides that allow it to ensure good practices in the design, development, and manufacturing of medical devices, including exoskeletons in any of their types and applications. The scientific rigor and the formalization of solutions that make it possible to offer high-quality exoskeletons to the market are supported by standardization systems. This chapter focuses on the standards that allow entities to regulate health risks, such as the Food and Drug Administration (FDA) in the case of the USA, and the Federal Commission for the Protection against Sanitary Risk (COFEPRIS) in the case of Mexico. ISO standards for user-centered design and risk management are also presented. Regulatory entities allow the evaluation of good manufacturing and quality practices, among others, issuing verification certificates through certifying bodies, accreditation entities, and techno-vigilance units. This chapter covers the rules for user-centered design, risk management, and standardization bodies.

6.2 NORMATIVITY

When the regulatory bases required for the evaluation of medical devices are established, the classification of the device is carried out, which determines the type of device, functionality, nomenclature, and level of risk that may occur for the patient, taking into account that the level of risk will generally be presented by the manufacturer based on a previously conducted risk analysis for their product [1].

Medical devices are classified as follows: Class I, which are those inputs known in medical practice and whose safety and efficacy have been proven and, generally, are not introduced into the body; Class II, which are those inputs known in medical practice and that may have variations in the material with which they are made or in their concentration and, generally, are introduced into the body for less than 30 days; and Class III, which are those inputs recently accepted into medical practice or that are introduced into the body and remain in it for more than 30 days [2].

Another classification is based on the function and purpose of use of the medical device, highlighting six large groups [2]: medical equipment; prosthesis, orthosis, and functional aids (**exoskeletons**); diagnostic agents; supplies for dental use; surgical and healing materials; and hygienic products.

The FDA has developed a regulatory cycle model that follows the device lifecycle in parallel to facilitate the process of design, commercialization, and use of the devices and at the same time allow the surveillance and traceability of the products and intervene if incidents with the devices occur and are reported.

DOI: 10.1201/9781003261995-6

The FDA places special importance on the design phase, as the quality, safety, and effectiveness of a device are validated during this phase. Design controls are required, some of the main requirements of the regulation are to establish written procedures for design control; perform design review, verification, and validation; and document the entire device design process in the design history file [1]. The idea or concept of the product is specified in the design and construction of an experimental physical model. In the experimental stage, and through laboratory tests and preclinical tests, its operation and the effectiveness of the function for which it was designed are verified. This part of the process includes compliance with security, quality, and connectivity or interoperability standards. Through testing and design adjustment of the prototype, the feasibility of the product is determined in its clinical and economic parts. The technical specifications of the product are established, the algorithms are validated in the computer programs, and the need for accessories or consumable parts is defined. The physical characteristics of the materials used for the construction of the device are specified [3].

During the manufacturing process, norms and standards must be applied and metrology measures must be carried out to guarantee the safety, quality, and conformity of the products with the respective norms. One of the critical aspects during production is the verification of compliance with standards, both for manufacturing processes and for final products [2]. Some of these rules are NOM-240-SSA1-2012, NOM-137, NOM-241-SSA1-2012, ISO-14971, IEC-60601, IEC-62353, IEC-80001, and ISO-13485.

NOM-240-SSA1-2012: Installation and operation of Technovigilance. NOM-137 has to do with the labeling of medical devices and establishes the minimum requirements, which serve to communicate the information to users, which must contain the labeling of medical devices (exoskeletons). NOM-241-SSA1-2012: Good manufacturing practices for medical devices has to do with establishing the requirements that the processes must meet (from design, development, production, assembly, handling, analysis, control, storage, and distribution) and has to ensure that they meet the quality and functionality requirements to be used by the final consumer or patient. The ISO-14971: standard for risk management in medical devices is designed to determine the safety of a product throughout the product lifecycle (design and manufacturing). The IEC-60601 outlines safety requirements for electrical systems. The IEC-62353 outlines recurrent tests after the repair of medical equipment. The IEC-80001 deals with risk management for information system networks incorporating medical devices. ISO-13485 specifies the requirements of a quality management system in the medical device industry. It is intended for use by organizations for design and development, production, installation, service, and sales. Among the important points mentioned in the standard are [4]:

- In design and development planning, the organization must maintain and update documentation such as design and development processes. In addition, design and development planning must be documented. This includes methods to ensure the traceability of design and development outputs concerning design and development inputs and the resources that were required.

- Design and development verification and validation; these clauses include requirements to document the verification and validation plan, methods, acceptance or rejection criteria, justification of sample sizes, and the risks associated with those sample sizes, along with verification and validation of the device interface.
- Design and development transfer focuses on transfer plans concerning suppliers, which includes manufacturing and its environments, personnel, and equipment installation.
- Design and development change control will control changes in the design and development of the established processes. The process shall include the means to determine the significance of the changes to the operation, performance, and safety of the product and the applicability of the regulatory requirements to the intended use and what actions should be taken.
- Design and development records require that all design and development records be maintained and correctly identified (processes, product type, manufacturing, etc.) for each device or family of devices.

The safety of medical devices concerning the patient is of vital importance by the health jurisdiction of different countries. For the design of robotic devices for rehabilitation, standards and certifications are applied according to the case.

Several legislations require the establishment of specifications so that the use of the device is intended and risks have been identified for their minimization. This process must also be iterative. Clearly, this has design implications since new requirements will be added not only in the initial phase of analysis but in subsequent iterations.

The study of usability and ergonomics in the design of a product is also known as human factors. The FDA has several documents that specifically deal with the study of human factors for such devices [5].

There is a wide range of standards that are prepared for specific devices and others of a more general nature that must be considered in the design and testing of products. In addition to global standardization organizations, there are another series of organizations that develop standards and protocols that apply to medical devices or their connection to information systems, such as the Institute of Electrical and Electronics Engineers (IEEE) and the Association for the Advancement of Medical Instrumentation (AAMI), among others.

An existing international standard, ISO 13482:2014, Robots and robotic devices—Safety requirements for personal care robots, addresses safety requirements for personal care robots, some of which may be considered exoskeletons. While exoskeletons have the potential to improve certain human abilities and protect worker safety, their use may also introduce new hazards. The potential risks of using exoskeletons include friction and injury from direct contact between the exoskeleton and the user, joint hyperextension, unintended contact, collision, vibration exposure, overexertion, and worker instability. Exoskeletons may also apply uncomfortable pressure on the body or be too heavy for workers to wear comfortably.

Some exoskeletons redistribute forces to other parts of the body so workers can hold a posture longer. It is important to make sure that the force redistribution does not cause new health hazards to other parts of the body. Exoskeletons can be considered a type of personal protective equipment (PPE). As with all PPEs, exoskeletons should not be the only control measure considered. Following the hierarchy of controls, PPEs should only be used when other controls such as elimination, substitution, engineering controls, and administrative controls are not possible or to supplement the protection of other control measures [6].

6.2.1 ASTM F48 COMMITTEE

The F48 committee of the American Society for Testing and Materials (ASTM) International was formed in 2017 [7]. It is currently working on the proposed exoskeleton and exosuit standard, WK68719. The WK68719 provides a test methodology for exoskeleton researchers and intermediate parties to conduct a cognitive analysis on the use of an exoskeleton, including the user's intent to abandon or use the exoskeleton for work in the future as well as the exoskeleton's cognitive fit with the user [8]. Six subcommittees have about 150 members, including startups, government agencies, and enterprises such as Boeing and BMW [9]. By providing a common and consistent lexicon, the purpose of this terminology is to facilitate communication between individuals who may be involved in the research, design, deployment, and use of exoskeletons and exosuits in applications, including but not limited to industrial, military, emergency response, recreational, and medical areas [10].

ASTM International published its first two standards documents, which are intended to provide consensus terminology (F3323) and set forth basic labeling and other informational requirements (F3358) [9]. In the early 2000s, the U.S. Defense Advanced Research Projects Agency (DARPA) began the development and demonstration of "critical technologies such as power, control, and actuation that will lead to a self-powered external structure to enable a Soldier to carry over 100 pounds of additional weight effortlessly" [DARPA, 2006]. The results of these efforts were transitioned to the U.S. Army Natick Soldier Research, Development, and Engineering Center (NSRDEC) in 2007. In 2014, NSRDEC invited representatives from the National Institute of Standards and Technology (NIST) to participate in an Augmentation Round Table to discuss the challenges and future directions of this technology. In 2015, the National Institute for Occupational Safety and Health (NIOSH) contacted Department of Defense (DOD) agencies after receiving a series of inquiries from industry stakeholders and product developers about the capabilities and efficacy of the technologies in industrial/occupational applications. These common interests and discussions led to the formation of an ad-hoc workgroup among these, and several other, U.S. federal and DOD agencies with interests in standards and/or best practices for the use of wearable human augmentation technologies (exoskeletons) [11].

In 2016, NIST hosted a preliminary meeting of the federal (Department of Energy, Department of Homeland Security, FDA, NIOSH, Occupational Safety and Health Administration), and DOD (U.S. Army Research Lab, U.S. Army Research Institute of Environmental Medicine, U.S. Army Clinical and Rehabilitative Medicine Research Program, U.S. Army Communications-Electronics Command, U.S. Special Operations Command, U.S. Navy, U.S. Air Force) agencies to discuss the current state of standards within the exoskeleton and wearable robotics space and to identify gaps in standards for safety, performance, interoperability, ergonomics, and cybersecurity. In follow-up, an open public technical interchange meeting was held in 2017, which was broadly inclusive of stakeholders across the military, medical, and industrial spaces and the academic community. Meeting objectives were to 1. identify opportunities to transfer knowledge and technologies from medical and military applications to industrial applications; 2. identify the key framework elements for a body of knowledge and a community of practice on human-wearable augmentation devices; 3. identify federal agencies and their respective interests, initiatives, projects, and deployments of human-wearable augmentation devices for industrial applications; and 4. discuss terminology and standards needs among industrial end users, government industrial program leaders, insurance representatives, and the testing and standards community. A key outcome of this meeting was a vote to move forward with ASTM International as the standards development organization for exoskeletons [7].

F48 now broadly addresses active, passive, and quasi-active/passive exoskeletons and classifies their general use cases according to the following: medical: amputee, injured, and/or physically disabled patients wearing exoskeletons can experience increased mobility and stability and enhanced physical therapy; industrial: employees working in logistics, warehouse, and factory settings could utilize exoskeletons for overhead, load carrying, tool-use, mobility, and squatting activities, allowing them to have higher performance for a longer duration with less impact on the body, while also decreasing the risk of injury; military: soldiers may benefit through the use of exoskeletons that can allow them to march farther with less fatigue, move logistical loads more easily and safely, and carry more supplies or weaponry which may otherwise prove too heavy or burdensome on the body; public safety: first responders may benefit from exoskeletons that can allow them to move larger objects when searching for victims within collapsed structures and to carry more equipment such as extra air bottles for firefighters and heavy bomb suits for explosive ordinance disposal technicians; and consumer/recreational: consumers may benefit from exoskeletons for personal use, recreational sports, home and yard work, and other physically demanding tasks [11].

The first official F48 meeting was held in February 2018 when subcommittee scopes were approved. As of August 2018, 18 task groups have been proposed within the subcommittees to draft specific standards, with a terminology standard that has passed the ballot as ASTM F3233, and further terminology and product labeling work items are currently in pre-ballot form.

Design and Manufacturing (F48.01)—The F48.01 subcommittee is focused on exoskeleton design, validation, and manufacturing and is specifically targeting standardization of structural function, such as mechanical and electrical components, embedded components, energy systems, cooling and fluid power systems, software, and user experiences. In addition, F48.01 is working to provide guidelines on active and passive systems and to define system needs, especially for energy storage and transportation.

Human Factors and Ergonomics (F48.02)—Based on the disciplines of human factors, ergonomics, and safety, the F48.02 subcommittee is focused on user-centered design and the selection of exoskeletons. More specifically, this subcommittee is working to develop physical-activity-based and anthropometric-based standards (excluding strength and mobility) for applications relevant to users from the consumer, industrial, medical, military, and emergency management sectors, while incorporating key human factors and ergonomic aspects such as 1. design for population accommodation, 2. assessment of system usability, 3. assessment of system ergonomics, 4. assessment of system safety, and 5. assessment of system training. This subcommittee is also considering anthropometric variables.

Task Performance and Environmental Considerations (F48.03)—The F48.03 subcommittee is targeting task performance and environmental considerations for consumers, public safety personnel, industrial/occupational users, and military personnel. This subcommittee is also working to generate a guide that maps applications to tasks, to provide a baseline on how the standards should be implemented. In addition, F48.03 is using F3218-17 (ASTM F3218-17, Standard Practice for Recording Environmental Effects for Utilization with A-UGV Test Methods) to understand possible analogous applications in recording and analyzing the effects of the environmental factors, particularly during exoskeleton utilization and testing.

Maintenance and Disposal (F48.04)—The F48.04 subcommittee is currently working to develop standards that consider the decontamination and/or disposal of exoskeleton systems following exposures in radioactive and chemical environments, as well as maintenance guidelines and general disposal procedures, including, exoskeleton system consumables and components.

The F48.05 subcommittee is presently involved in formulating guidelines for the implementation of security and privacy measures to safeguard the data related to the exoskeleton system, along with devising suitable techniques for testing the protocols.

On the other hand, the F48.91 subcommittee is responsible for maintaining the F48 terminology standards and is collaborating with representatives from all F48 subcommittees to develop coherent and comprehensible definitions and terms. This subcommittee also acts as an editorial support system for other subcommittees, assisting them in eliminating redundancies, reconciling variations, clarifying meanings, and standardizing definition formats.

The community of interests relevant to human augmentation, wearable robotics, and exoskeletons across medical, military, industrial, public safety, and consumer spaces is multidisciplinary and diverse. ASTM F48 has been establishing liaisons with relevant professional societies, technical committees, consortia, and stakeholder groups. Some of the key groups currently include the Human Factors and Ergonomics Society (HFES), Biomedical Engineering Society (BMES), IEEE Technical Committee on Wearable Robotics, American Society of Mechanical Engineers (ASME), ISO Technical Committee (TC) 299, Materials Handling Institute, NATO Committee HFM-266 (3D Scanning for Clothing Fit and Logistics), American Industrial Hygiene Association, International Society of Biomechanics, NextFlex Alliance on Flexible Hybrid Electronics (FHE), and European Cooperation in Science and Technology. There have also been interactions with newly forming specialized exoskeleton interest groups such as the North American AExG (Automotive Exoskeleton Group) and insurance providers focused on workers' compensation and return to work [11].

ASTM F3444/F3444M-20 is a standard practice for training exoskeleton users. This practice establishes the minimum training requirements, including general knowledge, skills, and abilities, for personnel who use an exoskeleton as part of their duties It is recognized that organizations and job responsibilities vary widely among military, medical, industrial, and emergency response communities. It is the responsibility of the user of this practice to identify the appropriate subject matter for its program and its specific needs. Users of this practice should consult with the exoskeleton manufacturer to ensure they have the latest and most relevant information on the exoskeleton. In addition, all training should comply with laws and regulations regarding user safety and health as well as the safety of individuals close to the user. The values stated in either SI units or inch-pound units are to be regarded separately as standard. The values stated in each system may not be exact equivalents; therefore, each system shall be used independently of the other. Combining values from the two systems may result in non-conformance with the standard [12].

6.2.2 ISO AND JAPANESE STANDARDS ASSOCIATION (JSA) STANDARDS

An existing international standard, the International Organization for Standardization (ISO) 13482:2014, addresses safety requirements for personal care robots, some of which are considered exoskeletons. Portions of ISO 13482 apply to a subset of exoskeletons, but much of the exoskeleton space is outside of the scope of ISO 13482. ISO 13482 does not apply to robots as medical devices nor to military or public force application robots, both of which were intended to be within the scope of ASTM F48. ISO 13482:2014 applies to wearable physical assistant robot exoskeletons that may be used in the workplace. These technologies may enable increased work capacity or reduce biomechanical loads and/or worker fatigue and overexertion risk, among other use cases. ISO 13482 recognizes that while physical assistant robots may augment certain human capabilities, their use introduces potential new hazards. Some of these hazards result from the fastening and direct contact of the robot device with the user, while other hazards are similar to those of robots operating in the environment. The ISO standard emphasizes the need for risk assessment and hazard identification analysis for the safe design and operation of these technologies. ISO Technical Committee (TC) 299 work groups are developing two test methods: 1. a skin stress test method for exoskeletons that looks at the possible maximum load on a user's skin using a simulation device and 2. a test method for visible fracture, deformation, disengagement of parts, and functional damage of a robot, including those worn by a person, for durability assessment [13]. A second existing standard, Japanese Standards Association (JSA)-Japanese Industrial Standards (JIS) B 8456-1, Personal Care Robots—Part 1: Physical Assistant Robots for Lumbar Support (in Japanese) "specifies performance requirements, safety requirements and indication requirements of wearable robots for lumbar support based on a consensus between manufacturers, consumers, and other neutral bodies" [14].

Exoskeletons have demonstrated the potential to improve individual well-being and quality of life. Examples in the medical space are lower extremity exoskeletons improving standing, walking, and sitting ability for some multiple sclerosis patients [15] and positive impact on the ability to walk [16], quality of life, cardiovascular endurance, and motor neurological status in spinal cord injury patients [17]. While the medical exoskeleton market share has, to date, well exceeded that of the industrial market, a 2015 market research report projected the industrial market share to surpass the medical market by 2021. The promise of industrial exoskeletons and exosuits to the fully physically-abled embodies both productivities for the organization and injury prevention for the individual user. The technologies are intended to augment a worker's physiologic capabilities (stability, force, and power production) in industrial task performance to increase work capacity or reduce biomechanical loads and/or worker fatigue, thus mitigating overexertion risk [11].

Exoskeletons address a mismatch between workplace physical demands and human strength/endurance capabilities, consistent with any other ergonomic equipment intervention. However, by their wearable nature, exoskeletons have some characteristics of personal protective equipment (PPE). As such, in the technical interchange meetings described in Section 6.2, it was proposed that exoskeletons represent an emerging new class of PPE. A National Science Foundation program solicitation (NSF 18-518) under the National Robotics Initiative 2.0: Ubiquitous Collaborative Robots describes interest in "wearable, prosthetic-like, exoskeletal, bionic, and other attachable human assistive robotic devices that can serve the workforce by functioning as smart personal protective equipment (PPE) and performance augmentation and amplification devices (PAADs)". As an alternative to the PPE characterization, exoskeletons have been likened to other forms of work aid, material handling equipment, or tooling/equipment modifications that reduce the user/operator's physical effort in executing a task, consistent with an engineering controls approach. However, the wearable nature of these devices that involve attachment, fitting/adjustment, and donning/doffing may be more akin to PPE use concerning acceptance by industrial workers. Traditional PPE (e.g., respirators, protective eyewear, hearing protection devices, head protection) is generally characterized by a physical barrier between the worker and the physical agent or hazard. PPE adoption is part of a safety management system but is also persuaded by regulatory requirements and mandated use in environments where hazards cannot be eliminated, substituted, or mitigated with other engineering or process design approaches. Traditional PPE equipment has established certifications and test methods that communicate and/or certify protectiveness [11].

Exoskeletons protect the user through the reduction of internal biomechanical loads across the user's joints, muscles, and soft tissue or by reducing their metabolic exertion. One challenge to standards development for exoskeletons will be to establish test methods and certifications to communicate this protectiveness in a manner analogous to PPE protectiveness while also recognizing the ability of exoskeletons to augment capabilities that traditional PPE does not. This will likely involve multiple test methods given the range of tasks and functions of these systems in industrial applications. Employers and workers (users) may be more confident in adopting these technologies if standards exist for certifying and communicating their protectiveness like PPE [11].

6.2.3 ANSI/ASSE A10.40-2007

Forthcoming exoskeleton standards that address device capabilities toward overexertion/musculoskeletal injury prevention in the workplace should be applied consistently with industrial hygiene principles and consensus standards. For example, in the construction industry, per ANSI/ASSE A10.40-2007, solutions for jobs/tasks with risk factors for musculoskeletal disorders should be based on the hierarchy of controls, prioritized as 1. elimination, 2. substitution, 3. engineering controls, 4. administrative changes, 5. work practice changes, 6. training, 7. protective equipment, and 8. assessment of individual physical capabilities. Deployment of exoskeletons to protect employees from overexertion and/or cumulative trauma injury risks should consider the potential for overreliance on the technology. One way in which this has been addressed is with policies stating that exoskeleton deployment should not be an opportunity to increase throughput or workload that might negate a margin of safety afforded by the exoskeleton. In addition to standards for safe design and use, to minimize any new workplace risks introduced by exoskeletons, future work might emphasize test methods whereby exoskeletons can be evaluated in terms of the degree to which they mitigate user overexertion and musculoskeletal risk. The ability to standardize testing of an augmentation "multiplier", that is, the extent to which the device increases an occupationally relevant specific capability or tolerance to external loading, is needed to comparatively assess similarly purposed devices [11].

6.2.4 STANDARDS APPLICABLE TO EXOSKELETONS

The standards are mainly from ISO, with relevant ones from IEC, SS, JIS, IEEE, and ASTM, which include the common requirements for robots. Some standards are the following [18, 19, 20]:

ISO 14971:2019—Medical devices: Application of risk management to medical devices
ISO/DIS 5363—Test methods for Exoskeleton-type Walking RACA Robot
ISO TC 299—Robotics
WG1: Robot vocabulary and characteristics
WG2—Personal Care Robot Safety
ISO 13482:2014—Robots and robotic devices—Safety requirements for personal care
ISO/DTR 23482-1—Application of ISO 13482—Part 1: Safety-related test methods
ISO/TR 23482-2:2019—Application of ISO 13482—Part 2: Application guidelines
WG5—Medical Robot Safety—JWG9: MEE & MES using robotic technology, and JWG36: Medical robots for rehabilitation
WG6—Modularity for service robots—Modularity for service robots—Part 1: General requirements
ISO 8373:2012—Defines terms used concerning robots and robotic devices operating in both industrial and non-industrial environments; adopted as Singapore Standard: SS ISO 8373:2017—Robots and robotic devices (Vocabulary)
ISO 9787:2013—Adopted as Singapore Standard: SS ISO 9787:2017—Robots and robotic devices—Coordinate systems and motion nomenclatures

ISO 11161:2007—Safety of Machinery: Integrated Manufacturing Systems—Basic Requirements

ISO 12100:2010—Safety of machinery—General principles for design—Risk assessment and risk reduction

ISO 13849-1:2015—Safety of machinery—Safety-related parts of control systems—Part 1: General principles for design

ISO 13849-2:2012—Safety of machinery—Safety-related parts of control systems—Part 2: Validation

ISO/TS 15066:2016—Adopted as Singapore Standard: TR ISO/TS 15066:2016—Robots and robotic devices—Collaborative robots

ISO 19649:2017—Adopted as Singapore Standard: SS ISO 19649:2017—Mobile robots—Vocabulary

ISO 25000:2005 (Replacing ISO-9126 and ISO-14598)—Software Engineering—Software product Quality Requirements and Evaluation (SQuaRE)—Guide to SQuaRE Industrial Robots

ISO 9283:1998—Manipulating industrial robots—Performance criteria and related test methods

ISO 9409-1:2004—Manipulating industrial robots—Mechanical interfaces—Part 1: Plates

ISO 9409-2:2002—Manipulating industrial robots—Mechanical interfaces—Part 2: Shafts

ISO 9946:1999—Manipulating industrial robots—Presentation of characteristics

ISO 10218-1:2011—Adopted as Singapore Standard: SS ISO 10218-1:2016—Robots and robotic devices—Safety requirements for industrial robots—Part 1: Robots

ISO 10218-2:2011—Adopted as Singapore Standard: SS ISO 10218-2:2011—Robots and robotic devices—Safety requirements for industrial robots—Part 2: Robot systems and integration

ISO 11593:1996—Manipulating industrial robots—Automatic end effector exchange systems—Vocabulary and presentation of characteristics

ISO/TR 13309:1995—Manipulating industrial robots—Informative guide on test equipment and metrology methods of operation for robot performance evaluation following ISO 9283

ISO 14539:2000—Manipulating industrial robots—Object handling with grasp-type grippers—Vocabulary and presentation of characteristics

ISO/TR 20218-1:2018—Robotics—Safety design for industrial robot systems—Part 1: End-effectors

ISO/TR 20218-2:2017—Robotics—Safety design for industrial robot systems—Part 2: Manual load/unload stations

ISO 18646-1:2016—Adopted as Singapore Standard: SS ISO 18646-1: 2017—Robotics—Performance criteria and related test methods for service robots—Part 1: Locomotion for wheeled robots

ISO 18646-2:2019—Robotics—Performance criteria and related test methods for service robots—Part 2: Navigation, Service Robots (Exoskeleton)

ISO 13482:2014—Adopted as Singapore Standard: SS ISO 13482:2017—Robots and robotic devices—Safety requirements for personal care robots

ISO/TR 23482-1:2020—Robotics—Application of ISO 13482—Part 1: Safety-related test methods

ISO/TR 23482-2:2019—Robotics—Application of ISO 13482—Part 2: Application guidelines

ISO 9241-220—Ergonomics of Human-System Interaction Part 220: Processes for Enabling, Executing and Assessing Human-Centered Design within Organizations

IEC TR CD 60601-4-1—Medical electrical equipment—Part 4–1: Guidance and interpretation—Medical electrical equipment and medical electrical systems employ a degree of autonomy

IEC 60204-1:2016—Safety of Machinery—Electrical equipment of Machinery—Part 1 General Requirements

IEC 60335-2-2:2019—Household and similar electrical appliances—Safety—Part 2–2: Particular requirements for vacuum cleaners and water-suction cleaning appliances

IEC 62061:2005—Safety of Machinery: Functional Safety of safety-related electrical, electronic, and programmable electronic control systems

IEC 60335-1:2020—Household and similar electrical appliances—Safety—Part 1: General

IEC/TR 60601-4-1:2017—Medical electrical equipment—Part 4–1: Guidance and interpretation—Medical electrical equipment and medical electrical systems employ a degree of autonomy

IEC 80601-2-77:2019—Using Standard IEC 80601-2-78 for the Testing of Medical Exoskeletons and other RACA; Medical electrical equipment—Part 2–77: Particular requirements for the basic safety and essential performance of robotically assisted surgical equipment

IEC 80601-2-78:2019—Medical electrical equipment—Part 2–78: Particular requirements for basic safety and essential performance of medical robots for rehabilitation, assessment, compensation, or alleviation

IEC/FDIS 80601-2-78—Medical electrical equipment—Part 2–78: Particular requirements for basic safety and essential performance of medical robots for rehabilitation, assessment, compensation, or alleviation

IEEE 730-2014—Software Quality Assurance Processes

IEEE 1059-1993—Guide for Software Verification and Validation (V&V) Plans

IEEE 1012-2016—Software, and Hardware Verification and Validation

JIS B 0138-1996—Industrial robots—Graphical symbols of mechanism

JIS B 8439:1992—Industrial robots—Programming language slim

JIS B 8440-1995—Industrial robots—Intermediate code STROLIC, Service Robots (General)

JIS B 8446-1:2016—Safety requirements for personal care robots—Part 1: Static stable mobile servant robot with no manipulator

JIS B 8446-2:2016—Safety requirements for personal care robots—Part 2: Low power restraint-type physical assistant robot

JIS B 8446-3:2016—Safety requirements for personal care robots—Part 3: Self-balancing person carrier robot

JIS B 8456-1:2017—Personal care robots—Part 1: Physical assistant robots for lumbar support

ASTM F3323—Standard Terminology for Exoskeletons and Exosuits Practice for Labelling and Information on Exoskeletons and Exosuits

ASTM F3358—Standard Practice for Labelling and Information on Exoskeletons and Exosuits

ASTM WK65295—New Test Method for Load Handling When Using an Exoskeleton

ASTM WK65296—New Practice for Recording Environmental Conditions for Utilization with Exoskeleton Test Methods

ASTM WK65346—New Guide for Safety Considerations in Designing and Selecting Exoskeletons for Industrial, Medical, and Military Applications

ASTM WK65347—New Guide for Utilization of Digital Human Modeling

ASTM WK65587—New Guide for Assessing System Training—Service Robots (Healthcare)

ASTM WK77587—Revision of F3323-20 Standard Terminology for Exoskeletons and Exosuits; the rationale is designed to define the terms surrounding the domain better; a Work Item (WK) is a proposed new standard or a revision to an existing standard that is under development by a committee

ASTM F3358-18—Standard Practice for Labeling and Information for Exoskeletons

ASTM F3323-19—Standard Terminology for Exoskeletons and Exosuits

ASTM F48.01—Design and Manufacturing

ASTM F48.01: WK62649—Labeling and Information for Exoskeletons and Exosuits

ASTM F48.02—Human Factors and Ergonomics

ASTM F48.02: WK65346—Safety Considerations in Designing and Selecting Exoskeletons for Industrial, Medical, and Military Applications

ASTM F48.02: WK65347—Utilization of Digital Human Modeling

ASTM F48.02: WK65587—Assessing System Training

ASTM F48.03—Task Performance and Environmental Considerations

ASTM F48.03: WK65295—Load Handling When Using an Exoskeleton

ASTM F48.03: WK65296—Recording Environmental Conditions for Utilization with Exoskeleton Test Methods

ASTM F48.04—Maintenance and Disposal

ASTM F48.04: WK67755—Exoskeleton Wearing, Care, and Maintenance Instructions

ASTM F48.91—Terminology

ASTM F48.91: WK60882—Exoskeletons and Exosuits

ANSI/AAMI HE75:2009—Human Factors Engineering: Design of Medical Devices

ANSI/HFES 100-2007—Human Factors Engineering of Computer Workstations

APA—Handbook of Human Systems Integration (2015)

HF-STD-001—FAA Human Factors Design Standard

HFES 200-2008—Human Factors Engineering of Software User Interfaces

HFES 300-2004—Guidelines for Using Anthropometric Data in Product Design

HF-STD-001—Human Factors Design Standard (Federal Aviation Administration)
Mil-Std-1472H—Department of Defense Design Criteria Standard: Human Engineering
Mil-Std-882—Department of Defense Standard Practice: System Safety
NASA-STD-3001—Volumes 1 and 2, NASA Space Flight Human System Standards
NUREG-0700—Human-System Interface Design Review Guidelines
SAE6906—Standard Practice for Human Systems Integration
ANSI/ASSE. A10.40-2007 (R2013)—Reduction of musculoskeletal problems in construction American Society of Safety Engineers (ASSE)

6.3 NORMATIVITY IMPLEMENTATION

6.3.1 RISK MANAGEMENT AND REGULATIONS FOR LOWER LIMB MEDICAL EXOSKELETONS

Gait disability is a major healthcare problem worldwide. Powered exoskeletons have recently emerged as devices that can enable users with gait disabilities to ambulate in an upright posture and potentially bring other clinical benefits. In 2014, the FDA approved the marketing of the ReWalk Personal Exoskeleton as a class II medical device with special controls. Since then, Indego and Ekso have also received regulatory approval. With similar trends worldwide, this industry is likely to grow rapidly [21].

Upper limb exoskeletons are typically considered safer than lower limb ones because they are stationary and do not pose the risk of falling. The FDA identifies a powered lower extremity exoskeleton as "a prescription device that is composed of an external, powered, motorized orthosis that is placed over a person's paralyzed or weakened limbs for medical purposes" (Regulation 21 CFR 890.3480) [22]. On the other hand, all current FDA-cleared exoskeletons are recognized under product code PHL, which describes a powered lower extremity exoskeleton as "a prescription device that is composed of an external, powered, motorized orthosis used for medical purposes that are placed over a person's paralyzed or weakened limbs to provide ambulation". The ability to provide over-ground ambulation is a distinct feature compared to stationary robotic devices that are generally attached to treadmills. Ambulation also imposes significant challenges and risks in terms of maintaining balance and preventing falls [21]. In treadmill-based systems (e.g., Lokomat of Hocoma), a body weight support tether is often used as an easy and robust countermeasure to prevent falls. Lokomat is categorized by the FDA as an isokinetic evaluation and testing system under Regulation CFR 890.1925.26 [23].

Currently, three devices in the USA have been cleared by the FDA since this device category was established in 2014: ReWalk Personal (Argo Medical Technologies, Israel), Indego (Parker Hannifin, USA), and Ekso GT (Ekso Bionics, USA) [21].

6.3.1.1 ReWalk

ReWalk was cleared for marketing in the USA as a Class II medical device by the FDA in 2014 and became the first of its kind. Indego was confirmed to be substantially equivalent (SE) to ReWalk in March 2016 by the FDA, and therefore also cleared for marketing in the USA [24]. Ekso was approved by the FDA in the same manner shortly after [25].

ISO is the world's largest developer of voluntary international standards, and many ISO standards are recognized by the FDA. The FDA recognizes the standard for risk management in medical devices (ISO 14971), which was last revised in 2007. In 2012, the European Committee for Standardization (CEN) adopted a harmonized version of the ISO standard as EN ISO 14971:2012 (applies only to manufacturers with devices intended for the European market). Compliance with ISO 14971 and EN ISO 14971:2012 is an integral step in the process of bringing a medical device to the U.S. and the European consumer markets. ISO 14971 outlines the process of risk management and provides guidelines for evaluating, reducing, and documenting risks [26]. The FDA has formally recognized powered lower extremity exoskeletons as a Class II medical device with special controls [27].

ReWalk is the first exoskeleton cleared by the FDA for both personal use as well as use in a rehabilitation setting in the USA. FDA issued Order PS140001 [28], requiring postmarket surveillance because the device's failure to prevent a fall would be reasonably likely to cause serious injury or death to the users and assisting individuals [29]. Argo Medical Technologies Ltd received a warning letter from the FDA after failing to conduct such a postmarket surveillance program regarding the risk of falls [30]. ReWalk announced the launch of the required postmarket study in August 2016 [31]. In addition to commonly accepted ISO standards and FDA guidelines to mitigate risks, ReWalk features the following safety measures concerning software and hardware [29]:

- "Graceful collapse/sitting": In the event of a major system failure, such as complete loss of power, the weight of the patient causes the ReWalk unit to enter a graceful collapse, i.e., the body's weight rotates the inner rotor of the motor and moves the exoskeleton joints into a slowly achieved collapsed sitting position.
- Battery: The main battery is a lithium-ion battery that allows the user to walk continuously for >2 hours on a charge. The secondary is a lithium-polymer battery that allows at least an additional 15 minutes of continuous walking. The user is alerted when the charge of the battery is low by a short vibration (buzz) repeated every 10 seconds. Warnings are provided to the user not to use the device while charging.
- Excessive joint angles: There is a threshold in the software that limits the movement through a safe range of motion and a fixed mechanical stop, which also prevents movement beyond a safe joint angle trajectory.
- Software: The system does a self-check at start-up and disables the system until the problem is corrected. The system will default over to manual control when a main computer failure occurs.
- Misstep or obstacle: If the user contacts an obstacle with one of the limbs, the movement restriction generates excess torque. A torque threshold limit and alert are issued by the buzzer and vibrator, and the leg then moves back to a standing position.

- Loss of communication between remote and main computer: The system can enter a bypass mode where the device can be controlled with buttons on the hip actuation unit.

ReWalk has been tested in several clinical studies to examine its efficacy and safety [32, 33]. It has received mixed reviews. Positive opinions include that ReWalk is a safe device for in-hospital ambulation [34] and that it provides potential for functional gain and improved fitness because of higher heart rate and oxygen demand than standing or sitting [35]. There are no reports of serious adverse events, and participants had generally positive opinions regarding the use of the system [3]. ReWalk has been the most studied powered exoskeleton for the SCI population. However, one study 21 reported a high incidence of skin aberrations when using the ReWalk exoskeleton: five out of ten enrolled subjects experienced at least one mild skin aberration, and two of them were withdrawn from the study owing to recurring skin breakdown. Also, one subject had a hairline fracture of the talus after using the device, possibly because of inaccurate joint alignment. No further treatment was needed, but the subject was excluded for the rest of the study because of this near serious adverse event. The administrators of that study recommended prescreening subjects with osteopenia or osteoporosis in future studies [33].

6.3.1.2 Indego

The Indego exoskeleton is deemed SE to ReWalk, and thus, most of its identified risks and associated risk mitigation approaches are similar [24]. It has passed various tests such as durability testing and software verification. There are some differences when compared to ReWalk. Small variations exist in the size of components, weight, allowable height and weight of users, control method, and battery, all of which are deemed similar without additional safety or efficacy concerns.

Of interest is Indego's fall detection feature: it detects forward, backward, and sideways falling as it is happening, with the device adjusting during the fall to position the user for minimal risk of injury. In the event of power failure, the knees become locked and the hips free. This mechanism allows the user to remain standing in the event of a malfunction. There are a few clinical studies to date that utilize Indego. It is reported that Indego outperforms a knee-ankle-foot orthosis [36], enables acute cardiorespiratory and metabolic responses, and enabled persons with tetraplegia and paraplegia to learn to use it quickly. No adverse events have been reported [37].

6.3.1.3 Ekso

Similar to ReWalk and Indego, Ekso also has bilateral powered hip and knee joints in the sagittal plane. However, it is the first and, currently, the only exoskeleton cleared by the FDA for use by stroke patients. After the announcement that the FDA would regulate exoskeletons as Class II medical devices with special controls, Ekso Bionic filed a notification to the FDA in December 2014. In the meantime, the company was allowed to continue marketing under Class I registration while the application was under review. The company received clearance for marketing from the FDA in April 2016, on the basis that it is SE to ReWalk [25].

Ekso has been evaluated in several clinical studies and has been shown to improve the gait speed and step length of SCI subjects after 20 sessions of training. A pilot study explored incorporating transcutaneous spinal cord stimulation in daily training with Ekso. In a study using a prototype version of Ekso, multiple falls were recorded without any physical adverse conditions. An overhead tether was used in this study to prevent actual falls. A "fall" was therefore defined as an event when the tether was triggered to function, not when the user fell. In particular, a faulty feature that was initially designed to help trigger steps via contact sensors on the crutch was removed in later versions of the device because of frequent malfunctioning. There are six adverse events registered in the Manufacturer and User Facility Device Experience (MAUDE, an FDA database of device-related adverse events: www.accessdata.fda.gov/scripts/cdrh/cfdocs/cfmaude/search.cfm) database.

None of them resulted in the injury of users or anyone else. All are mechanical issues, such as a footplate separating from the device and a broken epoxy bond allowing the ankle joint to rotate [21].

6.3.1.4 HAL

HAL for Medical Use (Lower Limb Type) is a bilateral lower limb exoskeleton with two active degrees of freedom at the hip and knee and a passive degree of freedom at the ankle joint of each leg. Its control system processes data from surface electromyography (EMG) sensors, angle/acceleration sensors, and force sensors to estimate the necessary forces to assist as needed the user's intended actions. The use of EMG signals in HAL's shared control system to help detect the user's intent represents a type of hybrid peripheral neural interface [38].

Its European model has been certified under the European Medical Device Directive (CE 0197). HAL was approved to manufacture and sell Japan's first robot therapeutic device, HAL for Medical Use (Lower Limb Type), by the Japanese Ministry of Health, Labor, and Welfare on November 25, 2015. In December, the company applied for national health insurance coverage for HAL for medical use [39].

HAL has been widely tested in clinical trials. A systematical review of clinical applications of HAL for gait training for 140 subjects with stroke or SCI suggested that minor and medical transient side effects occurred, but no serious adverse events were reported. HAL is thus considered safe and feasible for stroke patients to use. One study examined the feasibility and safety issues of using HAL in acute-phase rehabilitation after a stroke [40]. Though no serious incident happened, four of the subjects experienced orthostatic hypotension (orthostatic hypotension was defined as a decrease in systolic blood pressure of >20 mmHg immediately after sitting or standing.), resulting in one subject withdrawing from the experiment [21].

This is noteworthy because blood pressure responses after using exoskeletons are usually not measured or are reported as within normal limits in other studies. A similar acute-phase rehabilitation feasibility and safety study recruited eight patients and thoroughly reported all adverse reports from the participants. Moderate discomfort from tight straps and the heavy weight of the device was reported by several subjects, although these did not last after the training.

Moderate pain due to pressure was reported at the cuff over the knee and the malleolus. This was solved by readjusting the device. Although minor and solvable, this adverse effect highlighted the importance of proper alignment of the device. Chafed feet were reported in one subject due to the wrong shoe size. This was not a technical error, but better labeling and rigorous staff training will minimize the chance of user errors. Stumbling due to impaired weight shifting occurred from time to time. Subjects were secured by an overhead tether and also supported by two therapists when needed [21].

6.3.1.5   Rex

The Rex of Rex Bionics from New Zealand carries the CE mark and is available in the EU market. It distinguishes itself from other exoskeletons because it can self-balance, albeit under restricted conditions, without the need for any extra balancing instruments (cane or walker). Rex thus offers a "hands-free" experience to users.

To date, there are no published clinical trials to demonstrate the clinical effectiveness and risks of Rex. However, a serious adverse event was reported to the MAUDE database [41]. One user with SCI suffered bilateral symmetrical fractures after finishing a supervised session. The patient noticed swelling in the ankles and knees in the evening. An appointment was organized for the following day, and bone fractures were identified by X-ray. According to the manufacturer, there are three likely contributing factors: 1. the patient was found to have osteoporosis; 2. the patient had a spasm, and so inadvertently kicked the heel stops back, resulting in misaligned ankles and knees; or 3. two ankle braces were used to support the user's ankles. They restricted the range of motion such that the user no longer met the required range of motion specified for the device. This adverse event highlights the possibility of bone fracture due to the misalignment of joints. The event was probably the result of a series of unfortunate mistakes: poor, or lack of, training of physiotherapists; lack of clarity in the exclusion criteria; and lack of countermeasures for unsecured joints [21].

Several data were consulted from ClinicalTrials.gov (https://clinicaltrials.gov/), an online NIH database that compiles information on clinical studies involving human participants.

6.3.2   Reported Adverse Events

An adverse event is defined by ISO 62366–2 as an event associated with a medical device that led to death or serious injuries of a patient or may lead to such if the event recurs [21].

6.3.2.1   Identified Risks

The FDA identified nine risks when it reviewed ReWalk's de novo application [29]. Similar risks likely exist in other devices as well since they usually claim to be SE to ReWalk. Potential risks of using exoskeletons include friction and injury from direct contact between the exoskeleton and the user, joint hyperextension, unintended contact, collision, vibration exposure, overexertion, and worker instability [21].

6.3.2.2   Falls

Injuries resulting from falls are a major public health concern for the elderly, representing one of the main causes of long-standing pain, functional impairment, disability, and death in this population. Using exoskeletons impose an additional risk of falls on users who already suffer from a motor deficiency. When a person walks freely, the body interacts with the environment (ground), which is predictable unless obstacles catch the person off guard. When the person uses an exoskeleton, however, this direct interaction is reduced or distorted. Feedback is inevitably distorted because of the extra layer of media. Sometimes, there are additional sources of feedback such as vibrations and sound. Users may need some time to adjust to these extrinsic stimulations. Additionally, users may attempt to execute certain movements, yet cannot correctly achieve them because of the physical constraint imposed by the exoskeleton. Finally, depending on the control scheme, the exoskeleton may incorrectly react to body movement, resulting in the triggering of an unexpected command that may contribute to the occurrence of a fall [21].

ReWalk, Indego, and Ekso all have their strategies to mitigate the risk of falls, summarized in three categories: 1. to detect and actively mitigate falling, 2. to seek minimal damage should power failure and/or a fall become inevitable, and 3. to deploy assistants who stand beside the user according to indications for use. Indego is the only device that has an active fall detection and mitigation feature: it detects falls and adjusts itself.

The method by which Indego detects falls, its responsiveness, and what kind of adjustments are to be made during the fall are unclear. Nonetheless, such a feature is important in controlling an exoskeleton. In the unlikely event of a power failure when falling is inevitable, ReWalk will collapse to a sitting position slowly, which is called "graceful collapse" [29].

Indego and Ekso lock the knee joint and allow free movement of the hip when a power failure occurs. Although it provides a better solution if the user is in a standing posture when power fails, it is still risky to lock the knee should a power failure occur during the swing phase. Another difference between the three devices is their indications for use. All require a trained person to stand beside and always supervise the user. While ReWalk and Indego offer training programs and certificates. The FDA has requested ReWalk to conduct a postmarket surveillance program to further monitor and study the risks of falls [21].

6.3.2.3 Skin and Soft Tissue Injury

Skin and soft tissue injury is the most frequent type of injury. It is universal, as it occurred with all listed devices and is repetitive, happening to several subjects in the same study. In some cases, skin damage happened repeatedly to the same subject, suggesting that the researchers could not avoid this problem even after noticing its occurrence [33].

Despite the prevalence of this type of injury, it has attracted little attention. Only half of the clinical trials considered skin conditions as an exclusion criterion. Skin and tissue injuries were usually dismissed as minor issues and did not affect the safety evaluation of exoskeletons.

It is important that manufacturers systematically examine the cause and location of skin and soft tissue damage. Currently, it is difficult to summarize any pattern of skin and tissue damage given the information available and the lack of sensors in padded braces that could monitor forces at the physical interface. Even in the studies that do report them, they are usually briefly mentioned without specifying the frequency, cause, location, and seriousness of the damage. Sensors have been proposed as a novel method to prevent skin injuries related to excessive pressure in mobility-impaired exoskeleton users. Therefore, it is important to place force detecting sensors on the joints of the exoskeleton to give an alarm when excessive pressure occurs [21].

6.3.2.4   User Error

User error is defined in ISO 62366–1 as a user's unexpected action or lack of action that could lead to a different result than intended by the manufacturer or user. It can occur during normal use. For instance, a user may accidentally rotate their pelvis and shift their body weight. This may trigger false alarm movement in exoskeletons because they use such movements as a trigger to initiate a new gait cycle. Other possible errors include tripping over obstacles, wrong menu selection, and operating with low battery life [21].

Thus, it is important to design a human-machine interface that is friendly and robust, independent of the technological fluency or attentional state of the user. Caregivers and physical therapists accompanying the user during training may also make errors. They may choose the wrong commands in settings, incorrectly fasten straps, or fail to support the user when he or she loses balance. In a bone fracture accident, the manufacturer suspected that one of the causes was that the therapist did not correctly secure the user's ankles. Human factor validation testing is an important step in risk management according to FDA's guidelines for medical devices [42].

6.3.2.5   Bone Fracture

The exoskeleton must be precisely aligned with the user's joint so that there is minimal incorrect torque forced onto the joints. Misalignment can result in skin abrasion, sores, hairline fractures, or bone fractures. Currently, there are two reported bone fracture accidents. Both injured users had SCIs and therefore did not notice the fracture immediately and continued to finish their scheduled training sessions. They both reported the abnormal appearance of their legs later in the day and discovered bone fractures through X-ray exams on the following day [21].

Individuals using medical exoskeletons are at an increased risk of bone damage due to the prevalence of osteoporosis in patients with spinal cord injuries, making fractures more likely. Additionally, SCI patients do not have the pain feedback mechanism in their lower limbs to indicate when excessive torque is being applied, increasing the risk of bone fracture. Bone fracture is a severe potential risk associated with the use of exoskeletons. To mitigate this risk, potential strategies include developing better strap designs to minimize the chance of misalignment and implementing participant screening measures, such as requiring DXA scans and X-rays, to evaluate the severity of osteoporosis and exclude patients with a high risk of fracture.

6.3.2.6   Long-Term Secondary Effects

Exoskeletons have the potential to bring clinical change to users with disability. Studies suggest that recovery is observed after weeks of training in many studies. However, it is not clear how this change is compared to other traditional rehabilitation procedures. Meanwhile, other physical and mental conditions of the users may also change after using exoskeletons. Some subjects reported improvements in pain and bowel and bladder function after using ReWalk. One of the advantages of using exoskeletons for mobility rehabilitation is that they provide repetitive practice session after session. However, very few clinical studies have protocols longer than 6 months, so, it remains unknown what the long-term effect is of using an exoskeleton. A review of protocols of body weight–supported treadmill training interventions with robotic orthosis found that, in general, longer treatments provide better outcomes. A study found that there is neurological recovery after chronic SCI patients train with an exoskeleton for 12 months. However, osteoporosis/osteopenia is viewed as a relative contraindication for SCI patients being considered for exoskeleton ambulatory training because of a risk of bone fracture. Thus far, it is unclear what would happen when a person with low bone density repeatedly uses an exoskeleton. More studies are needed to understand how exoskeletons may change patients' neurological status and biomechanical condition over time [21].

6.3.2.7 Regulations and Standards

Exoskeleton manufacturers, users, and regulators are the three major players in the exoskeleton industry. "Manufacturers" are companies (ReWalk, Indego, Ekso, etc.), institutions, and many other labs and startups whose prototypes are still in early development. Currently, there are few evaluations across devices to compare their advantages and disadvantages.

"Regulators" consist of government agencies and third-party organizations that create and update industry standards. In the USA, this occurs mostly between the FDA and the ISO. The FDA has directly recommended many ISO standards. The FDA recognized the importance of patient-centric assessment and patient-reported outcomes in its recently issued guidance [42]. Systematic studies in a top-down approach to collect users' feedback across devices will help regulators and the industry to better understand the need and problems end users face [21].

The "user" group consists of individuals who use and potentially benefit from the device directly. There are also clinicians, who indirectly interact with the device and oversee its performance. Clinicians, especially physical therapists, benefit from the device as it decreases the amount of physical labor required by them, making their work less physically intense and decreasing their risk of injury. However, the benefit compared to the imposed risk for the exoskeleton user remains to be seen [21].

6.3.2.8 Global Overview of Medical Device Regulations

Several studies are focused on the USA market and regulations. The regulations in the FDA's counterparts in Europe and Japan are also summarized. Research labs in Europe have been developing several exoskeleton prototypes for years. It is also common for exoskeletons to obtain CE clearance in the EU before obtaining FDA clearance in the USA, as has been the case for ReWalk, Ekso, HAL, and Rex. Japan is famous for its innovation in various humanoid robots. HAL is arguably its most prestigious lower limb exoskeleton. Its mass production began before the founding of many other companies: more than 20 sets of HAL exoskeletons were in use at hospitals and rehabilitation centers in 2009 [43, 44]. As opposed to the USA and Europe, where exoskeletons are usually developed by labs and startups, there is a trend for industry giants in Asia to directly jump into this market [21].

Honda is developing its stride management assistive device that helps the rotation of the hip joint. It has gone through a clinical trial [45]. Samsung has applied for a US patent for their wearable robot that features EMG control [46]. Panasonic also announced the development of several assistive robots, with plans to use them in elder care [47].

In the USA, powered exoskeletons have been officially classified by the FDA as a Class II device with special controls. The special controls include 1. biocompatibility, 2. electromagnetic compatibility, 3. software validation, 4. geometry and material composition, 5. various nonclinical performance testing, 6. clinical testing, 7. training program, and 8. labeling. When a product is to be marketed in the USA, the company should first classify the device (Class II for exoskeletons) and prepare a pre-market submission (de novo if it is a new category or 510(k) to claim SE to a currently approved medical device) for the FDA to review. The product must wait for FDA clearance before marketing. In the EU, there is no central government organization to issue certificates. Instead, medical devices are required to obtain the CE mark. CE marking on a product is a manufacturer's declaration that the product complies with the essential requirements of the relevant European regulations. Products with CE can be legally placed on the EU market. The CE certificate of an exoskeleton can be obtained from a notified body, which is a third-party, independent group that specializes in the conformity assessment of a product. When looking at the procedures in the USA and the EU, except for the fact that certificates are issued by different bodies, their procedures are generally similar [48].

The Japanese Ministry of Health, Labor, and Welfare (MHLW) is responsible for the device classification and issuing marketing approval for medical devices in Japan. Pharmaceuticals and Medical Devices Agency (PMDA) is the technical branch that performs the actual review, examination, data analysis, and so on to help MHLW's measure. While third-party certification is allowed for low-risk medical devices, MHLW's approval is based on PMDA. When looking at procedures for obtaining medical device approval in the USA, EU, and Japan, the USA requires applications to be approved by a federal agency, namely the FDA, whereas the EU distributes the responsibility to many independent notified bodies. Japan's government reviews reliability of the manufacturers both on-site and via documents, while the USA and the EU leave that responsibility to the manufacturers themselves [49].

6.3.3 Standards for the Safety of Exoskeletons Used by Industrial Workers

According to the Research Framework Program of the European Commission, the goal of the Robo-Mate project is to develop an intelligent, easy-to-maneuver, and wearable body exoskeleton for manual handling work. Workers in the manufacturing industry are exposed to factors that increase their likelihood of developing musculoskeletal disorders (MSDs) [50].

The Robo-Mate industrial exoskeleton has been designed following best practice ergonomic principles to facilitate manual handling activities in multiple case study settings. At present, two exoskeletons have been developed, the Mate and Mate XT exoskeletons. An array of existing standards will be referenced in detail when designing the exoskeleton. As there is currently no standard that specifically targets the safety of exoskeletons for industrial workers, it is intended to use Robo-Mate results to promote such development. To facilitate this process, a roadmap outlining tasks and responsibilities was created. It details who oversees the process to promote and facilitate the further development of existing standards and ensure Robo-Mate results are targeted at suitable stakeholders. This was achieved on three levels. In Level 1, the information was directly communicated to standards-developing bodies, specifically ISO, CEN, and their members. In Level 2, assistance was sought from organizations with interests in industrial robotics to add support to Robo-Mate when seeking to use the project's results to develop standards. The project detailed was distributed to increase the awareness of the Robo-Mate project to the public, end users, manufacturers, and distributors of industrial exoskeletons [50].

It has long been recognized that work and working environments are associated with workers' ill health. MSDs, affecting muscles and joints, are one of the top causes of workplace absenteeism and early retirement due to workers' incapacity to carry out normal daily work tasks [51]. The prevalence of the disorders is increasing with workers in all occupations worldwide being affected. Consequently, affected individuals, their employers, and the economy experience a significant financial burden [52]. Risk factors associated with the disorders include manual handling of loads, particularly with heavier larger, or unwieldy loads, increased frequency or duration of manual handling activities, repetitive movements, and sustaining extreme or awkward postures such as bending, reaching, or twisting [53].

In an attempt to reduce workers' risk of developing MSDs, it is recommended that employers and designers implement a hierarchical duty of care when organizing work environments and when designing tools and equipment concerning the capacity and limitations of workers [54, 55]. To assist in manual handling activities, technological evolution has progressed from mechanized tools to automated systems, to collaborative interactive robots, and of late, to wearable exoskeleton devices. On international and local levels, legislation, standards, and codes of practice have been introduced to minimize the presence of hazards in the workplace and reduce their levels of associated risk [56]. However, advancements in technology, such as the introduction of industrial robots, collaborative robots, and exoskeleton robots can occur at a rate with which the creators of these guidance requirements cannot match.

The EU-funded research and development project, Robo-Mate, is bringing exoskeletons into the industrial workplace setting and creating a device that augments the capacity of workers involved in manual handling activities. Using an industrial exoskeleton can reduce the burden on workers' health while maintaining or increasing production efficiency in all work environments where manual handling activities are required. The three-year Robo-Mate project started in September 2013 and is funded by the European Commission under the 7th Framework Program for Research and Technological Development. Its consortium is comprised of 12 partners from seven countries, which includes end users from automotive and dismantling industries, industrial robotics/technology developers, a robotics integrator, and ergonomics research groups. The work carried out in the Robo-Mate project has resulted in the accumulation of scientific and technological knowledge and expertise concerning industrial exoskeleton development [50].

To ensure the safe design, manufacture, and use of industrial exoskeletons—a new concept for assisting workers in manual handling activities—it is crucial to establish standardized safety criteria. This will provide designers and users with an agreed-upon framework for ensuring the safety of these products. Incorporating recognized international or European standards in the design and manufacture of exoskeleton products, such as the Robo-Mate exoskeleton, can improve the product's reliability and safety. This, in turn, increases the likelihood of the product's sale in various industry settings worldwide and enhances the confidence of users and employers in the product.

Current related standards that FDA recommends for Class II medical devices and lower limb prostheses. According to the AAMI website, AAMI 6061-1 is identical to IEC 60601-1. These two standards are followed by Indego and ReWalk, respectively [21]. There are several standards for exoskeletons depending on their application, as is the case of exoskeletons for medical applications. In this context, Table 6.1 shows the standards that ReWalk and Indego exoskeletons meet, divided into electrical, mechanical, and general categories standards.

TABLE 6.1

Categories and Standards for Exoskeletons (ReWalk and Indego)

Category	Standard
Electrical	
Software (lifecycle)	IEC62304 Ed. 1.1 2015-06
EMC/EMI	AAMI/ANSI/IEC 60601-1-2:2014
Electrical safety testing	IEC 60601-1:2005 (ReWalk)
	ANSI/AAMI ES60601-1:2005/(R)2012 (Indego)
Medical electrical devices (home use)	ANSI/AAMI HA60601-1-1 1:2015
Mechanical	
Durability testing (used in prosthetics)	ISO 10328:2006
Cyclic loading testing (used in prosthetics)	ISO 22675:2006
Particle ingress	ANSI IEC 60529:2004
General	
Risk management	ISO 14971:2007
Quality management	ISO 13485:2003
Labeling	ISO 15223-1:2012
Biocompatibility	ISO 10993-1:2009
Human factors engineering	AAMI ANSI HE75:2009/(R)2013
Training	AAMI TIR49:2013
Application of usability	AAMI ANSI IEC 62366-1:2015
Lithium batteries	UL 1642 5th ed.

6.4 CERTIFIED EXOSKELETONS

Three kinds of exoskeletons are the main ones in the market. First, the industrial exoskeletons, later the healthcare exoskeletons, and finally, the military exoskeletons. Several industrial exoskeletons have been implemented in the production lines without any certification, and others with a few certifications such as Underwriters Laboratories (UL), CE, ISO, ASTM, AAMI, ANSI, EMC, NIST, and IEC.

At present, 20 healthcare exoskeletons have an FDA register. Among exoskeletons, trademarks with the FDA register include B-temia, Cyberdyne, Ekso Bionics, Exoatlet, ReWalk Robotics, and Suitx. Table 6.2 shows the FDA establishment registration and device listing for these companies.

On the other hand, some military exoskeletons are being developed and tested. However, there is still a lack of adequate standards for exoskeletons in tactical operation, which consider design criteria to be used in military activities, such as the risk management, military regulations and ballistic parameters. These design criteria must be developed at the same time as new tactical exoskeletons. There are two ways to include exoskeletons in the defense operation: Exoskeletons as personal protective equipment (Marine Mojo Exoskeleton) and augmentative exoskeletons with various tactical functions (HULC exoskeleton). Underwriter Laboratories is a global leader in applied safety

---

TABLE 6.2
FDA Establishment Registration and Device Listing

Item	Establishment	Device
1	Exoatlet, KR	ExoAtlet II Powered Exoskeleton
2	ReWalk Robotics, MA, USA	Powered Exoskeleton
3	ReWalk Robotics, USA	ReWalk Powered Exoskeleton
4	ReWalk Robotics, USA	ReStore Powered Exoskeleton
5	ReWalk Robotics, USA	ReWalk Personal Powered Exoskeleton
6	ReWalk Robotics, IL, USA	Powered Exoskeleton
7	ReWalk Robotics, IL, USA	ReWalk Rehabilitation Powered Exoskeleton
8	ReWalk Robotics, IL, USA	ReWalk Personal Powered Exoskeleton
9	ReWalk Robotics, IL, USA	ReWalk ReStore Powered Exoskeleton
10	SuitX, USA	Phoenix Powered Exoskeleton
11	B-temia, CA	Keeogo Dermoskeleton System Powered Exoskeleton
12	Cyberdyne, JP	HAL (Lower Limb Type) Device, Biofeedback
13	Cyberdyne, JP	HAL (Lower Limb Type) Powered Exoskeleton
14	Cyberdyne, JP	HAL for Medical Use Devices, Biofeedback
15	Cyberdyne, JP	HAL for Medical Use Powered Exoskeleton
16	Ekso Bionics, CA	Ekso GT Powered Exoskeleton
17	Ekso Bionics, CA	Ekso NR Powered Exoskeleton
18	Ekso Bionics, USA	Indego Powered Exoskeleton
19	Ekso Bionics, USA	Indego Powered Exoskeleton
20	Ekso Bionics, USA	Indego Powered Exoskeleton

science. UL Solutions transforms safety, security, and sustainability challenges into opportunities for customers in more than 100 countries. UL Solutions delivers testing, inspection, and certification services, together with software products and advisory offerings, that support their customers' product innovation and business growth. The UL Certification Marks serve as a recognized symbol of trust in their customers' products and reflect an unwavering commitment to advancing their safety mission [57].

Within the UL certification, it is possible to distinguish two marks: UL Listing, the one that applies to finished products and places on the market for their final use, and Recognized Component, which applies to components that will later form part of a product, both having the same prestige. The UL MX NOM Mark, a product safety Mark for Mexico, means that UL has evaluated representative samples of a product and determined that they meet the appropriate safety requirements contained in the official Mexican standards [58].

6.4.1 Indego Exoskeleton

In 2018 Parker Hannifin Corporation announced that the FDA had given additional clearance to market and sell the Indego exoskeleton for use in the treatment of individuals with hemiplegia due to stroke. By expanding on its original clearance for individuals with a spinal cord injury, this announcement makes Indego the most broadly available exoskeleton for gait therapy and personal use in the United States [59]. Figure 6.1 shows the Indego exoskeleton.

To ensure the safe design, manufacture, and use of industrial exoskeletons for workers involved in manual handling activities, it is necessary to establish standardized safety criteria to provide an agreed-upon framework for designers and users. Incorporating recognized international or European standards in the design and manufacture of exoskeleton products, such as the Robo-Mate exoskeleton, can improve the product's safety and reliability. This, in turn, can increase the product's likelihood of being sold in various industry settings worldwide and enhance the confidence of users and employers in the product.

Indego is a cutting-edge rehabilitation and assistive technology that enhances patient mobility and independence while providing clinicians with a meaningful therapy tool. The recent FDA clearance for Indego was granted after a large, multi-site clinical trial involving eight rehabilitation centers in the United States, where a diverse range of stroke patients received gait therapy using Indego and its therapy software suite. Indego has also received a CE Mark, allowing it to be sold commercially in Europe, and a UL Mark, which certifies the high standards of its design, function, and safety after extensive testing.

6.4.2 Atalante Exoskeleton

Wandercraft's gait-training exoskeleton device, Atalante, has been cleared by the U.S. Food and Drug Administration. Since 2020, the French company has deployed 22 of its Atalante exoskeletons in clinical settings and 5 in other research settings. Wandercraft has launched its commercial operations in the United States. The company expects to deliver the first Atalante exoskeletons during the first quarter of 2023 [60].

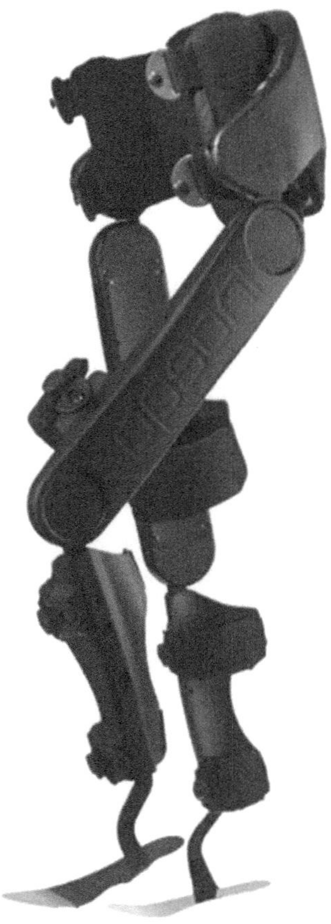

FIGURE 6.1   Indego exoskeleton.

(*Credit*: Parker)

Wandercraft was established in 2012, and its mission is to develop gait-improving technologies. The company commercialized the first version of the Atalante in 2019. In 2015 the device was CE-marked and has been used by hundreds of patients in European rehabilitation hospitals. As part of the certification process, the exoskeleton was subject to a series of tests designed to confirm its load capacity, durability, and safety. It was overloaded, pinched with heavy steel fingers, dropped to the ground, and tested for fire resistance/magnetic integration. It wasn't just the product, but also the manufacturing process that was subject to certification [61].

The ExoAtlet exoskeleton can be adjusted to each patient's proportions to make sure it fits perfectly. Once the device is activated, it helps the patient to put one leg in front of the other and walk in a close-to-natural pattern. ExoAtlet manufactures its exoskeletons in South Korea. Eventually, the manufacturer was granted the ISO-13485 certificate, a huge milestone on ExoAtlet's road to CE marking. In future work, one of the priorities is to evaluate the user-friendliness of the upgraded ExoAtlet exoskeleton, based on feedback from patients and medical practitioners in Europe [61].

6.4.3 CRAY X EXOSKELETON

The German Bionic Cray X exoskeleton has received TÜV SÜD certification, effective as of July 2022. It is now the world's first robotic exoskeleton to bear the "TÜV SÜD Safety Tested" certification mark. Extensive electrical and mechanical safety tests preceded the award of this certificate [62].

The certification confirms that the device meets high standards of safety, performance, usability, and features, including the IP54 protection class. Additionally, it ensures the product's production quality is consistently high and regularly monitored by the reputable TÜV SÜD testing and certification body.

6.4.4 GEMS EXOSKELETON

In 2020 Samsung's GEMS (Gait Enhancing and Motivating System) hip exoskeleton received the ISO 13482 certification from the Korea Institute for Robot Industry Advancement, becoming the first South Korean company to earn such accreditation [63].

The ISO 13482 certification outlines safety standards for three personal care bots: mobile servant robots, physical assistant robots, and person carrier robots. Samsung GEMS, a robotics wearable that assists users who have trouble walking, running, or standing up, was introduced last year. It currently has three models: the GEMS Hip, GEMS Knee, and GEMS Ankle [63]. GEMS Hip is an exoskeleton worn on the waist that reduces energy expenditure by 24% while walking and increases walking speed by about 14%. The GEMS Hip also earned the ISO 13849 certification, which applies to safety-related parts of control systems [64]

6.4.5 LAEVO FLEX EXOSKELETON

In 2022 the Laevo FLEX exoskeleton received official European Union certification as personal protective equipment (PPE), including the CE mark. This means that the Laevo FLEX exoskeleton meets the regulatory EU requirements proving particular safety functions and that the equipment is following all legal requirements of the EU market [65].

Laevo has sold thousands of exoskeletons for lower back pain (LBP) and learned a lot from the feedback of all their customers, not only in terms of improving the exoskeleton itself but also in terms of a successful implementation process in general. The Laevo FLEX has been tested against the intended use to reduce the risk of back injuries during work while bending forward, holding this posture, and returning upright, along with squatting and lifting weights. This also includes reducing the risk of back injuries during work and fatigue due to bending or lifting [65].

6.4.6 EksoNR Exoskeleton

In 2022, Ekso Bionics announced it had received clearance from the U.S. FDA to market its EksoNR robotic exoskeleton for use with multiple sclerosis (MS) patients, an indication that significantly expands the device's use to a broader group of patients. EksoNR is the latest-generation device of the most clinically used robotic exoskeleton on the market. It was previously cleared by the FDA for stroke and spinal cord injury rehabilitation in 2016 and acquired brain injury (ABI) in 2020. The device was the first of its kind to receive a stroke indication, is the only exoskeleton with an ABI indication, and now is the first to receive an indication for MS [66].

The certification verifies the device's safety and high standards of performance, usability, and features, such as the IP54 protection class, as well as its consistently high production quality. TÜV SÜD, an internationally recognized testing and certification body, regularly monitors and confirms this certification.

EksoNR has obtained both FDA clearances and a CE mark, making it available in Europe as well. With over 375 rehabilitation centers worldwide utilizing Ekso devices, patients have taken nearly 200 million steps thanks to the technology.

6.4.7 RoboGait Exoskeleton

A Turkish start-up company called Bama Technology produces the RoboGait walking rehabilitation robot. RoboGait has contributed to the treatment of walking difficulties since 2010. Turkey's example with the establishment and development of "start-up" companies from the Bama technology entrepreneurs was established with support from the state. The company quickly commercialized the product and successfully carried out import substitution in the domestic market and expanded abroad. RoboGait devices started to be used in clinics in Poland, Romania, and Hungary. RoboGait has recently succeeded in being included in the U.S. FDA Approved Medical Devices List [67].

RoboGait is a system for robot-assisted gait rehabilitation that aids in restoring and improving walking ability in patients with neurological or orthopedic conditions such as traumatic brain and spinal cord injuries, stroke, or loss of mobility. The RoboGait executive orthosis is suitable for both pediatric and adult patients, and pediatric connections do not require additional mechanisms to continue therapy. This allows therapists to use the same module for children and eliminates the need for tiring and power-based orthosis module replacement. By using a single module, therapists can treat more patients in less time.

6.4.8 Muscle Suit Every Exoskeleton

In 2021, Innophys received a CE Mark for the sale and distribution of the Muscle Suit Every exoskeleton in Europe. Innophys has clearance to be sold in 31 European countries—27 EU countries plus 4 member countries of the European Free Trade Association (EFTA). Innophys will partner with local sales agents in EU countries, including France, Germany, and Spain, to market its product after deeming that it

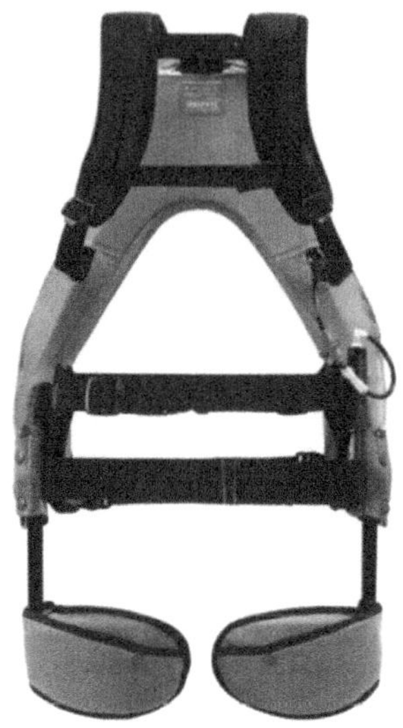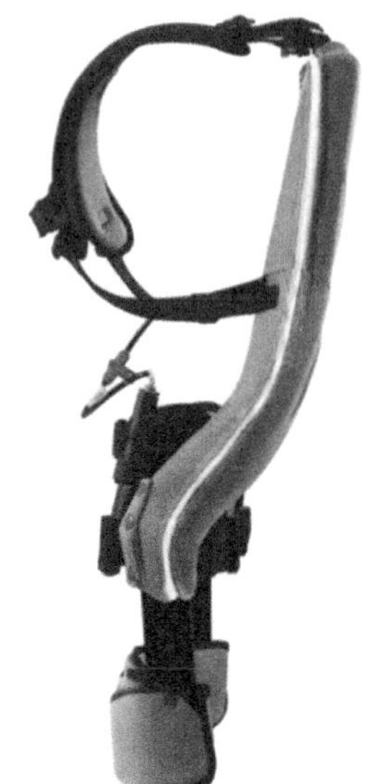

FIGURE 6.2   Muscle Suit Every exoskeleton.

(*Credit*: Innophys)

can expect demand in the region because its product can help prevent work-related accidents in the manufacturing and farming sectors and assist aging and nursing care workers [68]. Figure 6.2 shows the Muscle Suit Every exoskeleton.

6.4.9   MUSCULAR AIDING TECH EXOSKELETON (MATE)

The ESO-EAWS scientific research project was born from the collaboration of the Fondazione Ergo with the Alma Mater Studiorum University of Bologna and the Laboratory for Engineering of Neuromuscular System (LISiN) of the Polytechnic of Turin. The first aim of this project was to face one of the greatest open challenges in the field of industrial exoskeletons: to understand and quantify how the use of exo-skeletal systems can effectively reduce the biomechanical load for workers, assisting them in their postures and movements. In addition, the focus was on the impact of the biomechanical load calculation model of the Ergonomic Assessment Work-Sheet system (EAWS). This is also a tool for assessing the overall risk of biomechanical overload, generated by the use of the passive exoskeleton. Above all, the main result of ESO-EAWS project is the ESO-EAWS Form and the "addendum" to the user manual of the EAWS system, entitled "Exoskeletons Impacts on EAWS Evaluation". This ESO-EAWS version allows calculating the reduction of the ergonomic evaluation score of manual work activities achievable thanks to the use of a passive exoskeleton to which Fondazione Ergo gave a certification. EAWS is recognized by ISO and adopted globally by leading multi-national groups in the industrial manufacturing, automotive, and aerospace and defense sectors. Currently, there are two

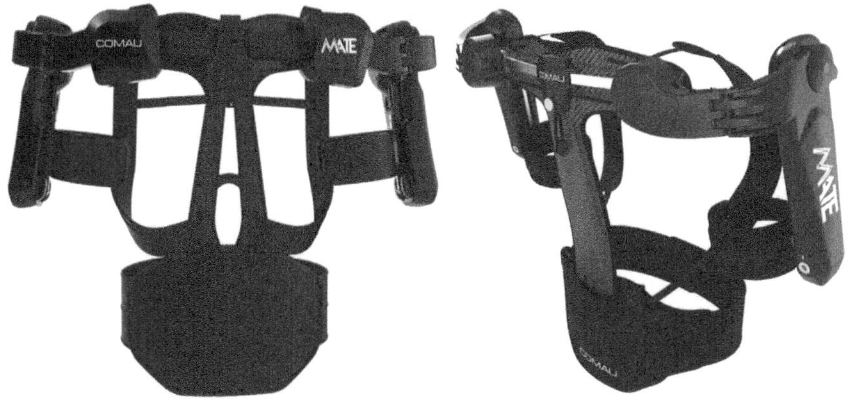

FIGURE 6.3   MATE (left) and MATE-XT (right) exoskeletons.

(*Credit*: IUVO/COMAU)

certified exoskeletons, which are the Muscular Aiding Tech Exoskeleton (MATE) and MATE-XT developed by IUVO-COMAU [69]. IUVO is a spin-off company of Scuola Superiore Sant'Anna (SSSA) in Pisa and its BioRobotics Institute. IUVO was founded on January 2015 by Prof. Nicola Vitiello and his colleagues at the Wearable Robotics Laboratory, which is part of the BioRobotics Institute of Scuola Superiore Sant'Anna in Pisa. IUVO has an agreement with SSSA for the exclusive license to commercially exploit patent applications and know-how of several wearable technologies. In August 2017, COMAU (an Italian company that is a member of the FCA Group and a leader in the field of industrial automation and robotics) and Össur (an Icelandic company that is a market leader in the field of prosthetics and orthotics) invested in IUVO through a joint venture, which holds the majority share of the company. The two investing companies have the goal to foster a wide adoption of wearable robotic technologies in daily life scenarios [70]. In addition, these exoskeletons have the certifications of ISO 13482:2014, CE marked (2006/42/EC), and TÜV Rheinland. Figure 6.3 shows the MATE and MATE-XT exoskeletons.

6.4.10   Paexo Exoskeletons

Paexo exoskeletons are made by Ottobock, a long-established company with 100 years of expertise in the development and production of biomechanical and orthopedic products. Since 2012, Ottobock has been researching innovative solutions to make jobs in industrials, logistics, and the trade sector more ergonomic. Its goal is to provide relief for people who perform physically demanding tasks, such as overhead work, thereby creating healthier working conditions. Ottobock Bionic Exoskeletons offers a broad range of exoskeletons and solutions for logistics, automotive and aviation assembly, maintenance and repair, painting, or construction. Its products are developed at its headquarters in Duderstadt, Germany. Paexo shoulder was certified by ESO-EAWS in July 2021 [71].

6.5   CLOSING REMARKS AND PERSPECTIVES

Some researchers and developers of exoskeletons think that the lack of exoskeleton standards is holding back their adoption in the workplace. In just 5 years, exoskeletons for industrial use have gone from virtually zero to approaching 10,000 commercially purchased units. Little by little, exoskeleton standards are emerging for best practices or guides and starting to have the first users using exoskeletons certified and with the emerging regulation. However, there is still no standardization of how exoskeletons are evaluated in the workplace. There is a lack of controlled tests to categorize exoskeletons and define which one is better than another. If a test is specified that includes a target list for medical exoskeletons, this test must assess that any medical exoskeleton can meet that target list. ASTM International has already published standards on exoskeleton technology (e.g., ASTM-F48), and ISO has also begun including exoskeletons in its standards, such as ISO 13482 Robots and robotic devices—Safety requirements for personal care robots.

Recommended areas of future work are, among others, as follows: assessment techniques for powered and passive exoskeletons, design techniques around human anthropometry, shapes, and job functions, system maintainability standards, system training standards, device certification criteria, third-party certification processes, augmented/extended reality, real-time health monitoring/risk assessment, access to big data systems, standards for artificial intelligence, machine learning safety, and performance enhancements. The market for exoskeleton technology has grown rapidly, and today, there are more than 80 companies around the world working with exoskeletons [72].

Evaluation activity. Please answer the next quiz.
https://forms.office.com/r/Qw67Adme8C

1. Which entity is in charge of regulating health risk in the USA?
   A. Food and Drug Administration (FDA)
   B. Federal Commission for the Protection against Sanitary Risk (COFEPRIS)
   C. International Organization for Standardization (ISO)
   D. International Electrotechnical Commission (IEC)

2. Regulatory entities allow the evaluation of good manufacturing and quality practices, among others, issuing verification certificates through certifying bodies, accreditation entities, and techno-vigilance units.
   A. True
   B. False

3. During the manufacturing process, norms and standards must be applied and metrology measures must be carried out to guarantee the safety, quality, and conformity of the products with the respective norms.
   A. True
   B. False

4. According to the FDA, how are medical devices classified?
   A. Class I, II, and III
   B. Class a, b, and c
   C. According to their risks
   D. None of the above

5. To which class does this description apply: Those inputs recently accepted into medical practice or that are introduced into the body and remain in it for more than 30 days?
   A. Class a
   B. Class B
   C. Class II
   D. Class III

6. NOM-241-SSA1-2012 corresponds to
   A. Good manufacturing practices for medical devices
   B. Standard for risk management in medical devices
   C. Safety requirements for electrical systems
   D. Risk management for information system networks incorporating medical devices

7. According to ISO 62366-1, how an error is described?
   A. Idea, opinion, or expression that a person considers correct but that is actually false or misguided
   B. Action that does not follow what is right, accurate, or true
   C. User's unexpected action or lack of action that could lead to a different result than intended by the manufacturer or user
   D. None of the above

8. The FDA has developed a regulatory cycle model that follows the device lifecycle in parallel to facilitate the process of design, commercialization, and use of the devices and at the same time allow the surveillance and traceability of the products and intervene in the event that incidents with the devices occur and are reported.
   A. True
   B. False

9. What is the other institution that generates relevant standards applicable to exoskeletons in this list: ISO, IEC, SS, JIS, IEEE, and?
   A. COFEPRIS
   B. ASTM
   C. TR
   D. ASSE

10. According to the Official Mexican Standard NOM-241-SSA1-2021, Good manufacturing practices for medical devices, and partially to international guidelines, the category of medical devices based on the function

and purpose of use of the medical device is divided into six large groups: medical equipment; prostheses, orthoses and functional aids (exoskeletons); diagnostic agents; supplies for dental use; surgical and curative materials; and hygiene products.

A. True

B. False

REFERENCES

1. Medina-Valdes, J.L., et al., Study to increase the TRL of exoskeleton ERMIS based on a methodology to the identification of real performance parameters. Applied Sciences, 2021.11(19): p. 9245.
2. FDA. Overview of medical device classification and reclassification, 2017; Available from: www.fda.gov/about-fda/cdrh-transparency/overview-medical-device-classification-and-reclassification.
3. Reifschneider, A., The New US FDA Regulations on Biocompatibility and Reprocessing for Medical Devices. Deutsche Gesellschaft für Regulatory Affairs, Bonn University, 2017: p. 95.
4. Badnjević, A., et al., Inspection of Medical Devices: For Regulatory Purposes. Springer, 2018.
5. Murff, H.J., J.W. Gosbee, and D.W. Bates, Human factors and medical devices. Making Health Care Safer: A Critical Analysis of Patient Safety Practices, 2001: p. 459.
6. CCOHS, Exoskeletons, 2022; Available from: www.ccohs.ca/oshanswers/safety_haz/exoskeletons.html.
7. ASTM, Committee F48 on exoskeletons and exosuits; Available from: www.astm.org/get-involved/technical-committees/committee-f48.
8. ASTM, New test method for standard test method using the user cognition and intent during exoskeleton use (UCI) assessment tool in the industrial domain, 2019; Available from: www.astm.org/products-services/standards-and-publications/standards/workitem-wk68719.
9. ASTM International proposes standards guide, center of excellence for exoskeletons. August 14, 2022, 2019; Available from: https://www.therobotreport.com/astm-proposes-exoskeleton-standards-center-excellence/.
10. ASTM F3323-21. Standard terminology for exoskeletons and exosuits, 2022; Available from: www.astm.org/f3323-21.html.
11. Lowe, B.D., W.G. Billotte, and D.R. Peterson, ASTM F48 formation and standards for industrial exoskeletons and exosuits. IISE Transactions on Occupational Ergonomics and Human Factors, 2019.7(3–4): p. 230–236.
12. ASTM F3444/F3444M-20 Standard practice for training exoskeleton users, 2020; Available from: www.astm.org/f3444_f3444m-20.html.
13. Bostelman, R. and T. Hong, Test methods for exoskeletons—lessons learned from industrial and response robotics. Wearable Exoskeleton Systems: Design, Control and Applications, 2018.13: p. 335–361.
14. Nabeshima, C., et al., Standard performance test of wearable robots for lumbar support. IEEE Robotics and Automation Letters, 2018.3(3): p. 2182–2189.
15. Kozlowski, A.J., et al., Feasibility and safety of a powered exoskeleton for assisted walking for persons with multiple sclerosis: A single-group preliminary study. Archives of Physical Medicine and Rehabilitation, 2017.98(7): p. 1300–1307.
16. Kozlowski, A., T. Bryce, and M. Dijkers, Time and effort required by persons with spinal cord injury to learn to use a powered exoskeleton for assisted walking. Topics in Spinal Cord Injury Rehabilitation, 2015.21(2): p. 110–121.

17. Raab, K., et al., Effects of training with the ReWalk exoskeleton on quality of life in incomplete spinal cord injury: A single case study. Spinal Cord Series and Cases, 2016.2(1): p. 1–3.
18. NIST. Standards related to exoskeletons, 2019; Available from: www.nist.gov/el/intelligent-systems-division-73500/exoskeletons-and-exosuits-research-and-standard-test-3.
19. NPR. Standards, Common requirements for robots; Available from: https://astar-nrp-staging.netlify.app/engineering/standards/.
20. Technical Standards, Human factors and ergonomics society, 2006; Available from: www.hfes.org/Publications/Technical-Standards.
21. He, Y., et al., Risk management and regulations for lower limb medical exoskeletons: A review. Medical Devices: Evidence and Research, 2017: p. 89–107.
22. FDA, 21 CFR 890.3480--Powered lower extremity exoskeleton; Available from: www.ecfr.gov/current/title-21/chapter-I/subchapter-H/part-890/subpart-D/section-890.3480.
23. FDA, §890.1925: Isokinetic testing and evaluation system; Available from: www.ecfr.gov/cgi-bin/text-idx?SID=a01aed88a2ea548118ec143023ae264d&mc=true&node=se21.8.890_11925&rgn=div8.
24. FDA, Indego 510(k) summary, 2016; Available from: www.accessdata.fda.gov/cdrh_docs/pdf15/K152416.pdf.
25. FDA, Ekso classification, 2016; Available from: www.accessdata.fda.gov/scripts/cdrh/cfdocs/cfpmn/pmn_template.cfm?id=k143690.
26. ISO 14971:2007. International Organization for Standardization.
27. FDA, Product classification: Powered exoskeleton, 2016; Available from: www.accessdata.fda.gov/scripts/cdrh/cfdocs/cfPCD/classification.cfm?ID=PHL.
28. FDA, 522 Postmarket surveillance studies, 2016; Available from: www.accessdata.fda.gov/scripts/cdrh/cfdocs/cfPMA/pss.cfm?t_id=347&c_id=2675.
29. Eguren, D. and J.L. Contreras-Vidal, Navigating the FDA medical device regulatory pathways for pediatric lower limb exoskeleton devices. IEEE Systems Journal, 2020.15(2): p. 2361–2368.
30. FDA, Warning letter to ARGO medical technologies, 2015; Available from: www.fda.gov/ICECI/EnforcementActions/WarningLetters/2015/default.htm.
31. ReWalk, ReWalk announces launch of 522 post-market study with Stanford University school of medicine as lead investigator site, 2016; Available from: https://rewalk.com/blog/rewalk-announces-launch-of-522-post-market-study-with-stanford-university-school-of-medicine-as-lead-investigator-site-2/.
32. Zeilig, G., et al., Safety and tolerance of the ReWalk™ exoskeleton suit for ambulation by people with complete spinal cord injury: A pilot study. The Journal of Spinal Cord Medicine, 2012.35(2): p. 96–101.
33. Benson, I., et al., Lower-limb exoskeletons for individuals with chronic spinal cord injury: Findings from a feasibility study. Clinical Rehabilitation, 2016.30(1): p. 73–84.
34. Yang, A., et al., Assessment of in-hospital walking velocity and level of assistance in a powered exoskeleton in persons with spinal cord injury. Topics in Spinal Cord Injury Rehabilitation, 2015.21(2): p. 100–109.
35. Asselin, P., et al., Heart rate and oxygen demand of powered exoskeleton-assisted walking in persons with paraplegia. Journal of Rehabilitation Research and Development, 2015.52(2): p. 147.
36. Farris, R.J., et al., A preliminary assessment of legged mobility provided by a lower limb exoskeleton for persons with paraplegia. IEEE Transactions on Neural Systems and Rehabilitation Engineering, 2013.22(3): p. 482–490.
37. Hartigan, C., et al., Mobility outcomes following five training sessions with a powered exoskeleton. Topics in Spinal Cord Injury Rehabilitation, 2015.21(2): p. 93–99.
38. Contreras-Vidal, J.L., et al., Human-centered design of wearable neuroprostheses and exoskeletons. Ai Magazine, 2015.36(4): p. 12–22.

39. The mechanical exoskeleton shaping the future of health care, 2017; Available from: www.thedailybeast.com/the-mechanical-exoskeleton-shaping-the-future-of-health-care.

40. Ueba, T., et al., Feasibility and safety of acute phase rehabilitation after stroke using the hybrid assistive limb robot suit. Neurologia Medico-Chirurgical, 2013.53(5): p. 287–290.

41. FDA, MAUDE adverse event report: Rex bionics ltd rex rehab. 2016; Available from: www.accessdata.fda.gov/scripts/cdrh/cfdocs/cfmaude/detail.cfm?mdrfoi__id=5793129.

42. FDA, Applying human factors and usability engineering to medical devices, 2016; Available from: www.fda.gov/ucm/groups/fdagov-public/@fdagov-meddev-gen/documents/document/ucm259760.pdf.

43. FDA, Factors to consider when making benefit-risk determinations in medical device premarket approval and de novo classifications; Available from: www.fda.gov/downloads/MedicalDevices/DeviceRegulationandGuidance/GuidanceDocuments/UCM517504.pdf.

44. IEEE, Exoskeletons are on the March, 2016; Available from: http://spectrum.ieee.org/robotics/medical-robots/exoskeletons-are-on-the-march.

45. Buesing, C., et al., Effects of a wearable exoskeleton stride management assist system (SMA®) on spatiotemporal gait characteristics in individuals after stroke: A randomized controlled trial. Journal of Neuroengineering and Rehabilitation, 2015.12(1): p. 1–14.

46. Roh, C.H., Wearable Robot and Method for Controlling the Same. Google Patents, 2020.

47. Panasonic, No more power barriers with Panasonic assists robots, 2016; Available from: http://news.panasonic.com/global/stories/2016/44969.html.

48. Food and H. Drug Administration, Medical devices; Physical medicine devices; classification of the powered lower extremity exoskeleton; Republication. Final order; republication. Federal Register, 2015.80(85): p. 25226–25230.

49. Tamura, A., Understanding Japanese medical device requirements. In 2011 AHC Workshop on Medical Devices: Implementation of GHTF Documents; Asian-Pacific Economic Cooperation: Seoul, Korea, 2011.

50. O'Sullivan, L., R. Nugent, and J. van der Vorm, Standards for the safety of exoskeletons used by industrial workers performing manual handling activities: A contribution from the Robo-Mate project to their future development. Procedia Manufacturing, 2015.3: p. 1418–1425.

51. Da Costa, B.R. and E.R. Vieira, Risk factors for work-related musculoskeletal disorders: A systematic review of recent longitudinal studies. American Journal of Industrial Medicine, 2010.53(3): p. 285–323.

52. Pierre Côté, D. and M. Marjan Vidmar, The prevalence and incidence of work absenteeism involving neck pain. European Spine Journal, 2008.17: p. 192.

53. Stattin, M. and B. Järvholm, Occupation, work environment, and disability pension: A prospective study of construction workers. Scandinavian Journal of Public Health, 2005.33(2): p. 84–90.

54. Riley, M.W., et al., Interactions between task repetition and psychosocial factors. Work, 2012.41(Supplement 1): p. 2392–2397.

55. Bosch, T., et al., The effect of work pace on workload, motor variability and fatigue during simulated light assembly work. Ergonomics, 2011.54(2): p. 154–168.

56. Karsh, B.-T., Theories of work-related musculoskeletal disorders: Implications for ergonomic interventions. Theoretical Issues in Ergonomics Science, 2006.7(1): p. 71–88.

57. UL Enterprise launches new brands, 2022; Available from: www.edie.net/partner-content/ul-enterprise-launches-new-brands/.

58. UL-MX NOM Mark; Available from: https://marks.ul.com/about/ul-listing-and-classification-marks/promotion-and-advertising-guidelines/ul-mx-nom-mark/.

59. Parker, Indego® exoskeleton receives U.S. Regulatory clearance for stroke treatment, 2018; Available from: https://rss.globenewswire.com/fr/news-release/2018/02/15/1348826/0/en/Indego-Exoskeleton-Receives-U-S-Regulatory-Clearance-for-Stroke-Treatment.html.

60. Tobin, J.J. and G. Walsh, Medical product regulatory affairs: Pharmaceuticals, diagnostics, medical devices. John Wiley & Sons, 2008.

61. ExoAtlet's Successful Journey to CE Marking; Available from: https://exoatlet.lu/news/exoatlets-successful-journey-to-ce-marking/.

62. Cray X: The world's first and only robotic exoskeleton with TÜV certification, 2022; Available from: https://germanbionic.com/en/cray-x-the-worlds-first-and-only-robotic-exoskeleton-with-tuev-certification/.

63. Samsung's GEMS exoskeleton earns ISO certification, 2020; Available from: https://en.yna.co.kr/view/AEN20200921003900320.

64. GCC, Samsung's Hip exoskeleton secures ISO certification, 2020; Available from: www.gccbusinessnews.com/samsungs-hip-exoskeleton-secures-iso-certification/.

65. Laevo FLEX 3.0 is the first-ever exoskeleton issued personal protective equipment PPE CE Mark, 2022; Available from: https://exoskeletonreport.com/2022/04/laevo-flex-3-0-is-the-first-ever-exoskeleton-issued-personal-protective-equipment-ppe-ce-mark/.

66. Ekso, Ekso bionics receives FDA clearance to market its EksoNR™ robotic exoskeleton for use with multiple sclerosis patients, 2022; Available from: https://d1io3yog0oux5.cloudfront.net/_2f1a1b4821dbd70e10d7275556e60806/eksobionics/news/2022-06-13_Ekso_Bionics_Receives_FDA_Clearance_to_Market_its__729.pdf.

67. Turkish firm to export robotic gait therapy system to US, 2021; Available from: www.dailysabah.com/business/tech/turkish-firm-to-export-robotic-gait-therapy-system-to-us.

68. CISION, Innophys to begin marketing "muscle suit every" in Europe on acquisition of CE certification showing it meets local safety standards, 2021; Available from: https://en.prnasia.com/releases/apac/innophys-to-begin-marketing-muscle-suit-every-in-europe-on-acquisition-of-ce-certification-showing-it-meets-local-safety-standards-309571.shtml.

69. ERGO, Exoskeleton certification; Available from: www.eaws.it/exoskeleton-certification/.

70. IUVO, Wearable technology, uplifted life; Available from: www.iuvo.company/.

71. Ottobock, Exoskeletons for the back; Available from: https://ottobockexoskeletons.com/?lang=en.

72. Sprinkle, T., Standardization news; Available from: https://sn.astm.org/features/future-exoskeleton-standards-.html.

7 Test Benches and Protocols

7.1 INTRODUCTION

The scheduling of the product development tasks includes critical activities, among which are the assessment of problems in the subsystem's design, the evaluations of the solution proposals, and the validation of said proposals, which allows the approval of each phase of the design of the exoskeleton. The scientific rigor and the precision of the results of the experimentation are fundamental in the decisions taken to increase the technological maturity of the design of the exoskeleton.

The experimental physical model is subject to the evaluation of the operating principle of the exoskeleton, for which a test protocol is established to carry out the experimentation in the test benches defined by experimental batches. There are companies that specialize in developing test benches with which the evaluations of the behavior of the experimental physical model are programmed, including the certifications of the approved tests.

The prototype is subject to the validation of a replicable product, which can be used for demonstration with users and in later stages for industrial demonstration, using pilot batches to verify its behavior with users in different real operating environments. This chapter addresses the design of test benches, and features, outlining of testing protocols, experimentation of subsystems, and the entire exoskeleton, considering the laboratory environment to evaluate the EPM and the real environment to evaluate the prototype.

7.2 STANDARDS FOR EXOSKELETONS TEST

ISO is a worldwide federation of national standards bodies (ISO member bodies). The work of preparing international standards is normally carried out through ISO technical committees. Each member body interested in a subject for which a technical committee has been established has the right to be represented on that committee [1]. ISO collaborates closely with the International Electrotechnical Commission (IEC) on all matters of electrotechnical standardization. The procedures used to develop this document and those intended for its further maintenance are described in the ISO/IEC Directives, Part 1 [2].

This chapter presents documents of test methods for the exoskeleton-type robot which is intended to move from one location to another, by making reciprocal motions having intermittent contact with the travel surface. The possible tests are positional accuracy test of each joint, repeated durability test of actuated applied part, and repeated durability test of support systems.

DOI: 10.1201/9781003261995-7

The possible tests are as follows: positional accuracy test of each joint of the Walking RACA robot, repeated durability test of actuated applied part, and repeated durability test of support systems of the Walking RACA robot. These tests can be used to verify the conformity of the requirements of IEC 80601-2-78. The following documents are referred to in the text in such a way that some or all of their content constitutes requirements [3]:

IEC 80601-2-78:2019—Medical electrical equipment—Part 2–78: Particular requirements for basic safety and essential performance of medical robots for rehabilitation, assessment, compensation, or alleviation.

IEC 60601-1—Medical electrical equipment—Part 1: General requirements for basic safety and essential performance.

ISO and IEC maintain terminological databases for use in standardization at the following addresses: ISO Online browsing platform: available at www.iso.org/obp and IEC Electropedia: available at www.electropedia.org/ [4].

The testing standards are mainly from ISO, with relevant ones from IEC, SS, JIS, IEEE, and ASTM, which include the common requirements for robots. Some standards are the following [5, 6]:

ISO 14971:2019—Medical devices: Application of risk management to medical devices.

ISO/DIS 5363—Test methods for Exoskeleton-type Walking RACA Robot WG2—Personal Care Robot Safety.

ISO 13482:2014—Robots and robotic devices—Safety requirements for personal care.

ISO/DTR 23482-1—Application of ISO 13482—Part 1: Safety-related test methods.

ISO/TR 23482-2:2019—Application of ISO 13482—Part 2: Application guidelines.

WG5—Medical Robot Safety—JWG9: MEE & MES using robotic technology, and JWG36: Medical robots for rehabilitation.

ISO 11161:2007—Safety of Machinery: Integrated Manufacturing Systems—Basic Requirements.

ISO 12100:2010—Safety of machinery—General principles for design—Risk assessment and risk reduction.

ISO 13849-1:2015—Safety of machinery—Safety-related parts of control systems—Part 1: General principles for design.

ISO 13849-2:2012—Safety of machinery—Safety-related parts of control systems—Part 2: Validation.

ISO 25000:2005 (Replacing ISO-9126 and ISO-14598)—Software Engineering—Software product Quality Requirements and Evaluation (SQuaRE)—Guide to SQuaRE Industrial Robots.

ISO 9283:1998—Manipulating industrial robots—Performance criteria and related test methods.

ISO 10218-1:2011—Adopted as Singapore Standard: SS ISO 10218-1:2016—Robots and robotic devices—Safety requirements for industrial robots—Part 1: Robots.

ISO 10218-2:2011—Adopted as Singapore Standard: SS ISO 10218-2:2011—Robots and robotic devices—Safety requirements for industrial robots—Part 2: Robot systems and integration.

ISO/TR 13309:1995—Manipulating industrial robots—Informative guide on test equipment and metrology methods of operation for robot performance evaluation following ISO 9283.

ISO 18646-1:2016—Adopted as Singapore Standard: SS ISO 18646-1:2017—Robotics—Performance criteria and related test methods for service robots.

ISO 18646-2:2019—Robotics—Performance criteria and related test methods for service robots—Part 2: Navigation, Service Robots (Exoskeleton).

ISO 13482:2014—Adopted as Singapore Standard: SS ISO 13482:2017—Robots and robotic devices—Safety requirements for personal care robots.

ISO/TR 23482-1:2020—Robotics—Application of ISO 13482—Part 1: Safety-related test methods.

ISO/TR 23482-2:2019—Robotics—Application of ISO 13482—Part 2: Application guidelines.

ISO 9241-220—Ergonomics of Human-System Interaction.

IEC 60335-2-2:2019—Household and similar electrical appliances—Safety—Part 2–2: Particular requirements for vacuum cleaners and water-suction cleaning appliances.

IEC 62061:2005—Safety of Machinery: Functional Safety of safety-related electrical, electronic, and programmable electronic control systems.

IEC 80601-2-77:2019—Using Standard IEC 80601-2-78 for the Testing of Medical. Exoskeletons and other RACA. Medical electrical equipment—Part 2–77: Particular requirements for the basic safety and essential performance of robotically assisted surgical equipment.

IEC 80601-2-78:2019—Medical electrical equipment—Part 2–78: Particular requirements for basic safety and essential performance of medical robots for rehabilitation, assessment, compensation, or alleviation.

IEEE 730-2014—Software Quality Assurance Processes.

IEEE 1059-1993—Guide for Software Verification and Validation (V&V) Plans.

IEEE 1012-2016—Software, and Hardware Verification and Validation.

JIS B 0138-1996—Industrial robots—Graphical symbols of mechanism.

JIS B 8439:1992—Industrial robots—Programming language slim.

JIS B 8446-1:2016—Safety requirements for personal care robots—Part 1: Static stable mobile servant robot with no manipulator.

JIS B 8446-2:2016—Safety requirements for personal care robots—Part 2: Low power restraint-type physical assistant robot.

JIS B 8446-3:2016—Safety requirements for personal care robots—Part 3: Self-balancing person carrier robot.

JIS B 8456-1:2017—Personal care robots—Part 1: Physical assistant robots for lumbar support.

ASTM F3323—Standard Terminology for Exoskeletons and Exosuits Practice for Labelling and Information on Exoskeletons and Exosuits.

ASTM F3358—Standard Practice for Labelling and Information on Exoskeletons and Exosuits.

ASTM WK65295—New test method for load handling when using an exoskeleton.

ASTM WK65296—New practice for recording environmental conditions for utilization with exoskeleton test methods.

ASTM WK65346—New guide for safety considerations in designing and selecting exoskeletons for Industrial, Medical, and Military applications.

ASTM WK65587—New Guide for Assessing System Training—Service Robots (Healthcare).

ASTM F48.02—Human Factors and Ergonomics.

ASTM F48.02: WK65347—Utilization of Digital Human Modeling.

ASTM F48.02: WK65587—Assessing System Training.

ASTM F48.03—Task Performance and Environmental Considerations.

ASTM F48.03: WK65295—Load Handling when Using an Exoskeleton.

ASTM F48.03: WK65296—Recording Environmental Conditions for Utilization with Exoskeleton Test Methods.

ASTM F48.91: WK60882—Exoskeletons and Exosuits.

ANSI/AAMI HE75:2009—Human Factors Engineering: Design of Medical Devices.

ANSI/HFES 100-2007—Human Factors Engineering of Computer Workstations.

HFES 200-2008—Human Factors Engineering of Software User Interfaces.

Mil-Std-1472H—Department of Defense Design Criteria Standard: Human Engineering.

Mil-Std-882—Department of Defense Standard Practice: System Safety.

7.3 TEST PROTOCOLS AND PRODUCT VALIDATION PROCESS

This chapter is focused on validating exoskeleton design. Previous chapters explained how the design process of exoskeletons includes the design methodology described in Chapter 3, the CAD modeling and CAE simulation shown in Chapter 4, and the CAM assessment and rapid prototypes depicted in Chapter 5. Likewise, Chapters 6, 7, 8, and 9 describe the standards, test benches, usability analysis, and intellectual property, respectively.

The validation of the exoskeleton is carried out through EPM in the test benches and the prototypes in emulation and testing in a real environment, using test protocols and usability metrics. Although there is a lot of information in the literature on exoskeleton design, a common mistake is to experiment without a test protocol or expected error metrics. A testing protocol is a guide to structure the experimentation according to case studies and tasks concerning DPs. Planning the study objectives, cases, tasks, materials, methods, and results report will help get reliable metrics and mitigate risk during design and manufacture. An external laboratory (outsourcing with a trusted partner) specialist in the test can be a good option to increase the readability of the test and to avoid workshop blindness. The design team task will be focused on the analysis of reported data. The test protocol serves for repeatability expectations, acceptance criteria, regulatory requirements, and applicable standards. Typical protocol sections are outlined as follows: scope, purpose, reference documents (test standards, regulatory guidance, previous test reports, and published

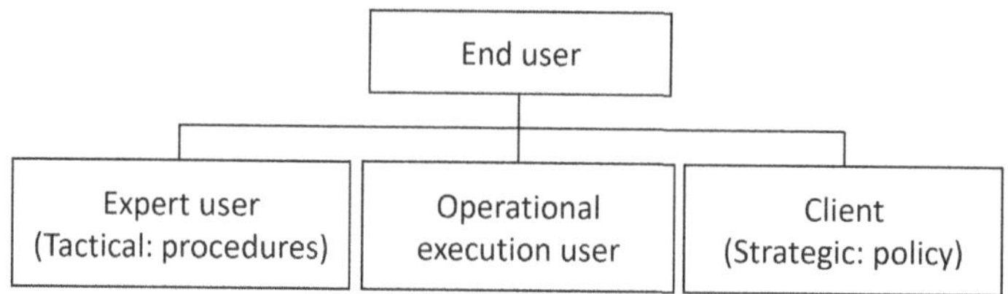

FIGURE 7.1 Classification of end users in exoskeleton design.

literature), test samples, materials and calibrated equipment, methods, acceptance criteria, exception conditions, data analysis, and documentation requirements, references, traceability, specimen preparation, test configurations, testing frequency, and target cycles. target load data or method for load selection, testing environment, testing rates, revision history, and signatures to ensure that all parties are aware of any changes and to get everyone on the same page. Any exceptions, changes, or modifications to the test protocol should also be noted to prevent confusion, set clear expectations, and preserve the necessary information for future reference and use [7].

In the validation stage the accomplishment of end-user requirements is verified, with the end users classified as an expert user who is aware of the tactical issues, which are the procedures for the correct use of an exoskeleton; the operational execution user (OEU), who performs the rehabilitation and assistive activities continually; and the client, who is the responsible for strategic planning and use policy. Figure 7.1 shows the classification of end users in exoskeleton design.

Currently, the approval process for exoskeleton products involves several techniques to ensure they meet end-user requirements, including verification, validation, and qualification. Verification is used to confirm that the exoskeleton has been developed following the required specifications. Validation, on the other hand, is focused on ensuring that the exoskeleton meets the expectations of end users in a real-world environment. Exoskeleton qualification or certification is a component of the product validation process that involves conducting performance and quality assurance tests to meet the criteria and regulations set by certification and accreditation bodies, contracts, or guidelines. Upon passing these tests, a declaration of conformity (DoC) or user satisfaction is issued.

The product approval process considers the FRs and DPs based on the axiomatic design analyzed in the third chapter, requirements to reach the TRL/MRL/IRL established in Figure 3.2, Kano model, usability testing, and UX research methods. Figure 7.2 shows a framework of the product approval process. In the framework, the starting dates are considered from the wide use of the methodologies, which have been maintained, updated, and increased in their impact until now. Through test protocols, the product approval methodologies (PAM) are implemented, reaching end-user expectations. Dr. Suh Nam Pyo developed the axiomatic design based on the independence (coupling, decoupling, and uncoupled FRs) and information (minimizing the information content of the design) axioms [2]. In 1990 several companies popularized the concept of "product platform", and researchers such as Meyer, Lenherd, Utterback, Cusumano, Ulrich, Sanderson, and Uzumeri further developed this concept. In 1995 John C. Mankins created the TRL scale; later, the TRL was

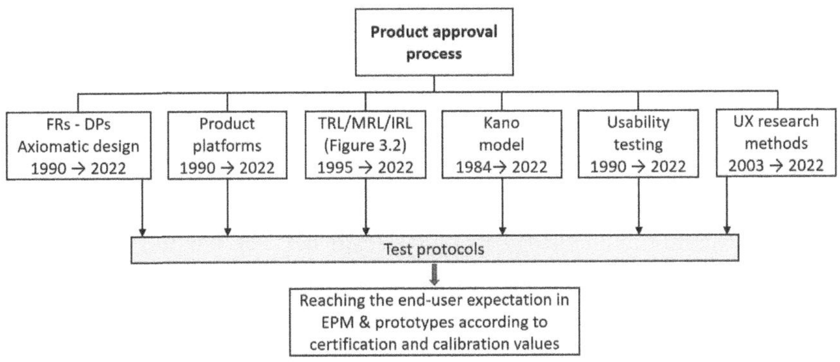

FIGURE 7.2 Framework of the product approval process.

adopted by the U.S. Department of Defense (DOD). In 1984 Noriaki Kano published the Kano model of product development and customer satisfaction, assigning the threshold (expected by the end user), performance (increasing the enjoyment but not essential to the end user), and excitement (surprise elements and delight the end user) attributes. In 1911, usability emerged with the calculation of times and movements during the manufacturing of products, to later reduce the work movement to smaller steps, teaching this method to soldiers to assemble and disassemble exoskeletons in the dark. Later, in 1936, usability was published as a feature of the new Frigidaire, then, in 1947, Bell Laboratories formed the Department of User Preferences, later renamed the Department of Human Factors, in 1957 the Human Factors Society was formed. In 1981, usability and usability testing were described, in 1985 the design for usability was disclosed, in 1986 the System Usability Scale (SUS) became the most used questionnaire for evaluating usability. In 1990, Shackel published a book chapter, as part of the book Human-computer Interaction, called: Human Factors and Usability, which defined usability in terms of efficiency, effectiveness, and satisfaction. These 3 concepts are part of the definition of usability of the ISO 9241 pt 11 standard. From these facts the usability concepts matured, giving way to UX [8]. In 2003 the common UX research methods were established, which include usability testing, user interviews, surveys, card sorting, tree testing, and field studies, among others, so to choose the right UX research method for exoskeleton design, we need to understand the problem and the required data to solve the problem [9].

The certification process can be summed up in the following steps: application (including testing), evaluation (exoskeleton meets qualification criteria), decision, and surveillance (exoskeleton in the marketplace continue to meet qualification criteria). Exoskeleton calibration sets value maximums and minimums by testing the operating principle systematically concerned with a reference standard.

7.4 EXOSKELETON USABILITY AND UX

Currently, the design of exoskeletons often involves the concepts of usability (UX) and customer experience (CX). Usability focuses on the ease of use of the exoskeleton, taking into account factors such as effectiveness (learnability, memorability, and error frequency), efficiency, and satisfaction. UX encompasses a broader range of aspects related to the end user's interaction with the exoskeleton, such as functionality, findability, trust, value, accessibility, and delight. On the other hand, CX is centered around attraction, awareness, advocacy, purchase, discovery, and cultivation.

The usability and UX testing are oriented to improve the exoskeleton performance, in the case of usability making solutions to make the user tasks easier and more intuitive, minimizing steps, removing roadblocks, and finding how and what the therapist does during the exoskeleton operation, while UX involves increasing the meaning and value of the task, emotional connection, and knowing how users feel. The goals of usability testing (UT) usually include identifying problems in the exoskeleton design, uncovering opportunities to improve, and learning about the target user behavior and preferences. The elements of UT are the facilitator, the tasks, and the participant [10].

Things that add cost include competitive testing of multiple designs, international testing in multiple countries, testing with multiple user groups, quantitative studies, and detailed analysis and reports about the findings; participant recruiting costs based on the requirements; expert review is another general method of usability testing. As the name suggests, this method relies on bringing in experts with experience in the field (possibly from companies that specialize in usability testing) to evaluate the usability of a product [11].

7.5 EXOSKELETON EPMS AND DEMONSTRATION PROTOTYPES

The design team previously defined the solution formulation reaching the design concept using mockups, now in the TRL3 the alpha exoskeleton is confirmed, which requires a test protocol that includes evaluating the following: operating principle, which is the inventive activity that refers to novelty, industrialization, and it not easily deductible by an expert in the field; initial materials and manufacturing implications, and the product feasibility regarding market demand, competitors, differential attributes, suppliers, and price estimate. The test protocol for TRL4 is focused on laboratory testing using an experimental pilot of EPMs, considering high safety conditions because performance is unknown due to uncertain variables. The validation of the TRL4 exoskeleton results in the obtaining of EPM approval.

In TRL5 involves the beta exoskeleton. It requires a test protocol that includes evaluating the following: prototype with parts of high reliability and experimental lot, including the demonstration pilot using the optimization due to communality and DFA index; analysis of manufacturing process developed with limited production; and competitive analysis.

7.6 TEST BENCHES AND STANDARDS TO EXOSKELETON PERFORMANCE

The test benches are experimentation platforms for assessment, evaluating, verifying, and validating exoskeleton systems, providing rigorous, transparent, and repeatable analysis of phenomena according to test protocols of standards and testing methods.

A test bench (TB) can be purchased or designed to specific testing requirements. Various instrumentation parts are used for TB design such as sensors, piezoelectric, strain gauges, servomotors, and data acquisition cards (DACs) controlled by a PLC or embedded systems or programming, for instance, in LabVIEW. When the TB design is required, there are two alternatives: either it is planned in parallel to the exoskeleton design, or it is planned once it gets an EPM. If the testing of a new exoskeleton reveals unexpected results, in this case, it is proposed a hypothesis to find the cause and repeat the critical result using destructive proofs.

Correct operation of exoskeleton test benches is as follows: laboratory accreditation and certification bodies, exoskeletons standards, and testing methods. The laboratory accreditation bodies are compliant with the ISO/IEC-17020 (specifies requirements for the competence of bodies performing inspection and for the impartiality and consistency of their inspection activities), ISO/IEC-17025 (enables all types of laboratories that performs testing, sampling, or calibration and providing reliable results), EN ISO-9001 (quality management systems) [12], Home Office Scientific Development Branch (HOSDB) [13], Allied Quality Assurance Publications (AQAP, AQAP-2110 NATO quality assurance requirements for design, development, and production), and codes for entities located outside the United States, which are called NATO Commercial and Government Entity (NCAGE) codes [14]. The accreditation bodies are the National Voluntary Laboratory Accreditation Program (NVLAP) [15] and the American Association for Laboratory Accreditation (A2LA) [16].

Standards and test customization are classified in regulations from organizations and test customization. Standards include the following: Standardization Agreement (STANAG is a NATO standardization document that specifies the agreement of member nations to implement a standard), Allied Engineering Publication (AEP) [17], MIL (for instance, MIL-STD and MIL-H), National Institute of Justice (NIJ) [18], technical guidelines (TR, German abbreviation, Technische Richtlinien), HOSDB, Centre for Applied Science and Technology, Governmental Standard (GOST, Russian acronym for Gosudarstvennyy Standart) [19], ASTM-F1233 (This is a test method for military devices, including military exoskeletons. This method provides a basis for comparative evaluation of ballistic resistance, focusing on factors of tooling, techniques, and duration of event.), ASTM-E3062-16, and ASTM-F48. Figure 7.3 shows the scheme of exoskeleton test benches, considering laboratories, standards, and clinical as well as industrial and military tests.

7.7 EXOSKELETON PROTOTYPES IN A REAL ENVIRONMENT

Version 1 of the exoskeleton prototype is achieved in TRL6, which requires a testing protocol that includes evaluating the following: testing of exoskeleton prototypes in the clinical area, including industrial demonstration using selected and created manufacturing technologies, reproducibility evaluations, and identification of the infrastructure and skills necessary for the component manufacturing process. Exoskeleton prototype version 2 is reached in TRL7, which requires a test protocol that includes evaluating the following: assembly groups validation in outdoor shooting using manufacturing refined and integrated with the risk management plan to test process, materials, and tooling still in development. The validation of the TRL7

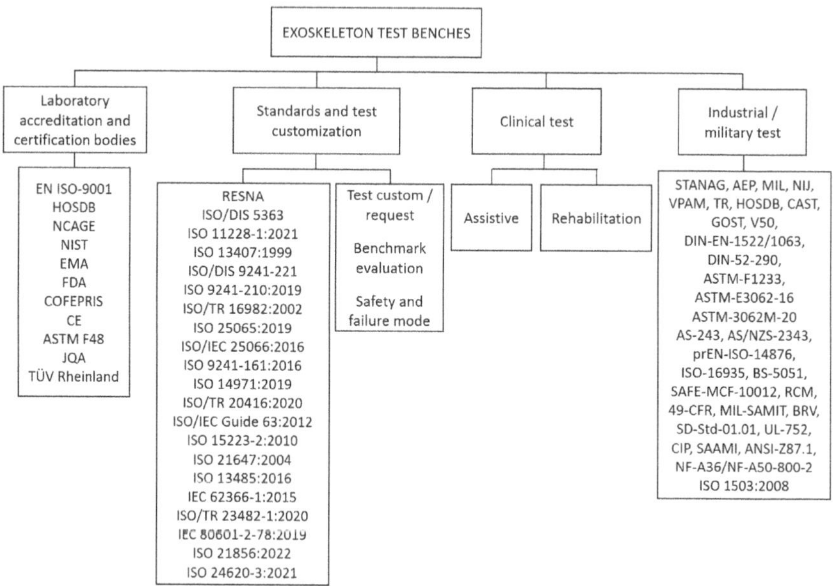

FIGURE 7.3 Test benches for medical, industrial, and military exoskeletons.

exoskeleton prototype results in the obtaining of MPV (low fidelity) approval with feedback from end users and potential clients in field testing with (clinical analysis) users and patients.

Later, to TRL7 a transition phase corresponds to validate the production by assembly groups according to the capability to produce the prototype version 2 reaching the MRL6. A certified exoskeleton (TRL8) requires a test protocol that includes evaluating the performance of certification bodies, pilot lines, final materials, user manual, technical support, and maintenance organization. So, an MPV (high fidelity) is reached with the declaration of conformity with FDA, CE, ISO, ASTM, IEC, ANSI, AAMI, and commercial clearances (ESWA, UL, etc.).

7.8 POLYMER EXOSKELETONS AND 3D-PRINTED PROTOTYPES

New exoskeleton design has been tested using new materials based on cost reduction by homogenizing the components' materials. Initially, the parts were made of steel, aluminum, other metals, or carbon fiber. Since then, several manufacturing processes have been integrated into exoskeletons, achieving today the functional use most of the components made of polymers, maintaining the critical parts made of steel, titanium, and aluminum. Between 1983 and 1986 were developed the first stereolithography (SLA) 3D printed parts in the patent (EP0535720B1) by Charles W. Hull, who in 1986 cofounded 3D Systems. This complemented the RPs manufacturing of exoskeletons, so exoskeleton parts were obtained, helping to design complex components and more attractive nonfunctional prototypes of exoskeletons due to low mechanical resistance of SLA material. Later, in 1988 and 1989 the fused deposition modeling (FDM) technology was developed as described in the patent (US00521329A) by Steven Scott Crump, who in 1989 cofounded Stratasys. This enhanced the RPs manufacturing of exoskeletons hugely, seeing as how the functional prototypes of exoskeletons could be manufactured with better mechanical properties in such a way that the design of the new exoskeleton using FDM and steel parts could be visualized to operate in test benches. Today EPM and RPs manufacturing is done using in the research stage: first SLA, later FDM, and finally, the rapid tooling to the exoskeleton prototype is integrated by steel, FDM (covers and parts except for mechanisms), and polyamide (ASTAMID and VESTAMID) parts. The polyamide parts obtained from RT are possible by the use of vacuum casting, and silicone mold technology has surged since 1970. The exoskeleton has been created using FDM 3D printers to get polymer and metal parts using plastic filament infused with metal powder or nearly full-metal filaments. The company's solid concepts (acquired by Stratasys in 2014) and several researchers and developers have created components for exoskeleton using DMLS technology, using, for instance, the EOSINT M270 Direct Metal 3D Printer.

7.9   EXOSKELETON PERFORMANCE CASE STUDIES

There are several case studies in scientific communications, patents, and more in the reports realized during the authors' experience of this book. Hence, a framework shown in Figure 7.4 on exoskeleton performance case studies (EPCE) has been consolidated to guide readers to an overview of the evaluation of EPMs and prototypes. The EPCE is classified into the following: usability and UX to get users' expected metrics.

The focus of usability and UX is on enhancing safety and performance, and to achieve this goal, desirable features include ergonomic design, adjustable settings, and grips. However, engineering challenges arise with clearances and tolerances when trying to strike a balance between cost-effective manufacturing by minimizing tolerances and incorporating self-adjusting mechanisms to tolerate wider tolerances.

7.9.1   IMPORTANT ASPECTS IN THE TESTING ASSESSMENT

The functional gait assessment (FGA) is a modification of the dynamic gait index (DGI) that uses higher-level tasks to increase the applicability of the test to people with vestibular disorders and to eliminate the ceiling effect of the original test. Three items were added to the DGI because these were noted to be difficult in people with vestibular disorders. The FGA is used to assess postural stability during various walking tasks [20].

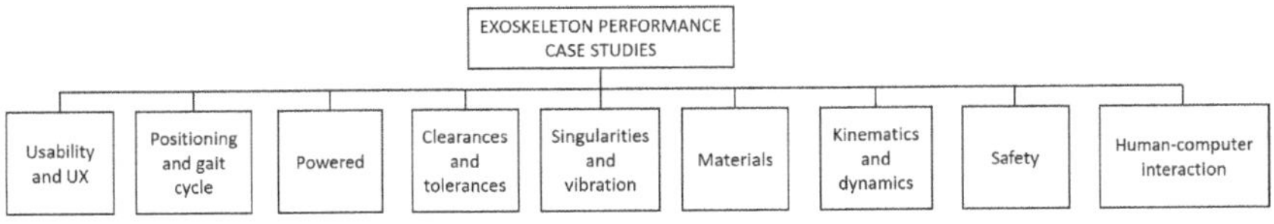

FIGURE 7.4   Framework of exoskeleton performance case studies.

An atypical gait is a common problem in ambulant children with cerebral palsy, making optimizing or improving the efficacy of gait a key orthotic treatment goal. The objective assessment must be equally thorough and include a range of tests, from oculomotor testing to dynamic visual acuity and gait/balance assessments [20]. Someone might have learned the theory of gait quite in detail, including but not limited to the phases, kinematics, kinetics, and EMG. Although, gait analysis practicalities are limited to observational gait analysis.

Gait can be analyzed using various methods—no equipment, minimal equipment, or in a completely equipped lab. The various methods of gait analysis can be broadly classified into two categories i.e., qualitative and quantitative methods. The clinician records the patient's gait using a camera and analyzes it through a slow-motion video. The analysis is done by replaying the video at a slower speed on a phone/computer and identifying abnormal gait patterns. Some examples of commonly used gait scales are The dynamic Gait Index, the Timed Up and Go Test, the and Edinburgh Visual Gait Score.

Quantitative methods of gait analysis include objective measurements of gait using various tools. The type of analyses that come under this category are kinematic analysis, which is the foundational element of every gait lab. This method involves the measurement of lower and upper body joint motion during gait. The assessment includes measurement of joint angles, range of motion (ROM), and spatiotemporal parameters (speed, stance phase). Kinetic analysis aims to understand the forces involved in joint motions. EMG analysis provides essential information on electrical activity and firing patterns of different muscles during the various phases of gait.

7.9.1.1   3D Gait Analysis

The 3D gait analysis is where the setup and analysis process of 3D systems is primarily similar to 2D. However, 3D systems require specialized equipment and infrastructure. Unlike many 2D systems, 3D systems also offer force plates and EMG integration options, increasing their applicability in research. Equipment required includes high-speed infrared cameras (three to eight cameras), retro-reflective markers, calibration frames, advanced computers with increased computational capacity, and force plate/EMG devices [21].

7.9.1.2   Electro-Goniometer/Potentiometer

An electrical goniometer is attached to a joint for measuring the range of motion data while walking. It can give faster data regarding joint angles. Equipment required includes an electro-goniometer, straps, and connection to electrical output [22].

7.9.1.3   Kinetic Gait Analysis

A force plate is a platform embedded with sensors usually placed in the middle of the walkway for gait analysis. As the patient walks over the platform, it provides the magnitude and direction of ground reaction force. Most platforms are submerged inside a cavity in the walkway to ensure a more natural gait pattern and are made invisible to the patient. Similar to a force plate, a pressure plate provides plantar pressure distribution in the feet while walking. Equipment required includes force plates, pressure plates, and photoelastic optical systems.

Another way is using pressure-detecting soles fitted in the shoes to measure plantar pressure, which are used to understand foot structure and function. Another alternative is using sensors placed on the body to record acceleration, angular velocity, and body orientation in space. The accuracy of many IMUs is comparable with 3D kinematic systems. Equipment required includes accelerometers and gyroscopes.

7.9.3.4 Electromyography (EMG) Analysis

Electrodes are placed over the skin, which receives input from a muscle's action potential. When the patient starts walking, the EMG provides information about electrical activity and firing patterns of different muscles during the various phases of gait. Equipment required includes EMG machine, headphones, electrodes, and gel [21].

7.10 CLOSING REMARKS AND PERSPECTIVES

Experimentation in test bench and field testing involves sensitive activities that are carried out using equipment of the latest generation as a recoil test bench. The developers of testing equipment have modernized its technology. The setup and design of the test bench should be viewed as a collaborative activity between vendors, scientists, and developers. Teradyne is a company dedicated exclusively to developing test stations for many areas, including medical devices, industries, defense systems, and the aerospace industry.

There are companies such as Teledyne DALSA, specialists in high-performance digital imaging and semiconductor technology, that fabricate and customize ultra-high-speed imaging systems with frame rates up to 100 million fps. The ultra-high-speed technology is suitable for analyzing the behavior of case studies with systems. Also, this technology allows stress analysis of exoskeleton components.

The instrumentation equipment has evolved to make the software more user friendly with industrial-strength code, libraries, and software development kit (SDK). High-performance 1D/2D CMOS and CCD cameras, 3D sensors of high accuracy laser profiling, stereo imaging and time of flight, image acquisition boards, smart cameras including vision tools with embedded software, uncooled long-wave infrared sensors for industrial and defense applications, and X-ray generators for nondestructive testing (NDT) are also available.

Evaluation activity. Please answer the next quiz.

https://forms.office.com/r/RubySjJQeV

1. The test benches are experimentation platforms for assessment, evaluating, verifying, and validating exoskeleton systems, providing rigorous, transparent, and repeatable analysis of phenomena according to test protocols of standards and testing methods.
   A. True
   B. False

2. What's the difference between validation and verification?
   A. Validation shows the right development of exoskeleton-related requirements; verification is focused on the right exoskeleton to meet end-user expectation in an operative environment.

B. Verification shows the right development of exoskeleton-related requirements; validation is focused on the right exoskeleton to meet end-user expectation in an operative environment.

C. Verification proves that an exoskeleton passed performance and quality assurance test according to outlines, regulations, or conditions of certification bodies, accreditation bodies, and contracts, emitting the declaration of conformity; validation shows the right development of exoskeleton-related requirements.

D. None of the above.

3. What are the types of end user?
   A. Expert user and client
   B. Expert and operational execution user
   C. Expert user, operational execution user, and client
   D. None of the above

4. All of the elements of the following list correspond to product approval processes: axiomatic design, product platforms, TRL, Kano model, usability testing, UX research methods.
   A. True
   B. False

5. What is the last step in the certification process?
   A. Evaluation
   B. Calibration
   C. Decision
   D. Surveillance

6. What covers a wider aspect of end-user interaction with the exoskeleton, including functionality, findability, trust, value, accessibility, and delight?
   A. CX
   B. UX
   C. Usability
   D. Kano model

7. What are the goals of usability testing?
   A. Identifying problems in the exoskeleton design, uncovering opportunities to improve, and learning about the target user behavior and preferences
   B. To cover a wider aspect of end-user interaction with the exoskeleton, including functionality, findability, trust, value, accessibility, and delight
   C. Certification of a product
   D. None of the above

8. The usability and UX testing are designed to improve the exoskeleton, in the case of usability developing solutions to make the user tasks easier and more intuitive, minimizing steps, removing roadblocks, and finding how and what the shooter do it during the exoskeleton operation, while UX is

about increasing the meaning and value of the task, emotional connection, and knowing how the user feels.
   A. True
   B. False

9. Which TRL results in MPV (low fidelity)?
   A. TRL7
   B. TRL8
   C. TRL9
   D. TRL10

10. An MPV (high fidelity) is reached with the declaration of conformity OTAN and commercial clearances.
   A. True
   B. False

REFERENCES

1. ISO, NEN-ISO 18629-43 Industrial automation systems and integration—Process specification language; Available from: www.nen.nl/norm/pdf/preview/document/112313/.
2. ISO, Directives and policies; Available from: www.iso.org/directives-and-policies.html.
3. ISO, 18646-4:2021 Robotics—Performance criteria and related test methods for service robots, Part 4: Lower-back support robots. International Organization for Standardization, 2021: p. 29.
4. ISO, ISO/IEC directives part 2, 2021; Available from: www.iec.ch/members_experts/refdocs/iec/isoiecdir2%7Bed9.0.RLV%7Den.pdf.
5. NIST, Standards related to Exoskeltons; Available from: www.nist.gov/el/intelligent-systems-division-73500/exoskeletons-and-exosuits-research-and-standard-test-3.
6. NRP, Standards, common requirements for robots; Available from: https://astar-nrp-staging.netlify.app/engineering/standards/.
7. Element, Importance of test protocol for medical device projects, 2022; Available from: www.element.com/nucleus/2018/test-protocol-for-medical-devices.
8. Sauro, J., A brief history of usability, 2013; Available from: https://measuringu.com/usability-history/.
9. Maze, Understan ding the top 9 UX research methods & techniques; Available from: https://maze.co/guides/ux-research/ux-research-methods/.
10. Moran, K., Usability testing, 2019; Available from: www.nngroup.com/articles/usability-testing-101/.
11. Standard, A., Standard terminology for additive manufacturing technologies. ASTM International F2792-12a, 2012: p. 1–9.
12. ISO, I., 13485 Management Systems of the Quality of Medical Equipment. ISO, 2016.
13. Boschert, S., C. Heinrich, and R. Rosen, Next generation digital twin. In Proceedings TMCE. Las Palmas de Gran Canaria, 2018.
14. Autiosalo, J., et al., A feature-based framework for structuring industrial digital twins. IEEE Access, 2019.8: p. 1193–1208.
15. Aviles, L.A.Z., et al., Systematic analysis of an IEED unit based in a new methodology for M&S. International Journal of Advanced Robotic Systems, 2010.7(4): p. 27.
16. Roderick, S. and C. Carignan, Designing safety-critical rehabilitation robots. Rehabilitation Robotics, 2007.1: p. 43–64.

17. Kiguchi, K. and Q. Quan, Muscle-model-oriented EMG-based control of an upper-limb power-assist exoskeleton with a neuro-fuzzy modifier. In 2008 IEEE International Conference on Fuzzy Systems (IEEE World Congress on Computational Intelligence). IEEE, 2008.

18. Kiguchi, K., Y. Kose, and Y. Hayashi, An upper-limb power-assist exoskeleton robot with task-oriented perception-assist. In 2010 3rd IEEE RAS & EMBS International Conference on Biomedical Robotics and Biomechatronics. IEEE, 2010.

19. Agrawal, S.K., et al., Design and optimization of a cable driven upper arm exoskeleton. Journal of Medical Devices, 2009.3(3).

20. Objective vestibular assessment. September 28, 2023; Available from: https://www.physio-pedia.com/Objective_Vestibular_Assessment.

21. Eddison, N., Introduction to gait analysis. In Technologies and Techniques in Gait Analysis; Past, Present and Future. The Institution of Engineering and Technology, 2022: p. 16.

22. Parati, M., et al., Video-based goniometer applications for measuring knee joint angles during walking in neurological patients: A validity, reliability and usability study. Sensors, 2023.23(4): p. 2232.

8 Usability Analysis

8.1 INTRODUCTION

Through years of experience, product development has led to the emergence of multiple tools to optimize the design process. Design optimization tends to generate solutions with a certain degree of uncertainty about the usefulness of the exoskeleton generated once it is launched on the market. The design is a balance between elegant solutions, described as simple, intuitive, and innovative. Product innovation is directly related to the assimilation and adoption of technology as quickly and accurately as possible. Therefore, designers try to describe user requirements in as much detail as possible. Once a prototype is obtained, they assess whether it meets user requirements relative to the priority of those requirements. This chapter presents the usability analysis from the assessment of requirements to the evaluation of the usability of the exoskeleton prototypes in the levels of technological maturity in which it is found. This usability analysis results in performance metrics of the exoskeleton prototypes, which allow designers to get satisfaction letters to refine the design. In addition, this chapter describes requirements and usability, usability metrics, methods, and case studies.

8.2 USABILITY

The ISO defines usability as the extent users can use a system, product, or service to achieve specified goals with effectiveness, efficiency, and satisfaction in a specified context. The specified users, goals, and context of use refer to the particular combination of them for which usability is being considered [1]. The word "usability" is also used as a qualifier to refer to the design knowledge, competencies, activities, and design attributes that contribute to usability, such as usability expertise, usability professional, usability engineering, usability method, usability evaluation, and usability heuristic [2].

Meyer et al. describe effectiveness, efficiency, and satisfaction of usability. Effectiveness reflects the accuracy and completeness with which users achieve specified goals; efficiency represents the resources (time, human effort, costs, and materials) used concerning the results achieved; and satisfaction is the extent to which the user's physical, cognitive, and emotional responses that result from the use of a system, product, or service meet the user's needs and expectation [3]. Figure 8.1 shows exoskeleton performance case studies for usability.

8.3 USABILITY METRICS AND METHODS

In the literature, metrics, measures, and key performance indicators (KPI) often overlap; however, they are different. A metric is a system or standard for measuring

DOI: 10.1201/9781003261995-8

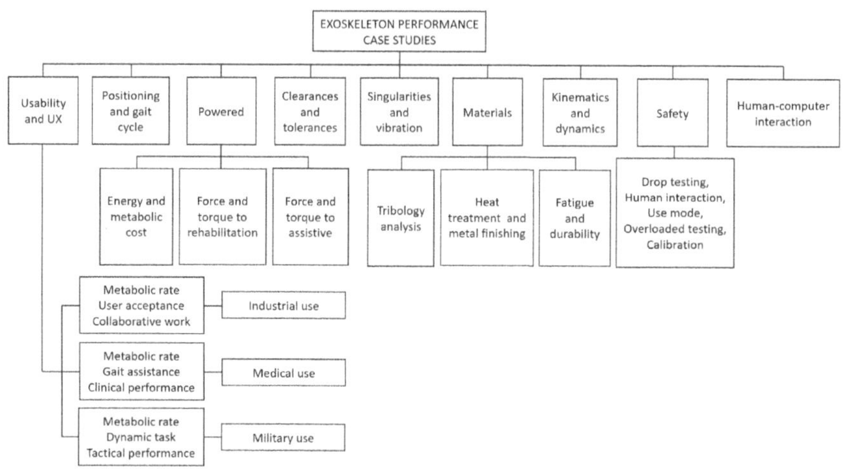

FIGURE 8.1　Exoskeleton performance case studies for usability analysis.

something: a value, number, or measure. KPIs are a subset of metrics, so all KPIs are metrics. A measure is a fundamental or unit-specific term. Then, a value is a number, a dimensional quantity with a measuring unit attached. Some authors refer to the usability implementation as usability metrics for user experience (UMUX), usability measurement, usability index, usability score, usability indicators, or usability values. This chapter uses usability metrics to include the remaining meanings.

The ISO TR 16982-2002 Ergonomics of human-system interaction—Usability methods supporting human-centered design provides an overview of existing usability methods that can be used on their own or in combination to support design and evaluation. Each method is described with its advantages, disadvantages, and other factors relevant to its selection and use. These include the implications of the project's stage in the lifecycle for the choice of method used to design and evaluate [4]. Such issues are dealt with more fully in ISO 9241-11 (Guidance on usability), which is complementary to this technical report and is aimed at system developers, specifiers, and purchasers of systems. Nonetheless, all parties involved in human-centered system development, including the end users of systems, should find the guidance in this technical report relevant. The selection of appropriate usability methods should also take into account the relevant lifecycle process. That technical report is restricted to methods that usability specialists and project managers widely use, so it does not specify the details of how to implement or carry out the usability methods described. Most methods require the involvement of human factor specialists. It may be inappropriate for them to be used by individuals without adequate skills and knowledge [5]. ISO TR 16982-2002 describes methods that imply the direct involvement of users, methods that imply the indirect participation of users (document-based methods), and model-based methods [4].

Adapted from the ISO TR 16982-2002, there are eight specific usability methods: 1. performance-related measurement (PRM), 2. questionnaire/survey, 3. interview, semi-structured (SemiS) or unstructured (Uns) oral feedback, 4. thinking aloud, 5. observation of users, 6. document-based method, 7 model/simulation-based focus, and 8. (usability) expert evaluation [2]. In addition, two usability methods are 9. Toronto Rehabilitation Institute Hand Function Test (TRI-HFT) and 10. experimental characterization [6].

TRI-HFT was developed to assess the gross motor function of the hands of patients with motor impairments and can be deployed to assess the usability of hand robotic exoskeletons for rehabilitation purposes. The test focuses on two main dimensions: the ability to manipulate and grasp strength [7]. Experimental characterization consists of a procedure involving probing and measuring a system's properties. It can be deployed to gauge the usability of a rehabilitative exoskeleton in terms of the torque and speed of the patient's movements [8].

Twenty-six measurements are presented in terms of neurophysiological measure, physiological measure, psychological measure, spatiotemporal metric, eye-tracking recording, and number of steps. Measurement includes standardized functional measures (SFM). This category includes the Upper Limb SFM Box and Block Test (UL-SFM-BBT), Jebsen-Taylor Hand Function Test (JTHFT), Action Research Arm Test (ARAT), Chedoke Arm and Hand Activity Inventory (CAHAI), Southampton Hand Assessment Procedure (SHAP), Assisting Hand Assessment (AHA), Smart Pegboard, Frenchay Arm Test (FAT), lower limb SFM 10 Meter Walk Test (LL-SFM-10MWT), 2 Minute Walk Test (2MWT), 6 Minute Walk Test 6MWT), Timed-Up-and-Go (TUG), General SFM Human-Robot Fluency Metrics (G-SFM-HRF Metrics), Assessment of Capacity for Myoelectric Control (ACMC), Thermography, Failure Mode and Effects Analysis (FMEA), ISO Regulation, Fit and Tolerance Assemblies, Assistive Torque Index (ATI) and Lumbar Compression Reduction (LCR) [3].

Thirty-six scales are presented, which are the Likert Scale (LS), Visual Analogue Scale (VAS), System Usability Scale (SUS), Numeric Rating Scale (NRS), NASA Task Load Index (NASA TLX), Quebec User Evaluation of Satisfaction with Assistive Technology (QUEST 2.0), modified System Usability Scale (mSUS), Raw Task Load Index (RTLX), After Scenario Questionnaire (ASQ), Perceived Usefulness, Perceived Ease of Use (PUEU), Perceived Rate Exertion (PRE), Assistive Technology Device Predisposition Assessment (ATD PA), Post-Study Usability Questionnaire (PSSUQ), Canadian Occupational Performance Measure (COPM), Usability Scale for Assistive Technology (USAT), Intrinsic Motivation Inventory (IMI), Usefulness, Satisfaction, Ease of Use Questionnaire (USEQ), Psychometric Scale to Assess the Satisfaction of Users with Assistive Technology (PYTHEIA), the Questionnaire for User Interaction Satisfaction (QUIS), Borg Scale of Perceived Exertion (BSPE), Michigan Hand Outcomes Questionnaire (MHOQ), Prosthesis Evaluation Questionnaire (PEQ), Psychosocial Impact of Assistive Device (PIAD), Questionnaire to Explore Human Factors and Their Technical Potential (QEHFTP), QuickDASH, SF-36, Telehealthcare Satisfaction Questionnaire—Wearable Technology (TSQ-WT), Trinity Amputation and Prosthesis Experience Scale (TAPXS), Usability Metric for User Experience (UMUX), Embodiment Questionnaire (EQ)

Ad hoc questionnaires, AttrakDiff, Self-Assessment Manikin, Heuristic evaluation, FUREO, SWAT, and ERPs [3]. Table 8.1 shows the 10 methods, 15 attributes/criteria, 26 measurements, and 36 scales.

TABLE 8.1

Usability Metrics and Methods

| Methods | Metrics | | |
	Attributes/ Criteria	Measurement	Scales
PRM Questionnaire/ Survey	Functionality	Neurophysiological measure	LS
Interview- SemiS-UnS	Ease of use	Physiological measure	VAS
Thinking aloud	Performance	Psychological measure	SUS
Observation of users	Safety	Spatiotemporal metric	NASA TLX
Document-based method	Comfort	Eye-tracking recording	QUEST 2.0
Model/simula- tion-based focus	Benefit	Number of steps	mSUS
Expert evaluation	Reliability	SFM:	RTLX
Focus group	Ergonomics	UL-SFM-BBT	ASQ
TRI-HFT	Technical req.	JTHFT	PUEU
Experimental characterization	Wearability	ARAT	PRE
	Adaptability	CAHAI	ATD-PA
	User needs	SHAP	PSSUQ
	Autonomy	AHA	COPM
	Feasibility	Smart Pegboard	USAT
	Intuitiveness	FAT	IMI
		LL-SFM-10MWT	USEQ
		2MWT	PYTHEIA
		6MWT	QUIS
		TUG	BSPE
		G-SFM-HRF Metrics	MHOQ
		ACMC	PEQ
		Thermography	PIAD
		FMEA	QEHFTP
		ISO regulation	QuickDASH
		Fit & Tol-Ass	SF-36
		ATI	TSQ-WT
		LCR	TAPXS
			UMUX
			EQ
			Ad hoc questionnaires
			AttrakDiff
			Self-Assessment Manikin
			Heuristic evaluation
			FUREO
			SWAT
			ERPs

TABLE 8.2

Measurement and Evaluation of Exoskeletons

Item	Exoskeleton Experiment	Evaluation
1	Maximal voluntary isometric contraction (MVIC)	Electromyography (EMG)
2	Change in calories	Energy expenditure
3	Changes in heart rate	Electrocardiogram (ECG, EKG)
4	Body kinematics	Motion capture
5	Physical demands	Rate of Perceived Exertion (RPE)
6	Physical discomfort	Discomfort Survey
7	Usability and acceptance	General feedback
8	Assistive torque index (ATI)	Instrumented human-shaped body dummy to simulate trunk movement
9	Lumbar compression reduction (LCR)	
10	Range of motion in the lumbar spine	Trunk movements for assessing ROM
11	Compressive spinal loads	Dynamic EMG-assisted spine model
12	Joint compression, muscle forces in the shoulder	Biomechanical model
13	Disc compression/shear forces; muscle forces	Biomechanical modeling and simulation
14	Deep tissue oxygenation	Circumferential compression testing
15	Peak and mean EMG in the back and leg muscles	Symmetric and asymmetric lifting
16	Algometry measures	Pressure tolerance testing
17	Number of errors; task completion time	Simulated overhead drilling task
18	User's movement; working postures	The simulated manual assembly task

Table 8.2 shows applications for exoskeleton experiments and evaluation, including methods, techniques, and devices.

8.4 CASE STUDIES

8.4.1 Usability Comparison of ReWalk, Ekso, and HAL Exoskeletons

Since the 1970s, research has been conducted to design exoskeletons to help people with paraplegia overcome limited mobility. Three different devices (ReWalk, Ekso, and HAL) were tested in the following study [9]. Two of these systems (Ekso and HAL) have been an integral part of the treatment of paraplegic patients at our center Bergmannstrost in Halle (Saale) since April 2014. The Ekso is used to treat complete and incomplete paraplegic patients; with a device called Variable Assist, it is possible to use remaining muscle function when paraplegia is incomplete. The HAL is used for therapy of paraplegic patients with a Janda strength level of at least 3/5 for hip flexion and knee extension. The results show that while exoskeletons can be used as therapy aids to supplement existing options, they are not an alternative to a wheelchair and should not be prescribed as orthopedic devices. The systems require further optimization to make them safe enough to be used as orthopedic devices.Every year, there are around 130,000 new cases of paraplegia worldwide. The consequence is usually permanent dependence on a wheelchair. In addition to the physical changes, those affected perceive the obviousness of their condition to be particularly unpleasant. Sitting in a wheelchair and "looking up" to other people combined with limited mobility, especially on uneven ground or when overcoming differences in height, such as stairs, are described as particularly stressful. To improve this situation and give a paraplegic individual the chance to stand and walk again, meet other people at eye level, and overcome the current limitations of mobility, there has been ongoing research into the development of exoskeletons since the 1970s. The study presented here tested the clinical feasibility of three different exoskeleton systems.

8.4.1.1   Methods

From January to June 2013, the ReWalk and Ekso exoskeletons were tested at the Centre for Spine Injuries of the occupational health and safety hospital in Halle (Saale), Germany. Exoskeleton therapy has been an integral component of treatment there since April 2014. In addition to the Ekso, the HAL is now also used for therapy. To date, 22 patients have received therapy with one of the exoskeletons. The level of the patient's lesions varied from C7 to L1, ASIA A. The patients' weights were between 55 and 100 kg, and their ages were between 34 and 62 years. The paraplegia had been present between 6 months and 29 years. All patients used an active wheelchair in their daily activities.

To test the time required for therapy, the times for converting and adapting the exoskeletons and putting them on and taking them off were measured. The length of each balance and gait training session was determined. The number of therapists required was also noted. The therapy period was between 2 and 10 weeks, and the number of therapy sessions per patient was between 2 and 30; a therapy session consisted of a maximum of 45 minutes of walking, including donning and doffing the exoskeleton. Parallel to various medical examinations, the practicality of each exoskeleton in clinical routine was tested. The goal was and is to discover indications and contraindications for exoskeleton therapy, develop a therapy algorithm, determine the physical and mental impact of therapy, and detect potential technical weak points.

8.4.1.2   ReWalk and Ekso

Computer-controlled motors assist in standing, walking, and standing up/sitting down. The desired program must be selected during therapy. The program is started by inclining the torso and thus shifting the center of gravity. Stride length, width, and duration must be set before therapy and adjusted during therapy as needed. Therapy must be interrupted for this.

For the ReWalk, the parameters must be determined on a trial basis; for the Ekso, there is a dimension sheet with recommendations depending on height and leg length. Patients with contractures greater than 10° in the hip or knee joint, leg length differences of more than 2 cm, or total hip replacements cannot use the exoskeleton. Hip flexion of approximately 130° is required to achieve the position for standing up. In patients with a total hip replacement, this can lead to dislocation. When walking, the hip joint is extended by the motor. If there are contractures, there is a risk of tendon avulsion. Flexion contractures in the knee joint lead to a functional difference in leg length. This means that the swing leg cannot be adequately relieved; walking is difficult.

For patients with rotational errors or axis deviations in the lower limbs, therapy can be attempted on a trial basis. However, the greater the deviation from normal anatomy, the greater the risk of putting excessive stress on the adjacent joints. The forearm crutches included must be placed far to the rear for standing up/sitting down. This requires good mobility in the shoulder girdle. It is not possible with either of these two devices to change stride height or width while walking. This means it is impossible to overcome obstacles or compensate for uneven ground. In the authors' opinion, they should therefore be used only on level ground and with a therapist's assistance. The patients agreed with this appraisal.

8.4.1.3 ReWalk

The torso is not secured in the orthosis, making active torso control necessary. The direct adaptation of patients to the orthosis using straps led to pressure points and skin abrasions in the trochanters, the fibular head, and the malleoli, especially the medial malleolus.

The straps do not allow patients, especially overweight patients, to be secured adequately. Unintended flexion occurs in the knee joints, resulting in a posterior shift of the body's center of gravity. This is compounded by the backpack containing the battery for the device. To counteract this situation and avoid falling backward, the torso had to be bent forward disproportionately, which put a very high load on the upper limbs. In some patients, this reactivated existing osteoarthritis. In addition, anterolateral shifting of the body's center of gravity was considerably more difficult, the swing leg could not be adequately relieved, and the stride could not be correctly initiated. Error messages and activation of the safety mode occurred frequently. The method of securing the lower limbs has since been modified. However, no data is available on any improvements this has led to.

The three-point gait pattern in the ReWalk is not physiological. Using stairs, which is possible according to the manufacturer, was tested but was shown to be associated with a very high risk of falling when ascending stairs, especially when descending stairs. The handrail and a crutch were used to ascend stairs. The torso must be shifted backward on the swing leg side and flexed toward the contralateral side after initiating a step to place the swing leg onto the next step of the stairs. When descending stairs, the height difference must be overcome, and the center of gravity is shifted far to the front. An attempt to descend stairs was broken off because it was deemed to be too dangerous. Because of existing instability, walking with forearm crutches was sometimes difficult for patients. When standing up/sitting down, the ringlike device for securing the forearm crutches exerts pressure at the bend of the elbow. This led to hematomas. According to the manufacturer, a modification will be made. In the authors' opinion, the ReWalk is suitable as a therapy device under a therapist's supervision for the following patients: maximum weight 100 kg; height 160 –190 cm; complete paraplegia with torso stability maintained; an attempt should be made to achieve a normal weight due to the problems described in securing the device.

8.4.1.4 Ekso

The torso is secured by a system of straps to a back plate that is firmly attached to the orthosis. The patient can be adequately stabilized in the orthosis with a wide abdominal strap; the center of gravity remains in the middle. The required battery is in a backpack; however, due to the back plate, it does not pull the patient backward as the back plate effectively secures the torso. The lower limbs are secured by a system of clamps attached to the orthosis itself at a certain distance. This ensures very high stability even for overweight patients. The center of gravity was not shifted backward in any of the patients. No pressure points were found. The reciprocal gait is similar to a physiological gait pattern. Patients can walk with the aid of a rollator or with forearm crutches. The rollator is perceived very positively by patients because it feels safer than forearm crutches, especially in the beginning.

Furthermore, with the Ekso there is the option of using the Variable Assist device. This allows the active use of any existing residual muscle function in the lower limbs; the motor power is adjusted accordingly. The necessity of adapting the stride cycle of the exoskeleton is described as difficult, as it cannot be actively controlled by the patient. In the authors' view, the Ekso is suitable as a therapy device under a therapist's supervision for the following: patients with complete and incomplete paraplegia and quadriplegia; maximum weight 100 kg; height 150–190 cm; active stabilization of the upper limbs, especially the elbows and wrists, must be possible; the patient must be able to use the walking aids safely. For incomplete paraplegia, the patient must adapt to the gait cycle of the device but can use his or her muscle strength with Variable Assist.

8.4.1.5 HAL

Unlike the ReWalk and Ekso, in the HAL, the stride is initiated and controlled by myoelectric potentials. To do this, electrodes that are connected to a computer are attached to the relevant muscle groups in the lower limb. Depending on the potentials detected, the computer coordinates the stride cycle and the required support of the respective muscle groups depending on the current phase of the cycle. This mechanism allows patients to control the stride on their own. The height and length of the stride can also be varied, which makes it possible to overcome obstacles. The patient can't rest using the fixed extension of the knee and hip joints during the resting phase. To allow the patient to rest, therapy must be conducted on the Woodway, or the patient must have enough strength on their own to maintain the extension of the hip and knee joints. These requirements mean that therapy with HAL is suitable for patients with incomplete paraplegia with a strength level of 3/5 on the Janda scale for hip flexion and knee extension. Alternative therapy options should be considered for levels below this. Patients can walk on a treadmill or, with the help of devices such as a rollator, on level ground. No tests have been conducted yet for walking using forearm crutches and walking without devices, however, both are considered to be possible under the appropriate circumstances. Using the Woodway, therapy is presumably also possible for patients with reduced torso control and strength in the upper limbs, but there is no practical experience with this. Therapy appears to be limited at this time by the standardization of the existing therapy devices. This standardization is based on an Asian standard that does not take adequate consideration of European patient populations. Regulating the width of the pelvic bar appears to be especially problematic. Another problem is the very short battery life during therapy.

During active use, the battery needs to be replaced after just 15–20 minutes. The authors' opinion is that the HAL is a suitable therapy device under a therapist's supervision for the following: patients with complete and incomplete paraplegia with a strength level of at least 3/5 on the Janda scale for hip flexion and knee extension; height from 150–190 cm; maximum weight 95 kg.

8.4.2 Usability Analysis in an Exoskeleton for Upper Limb Rehabilitation

According to the Handbook of Usability Testing [10], the main objective of these tests is to collect information on users' perceptions of design. There are different approaches when performing functionality tests. The objective of performing a usability test in this methodology is to analyze the perception that specialists have with the design of the exoskeleton. The usability analysis consisted of three phases [11]:

Pre-test: a survey focused on the academic level of the users and their workload during the rehabilitation sessions. Test: in this phase, the specialists analyzed the design of the exoskeleton and its components such as the screen, safety buttons, patient support, etc., and then a task was performed which consisted of simulating a rehabilitation session without a patient so that they could analyze the task analysis and device functionality. Post-test: in this phase, the specialists asked design engineers questions to know which aspects are intuitive and which require a prior introduction; they also made more specific comments on the design. The usability test consisted of six sections: The first section, "User Environment Profiling", takes into account issues such as interaction with the patient regarding a clinical environment. The second section, "Design", lets us know if the exoskeleton design is attractive, safe, and easy to use. The third section, "Interaction", encompasses factors such as the coupling of the exoskeleton to the body. The fourth section, "Ergonomic", analyzes the components of adaptability and the position of the patients and therapists. The fifth section tackles the task analysis considering factors such as the range of movement, mechanical stops, and safety. In the end, the sixth section covers the functionality evaluation to know if the device could be implemented in health centers to support physiotherapists. Each section contained five questions as answers to each question. The Likert scale suggested in [11] was used, which consists of the following options: strongly disagree, disagree, neutral, agree, and strongly agree. Each answer was assigned scoring criteria to make a statistical analysis of the positions of specialists regarding the design and use of the exoskeleton. This analysis was applied to 12 physiotherapists and three doctors. The highest score was given in the task analysis. Doctors and therapists considered this section the most important topic when evaluating a medical device because it determines the usefulness of the exoskeleton. The lowest score was given in the functionality area because this section is required to do experimentation with patients to establish the rehabilitation treatment. Overall, the evaluation result was acceptable getting an average of 4.015; for this reason, it was considered that the exoskeleton development can continue to the next stage, keeping its current technical specifications.

Two physiotherapists who approved the analysis of usability were invited to work on a pair of case studies (stage 12). It proposed a healthy patient emulate a rehabilitation protocol for shoulder-elbow and elbow-wrist to evaluate the tracking of ERMIS. The case studies were developed always under the guidance of the safety protocol established by the regulations inside [12, 13].

One of the most important points was that the physiotherapist in charge and one of the design engineers were present during the sessions of rehabilitation. Before the sessions, it was necessary to verify the presence and functionality of an emergency stop button and the electrical safety.

Depending on the protocol, the tasks, the intensity of the training, and the speed have been adapted individually [11]. Case study 1: a 39-year-old male performed a rehabilitation routine for shoulder-elbow, and the rehabilitation protocol simulated that the arm rotates like a rudder. The protocol included movements for the shoulder and elbow joints. At all times the training was supervised by a physiotherapist, who provided assistance and instructions for the patient, and a medical doctor in charge of documentation and supervision was present.

Case study 2: a 47-year-old female performed a rehabilitation routine for an elbow-wrist. The rehabilitation protocol included independent movements for each of the elbow and wrist joints. The procedure consisted of selecting the joint to be worked on (wrist) and immobilizing the rest of the joints of the arm by means of bandages or with the participation of a second therapist, but in this case, the therapy only uses the exoskeleton for immobilizing the rest of the joints (shoulder and elbow).

For stage 13, a summary of the previous stages is presented, with an emphasis on the cases of study and usability. A meeting was held with members of each team together with the team of specialists, and an opinion was issued stating that the exoskeleton works for passive rehabilitation, but the materials that were chosen are not the best. A budget is suggested to update mechanical elements with other types of materials. In addition, a recommendation for improving the interface design in HMI should be more intuitive for the therapist. It is suggested that a more extensive study be made regarding compatibility for patients of different sizes because the range of sizes that the exoskeleton can use is unknown.

This methodology is highlighted by the level of information that it manages from the perspective of the patient, therapist, and the clinical environment not only from the technological view but also includes the contextual view—this fact enabled the device to be accepted in 87.94% according to usability criteria. The methodology allowed to development of an EPM of an exoskeleton in 2 years with limited resources. The information is stored in a database and is embedded in a virtual environment inspired by the methodology of the digital twins. The use of technological know-how from other areas such as the industrial area allowed use of an industrial CPU within the medical area, which was robust enough to be able to perform rehabilitation therapy. The methodology integrates the validation of the exoskeleton through the analysis of the case studies. For the exoskeleton, it is demonstrated that is possible to reproduce the rehabilitation exercises in the patient in the same way as conventional therapy. For case study 1, the exoskeleton can follow 98.56% of the original trajectory, and for case study 2, 94.97% [11].

8.4.3 USABILITY ANALYSIS IN A WRIST TELEREHABILITATION ROBOTIC SYSTEM

The Wrist Telerehabilitation Robot System (WiTRoS) includes a wrist rehabilitation differential robot capable of generating the movements of flexion, extension, supination, pronation, ulnar and radial deviation. This system helps the physiotherapist adapt the rehabilitation protocol according to the needs of each patient, between passive rehabilitation and active rehabilitation, varying the time, the number of repetitions, and the range of motion for each exercise. The system has a control interface that is programmed by the physiotherapist from the clinic, then sends the data to a server. The robot downloads the package of parameters from the network, and it executes the exercises with the patient at home. The system has a mobile application (app) that provides visual feedback relating to the rehabilitation protocol through games. During the COVID-19 pandemic, it was observed that the rehabilitation medical could not be covered because of the lockdown. Hence, the telerehabilitation system was evaluated in ten patients, allowing the movement recovery protocol to continue. This work shows the usability study, where it is observed that the patients improved their range movement; also, it reduced the time for the therapy, and it was determined to have a score of 4.6 out of a total of 6.

Telecare is a technology for remote assessment and intervention in medicine [14], also more widely referred to as telepractice or telehealth; it is effective, efficient, affordable [15], and generally equivalent to caring for people [16]. Telerehabilitation is the term used for telehealth applied in rehabilitation [17]. Either it can be just a teleconference when the therapist tells the patient how to do the exercise, or it can use intelligent therapeutic robots that are supervised by the clinic or the therapist. The goal of telerehabilitation is to provide access for all and to help patients to face societal challenges by providing rehabilitation services.

Telerehabilitation platforms use different devices for motor and cognitive rehabilitation based on the neurorehabilitation process, which uses repetition. It develops the motor learning processes and promotes brain plasticity, but this repetition should lead to cortical connection as it creates some functional tasks [17].

Telerehabilitation is divided into three types by the kind of tools used. The first is the use of a virtual reality environment; the Ho Shin [18] study uses virtual reality rehabilitation for patients with damage to the upper limb after a stroke, and it shows the improvement results in patients who used the augmented reality (AR) system vs. patients who followed a conventional therapy, delivering better results patients who used AR. Caetano [19] describes the use of AR with disabled people who are training to drive a wheelchair; this AR system allows users to try scenarios that can help with the troubleshooting problems that arise in the operation of wheelchairs.

The second type of telerehabilitation is based on images which are characterized by maintaining a remote conference between the patient and the therapist. The work presented by Bragaglia [20] uses a Kinect joystick as a rehabilitation tool scanning the movements of the therapist; the system sends these movements to the patient, who follows the exercises through the help of another Kinect completing the rehabilitation protocol. This kind of telerehabilitation has a subdivision called postsurgical tele-training, which offers remote rehabilitation after a surgical process. Rehabilitation concentrates on regaining range of motion and strength and relieving sensitivity in the surgical area, as the work presented by Heuser [21] performs wrist rehabilitation work after tendon reconstruction surgery.

The third type is telerehabilitation based on sensors. Holst's [22] project applied the use of motion sensors to evaluate and perform therapy on patients who suffered a stroke that affected their motor capacity in their lower limbs; Serrano [23] has developed a sensory rehabilitation project in patients with upper limb damage performing therapies at home with a mat that includes an interface that relates texture with visual stimuli. In recent years we can observe the development of devices or applications in telerehabilitation. The lockdown caused by COVID-19 increased the need for tele-medicine when trying to cover the largest number of patients, and the sessions had a significant impact on improving mobility.

The usability analysis in telerehabilitation devices allows us to understand the impact on the patient and the therapist; this usability analysis determines the viability of the project. The viability of a telerehabilitation project is related to the impact that the patient generates on the ecosystem, considering indirect users such as the patient's assistant, who is the person that supports the rehabilitation sessions, and access to an Internet connection [24]. During the development of this project, the contribution of Michael Pramuka's [25] research in the analysis of accessibility and usability of rehabilitation devices was taken into account; it was designed under the analysis of factors such as the complexity of use, connectivity, cost, installation, synchronization, and interface.

Through a study with 27 patients, R. Maxime [26] demonstrates the advantages of using a robot in rehabilitation; it allows the necessary repetitions applying the same characteristics one after another, which improves neurorehabilitation. Therefore, it increases the range of motion. The analysis of 23 patients shows that the use of robots in rehabilitation therapies increases the range of motion by 30% while conventional therapies by only 21%.

In this context, the interest in performing wrist rehabilitation therapies was raised through the WiTRos, which consists of a database in the server, an app for smartphones, a robot, and a control interface that allows the therapist to monitor the results of the patient's sessions.

During the construction of the conceptual model, a usability study was carried out regarding the impact and analysis of therapists, who analyzed the design, the safety, the ease of use, and the range of movement to perform a complete rehabilitation protocol. The average score in each one obtained was 2.65/6.0, which is less than 50% approval of the design.

The system was reformulated considering the methodology for the design of rehabilitation devices [27] regarding the requirements and constraints analysis according to the characteristics of the rehabilitation, protocol, design criteria, and standards for medical device design. Also, it was created a simulation system in software in order to know the dynamics of the device.

The new robot version reaches 80° flexion, 80° extension, 80° supination, 80° pronation, 30° ulnar deviation, and 20° radial deviation, guaranteeing that the device allows 100% replication of the range's anatomical movements.

The telerehabilitation procedure is carried out first by logging a new patient into the database from the physiotherapist's computer. The app on the physiotherapist's computer contains the guide for the patient's rehabilitation training and manages the patient's rehabilitation protocol. It can distribute rehabilitation tasks to the wrist rehabilitation robot. It also displays the patient's rehabilitation data captured in the database, and it helps the physiotherapist understand the session's evolution and if the patient does the rehabilitation protocol correctly. The wrist rehabilitation robot is controlled by an embedded system that can connect to the Internet by ethernet cable and allows to download of the tasks that the therapist saved on the server. The network acts as a bridge to transmit the information between the server and the wrist rehabilitation robot. The rehabilitation robot saves training data in the server database, and the physiotherapist can see the results of the rehabilitation session at any time. As needed, enter the web application with the user name and password to see the databases.

The haptic device hardware is composed of a CPU based on the Arduino DUE board, two DC servo motors, two AS5041 magnetic encoders, and an emergency stop button. Also, the Arduino manages a w5100 Ethernet card and a Bluetooth transceiver.

For the clinical trial, five physiotherapists participated and invited and selected some affected patients in the follow-up of their rehabilitation sessions due to the confinement of the pandemic. The selection was made based on their pathologies so that they could benefit from the Wrist Telerehabilitation Robot System. Ten patients agreed to participate in the case studies. In the initial evaluation, the range of motion is measured for flexion-extension (F-E), pronation-supination (P-S), and radial deviation-ulnar deviation (UD-RD). These parameters will be compared with the values obtained at the end of the cycle of programmed sessions.

Two rehabilitation sessions were scheduled per week, and each patient had a different number of weeks scheduled according to their condition. Each therapy session lasted 1 hour, which includes the time in which the routine is connected and loaded, as well as putting the hand and securing it inside the Rehabilitator, adding the net time of the mobilization.

The Rehabilitator arrives at the patient's home through a logistics service; a briefcase containing the Rehabilitator, an Ethernet cable, and a power cable are delivered. The patient only has to connect the Ethernet cable to their modem and connect the cable power to its electrical outlet; then the patient puts the Rehabilitator on a table and opens the application with the patient's interface establishing a connection with a smartphone, where they enter their name and asks the Rehabilitator to download the routine that the therapist programmed. Meanwhile, the patient introduces his hand into the device and secures it. These operations can be done alone or if it is necessary, accompanied. When the session is loaded, the patient starts the device on the smartphone, and the mobilizer begins the rehabilitation routine. When the session is over, the telerehabilitation system uploads the collected data to the database. The system is repacked, and the logistics staff picks it up at the door of the house and sanitizes it to deliver it to the next patient. All the time, there is a technician who can remotely help the patient by answering any questions, either by the therapist or by the patient, and at the end of each working day to calibrate the device.

The analysis of the telerehabilitation system is divided into three parts; the first part analyzes the results of the impact that the rehabilitation sessions have on the patient, the second analyzes the impact on the work of the physiotherapist, and the third analyzes the feasibility and usability of the system of telerehabilitation.

8.4.3.1 Impact on the Patient

One of the aspects to be highlighted is that all the patients who participated completed their entire rehabilitation session. The abandonment of rehabilitation sessions is reduced with the use of remote therapies since it allows the patient not stay home, reducing the time and costs of the sessions [28]. For a specific analysis, the range of motion of each wrist joint is compared with the range of motion movement at the end of all programmed sessions; then the difference between each range value is calculated. It is known from previous studies [29] that patients with similar pathologies and following an equivalent therapy regimen present less increase in their range of motion in the same period in such a way that it is concluded that the remote rehabilitation system can improve the results of face-to-face therapies.

8.4.3.2 Impact on the Physiotherapist's Work

This analysis compared the way of working after and before confinement due to the pandemic for COVID-19. The therapist usually attended 23 sessions a week spread over a 6- to 8-hour shift for 5 days, which in total represents 35 hours a week; this data only refers to wrist rehabilitation. In the remote modality, with the help of the telerehabilitation system, the therapist schedules and programs the characteristics of the protocol of the ten patients for a week in half a working day. This includes the two sessions of each one; the rest of their day throughout of the week is dedicated to evaluating the data that is uploaded to the database at the end of each session. At the end of the week, the therapist can review the progress and decide which protocol each patient should follow the next week—that is, if the ranges in mobilizations are maintained or if they increase. The therapist has more time to monitor the progress of each one or to attend to more patients; in addition, he or she does not suffer physical wear and tear that comes with mobilizing the patient's wrist with their own force. Even more, The therapist does not put themself at risk by being in contact with the patients to avoid contracting or spreading COVID.

8.5 CLOSING REMARKS

With the growing trend of globalization and strict production demands, the modern exoskeleton industry is experiencing much greater pressure to attain high-quality exoskeletons at a low cost of production. While conventional machining processes continue to be used in the manufacturing of small exoskeletons, new technologies have been emerging over the years. These technologies range from the use of CNC machines, special casting processes, forming processes, injection processes, and powder metallurgy processes, to additive manufacturing processes (3D printing) capable of fabricating a three-dimensional object from an STL format file, which looks like a work of science fiction. Manufacturing processes are an integral part of the design of products, such that that they should be taken into account from the early stages of design. The selection of the appropriate technology and manufacturing process is necessary for the exoskeleton components to reach the expected requirements and to ensure that the entire exoskeleton works safely and reliably.

Evaluation activity. Please answer the next quiz.

https://forms.office.com/r/Fd0CHT0mLv

1. The ISO defines usability as the extent to which users can use a system, product, or service to achieve specified goals with effectiveness, efficiency, and satisfaction in a specified context.
   A. True
   B. False

2. The word "usability" is also used as a qualifier to refer to the design knowledge, competencies, activities, and design attributes that contribute to usability, such as usability expertise, usability professional, usability engineering, usability method, usability evaluation, and usability heuristic.
   A. True
   B. False

3. KPIs are a subset of metrics.
   A. True
   B. False

4. A metric is a system or standard for measuring something by means of a value, number, or measure.
   A. True
   B. False

5. Adapted from the ISO TR 16982-2002, the eight specific usability methods are 1. performance-related measurement (PRM), 2. questionnaire/survey, 3. interview, semi-structured (SemiS) or unstructured (UnS) oral feedback, 4. thinking aloud, 5. observation of users, 6. document-based method, 7. model/simulation-based focus, and 8. usability expert evaluation.
   A. True
   B. False

REFERENCES

1. Roto, V., Human-Centred design, 2019; Available from: https://mycourses.aalto.fi/pluginfile.php/951629/course/section/132657/1-HumanCentredDesign.pdf.

2. Koivusilta, T., Improving the initial user experience of the construction operations management app punchzee. In Faculty of Information Technology and Communication Sciences. Tampere, 2021: p. 72.

3. Meyer, J.T., R. Gassert, and O. Lambercy, An analysis of usability evaluation practices and contexts of use in wearable robotics. Journal of Neuroengineering and Rehabilitation, 2021.18(1): p. 1–15.

4. Technical report ISO/TR 16982; Available from: www.sis.se/api/document/preview/901955/.

5. A4BLUE, Report on the standardization landscape and applicable standards. 6.

6. Standard, I., Ergonomics of Human-System Interaction–Usability Methods Supporting Human-Centered Design. ISO Standard TR 16982: 2002. International Organization for Standardization, 2002.

7. La Bara, L.M.A., et al., Assessment methods of usability and cognitive workload of rehabilitative exoskeletons: A systematic review. Applied Sciences, 2021.11(15): p. 7146.

8. Vitiello, N., et al., Functional design of a powered elbow orthosis toward its clinical employment. IEEE/ASME Transactions on Mechatronics, 2016.21(4): p. 1880–1891.

9. Nitschke, J., et al., Comparison of the Usability of the Rewalk, Ekso and Hal Exoskeletons in a Clinical Setting. Orthopadie Technik, 2014.

10. Rubin, J. and D. Chisnell, Handbook of Usability Testing: How to Plan, Design and Conduct Effective Tests. John Wiley & Sons, 2008.

11. Cruz Martínez, G.M. and L.Z. Avilés, Design methodology for rehabilitation robots: Application in an exoskeleton for upper limb rehabilitation. Applied Sciences, 2020.10(16): p. 5459.

12. ISO, I., 13485 Management Systems of the Quality of Medical Equipment. ISO, 2016.

13. De Salud, S., NOM-241-SSA1-2012 Good Manufacturing Practices for Establishments. Norma Official Mexicana, 2012.

14. Rashid, L., Telemedicine and health care. Telemedicine Journal and e-Health, 2002.8(1).

15. Olson, C.A., et al., The current pediatric telehealth landscape. Pediatrics, 2018.141(3).

16. Shigekawa, E., et al., The current state of telehealth evidence: A rapid review. Health Affairs, 2018.37(12): p. 1975–1982.

17. Winters, J.M., Telerehabilitation research: Emerging opportunities. Annual Review of Biomedical Engineering, 2002.4(1): p. 287–320.

18. Shin, J.-H., H. Ryu, and S.H. Jang, A task-specific interactive game-based virtual reality rehabilitation system for patients with stroke: A usability test and two clinical experiments. Journal of Neuroengineering and Rehabilitation, 2014.11(1): p. 1–10.

19. Caetano, D.S.D., et al., The augmented reality telerehabilitation system for powered wheelchair user's training. Journal of Communication and Information Systems, 2020.35(1): p. 51–60.

20. Bragaglia, S., S. Di Monte, and P. Mello, A distributed system using ms kinect and event calculus for adaptive physiotherapist rehabilitation. In 2014 Eighth International Conference on Complex, Intelligent and Software Intensive Systems. IEEE, 2014.

21. Heuser, A., et al., Telerehabilitation using the Rutgers master II glove following carpal tunnel release surgery: Proof-of-concept. IEEE Transactions on Neural Systems and Rehabilitation Engineering, 2007.15(1): p. 43–49.

22. Holst, A., et al., Patients' experiences of a computerised self-help program for treating depression–a qualitative study of Internet mediated cognitive behavioural therapy in primary care. Scandinavian Journal of Primary Health Care, 2017.35(1): p. 46–53.

23. Vidrios-Serrano, C., et al., Integración de Un Sistema Robótico de Terapia Ocupacional para Extremidades Superiores con Estimulación Visual/Táctil de Los Pacientes. Revista Mexicana De Ingeniería Biomédica, 2018.39(2): p. 144–164.

24. Tanner, K., et al., Feasibility and acceptability of clinical pediatric telerehabilitation services. International Journal of Telerehabilitation, 2020.12(2): p. 43.

25. Pramuka, M. and L. Van Roosmalen, Telerehabilitation technologies: Accessibility and usability. International Journal of Telerehabilitation, 2009.1(1): p. 85.
26. Lum, P.S., et al., Robot-assisted movement training compared with conventional therapy techniques for the rehabilitation of upper-limb motor function after stroke. Archives of Physical Medicine and Rehabilitation, 2002.83(7): p. 952–959.
27. Cruz Martínez, G.M. and L. Z.-Avilés, Design methodology for rehabilitation robots: Application in an exoskeleton for upper limb rehabilitation. Applied Sciences, 2020.10(16): p. 5459.
28. Covert, L.T., J.T. Slevin, and J. Hatterman, The effect of telerehabilitation on missed appointment rates. International Journal of Telerehabilitation, 2018.10(2): p. 65.
29. Schmeler, M.R., et al., Telerehabilitation clinical and vocational applications for assistive technology: Research, opportunities, and challenges. International Journal of Telerehabilitation, 2009.1(1): p. 59.

9 Intellectual Property

9.1 INTRODUCTION

Scientometric and patentometric studies reflect that, unlike consolidated companies, most of the information on new exoskeletons only reaches a level of technological maturity of TRL3; furthermore, these exoskeletons are developed by universities and are not patented. This way of working is not convenient in the development of these medical devices, since the first images and relevant technical information of the development of the exoskeleton are disclosed, which means that later it cannot be patented due to that prior disclosure. Intellectual property comprises industrial property and copyright. This chapter is dedicated to presenting the background of intellectual property, the sections of the technical specification of the patent documents, and the structure and wording of the claims. Also, this chapter describes case studies of different kinds of exoskeletons.

9.2 INDUSTRIAL PROPERTY

The creation of new products such as exoskeletons is carried out with the constant work of covering needs and problems or taking advantage of opportunities. The needs are covered with the acquisition of one's own resources or investment projects, while the problems are solved through research projects according to an evaluation horizon. The opportunities are covered with usually short-term projects, which through intellectual property instruments allow technology transfers that are materialized through license agreements for use, and exploitation, with or without exclusivity, concessions, or franchises.

Industrial property includes patents, trademarks, and trade secrets. Patents include invention patents, utility models, industrial designs, and layout designs (topographies) of integrated circuits. Integrated circuit schematics are a three-dimensional arrangement of elements that make up an integrated circuit intended to be manufactured. This arrangement and order of elements obey the electronic function that said integrated circuit is going to perform. Industrial designs are figures of industrial property that guarantee originality, ornamentation, shape, and appearance; industrial designs include industrial models and drawings. Industrial drawings are a whole combination of figures, lines, or colors that are incorporated into an industrial product for ornamentation purposes and that give it a peculiar and unique appearance. Industrial models are made by any three-dimensional shape that serves as a type or pattern for the manufacture of an industrial product, which gives it a special appearance if it does not imply technical effects.

DOI: 10.1201/9781003261995-9

Utility models are objects, utensils, devices, or tools that, because of a change in their arrangement, configuration, structure, or shape, present a different function concerning the parts that make it up or advantages in terms of their utility.

An invention patent is an original product or process that can be manufactured at an industrial level and that contains an inventive step. The inventive step is the characterizing part that is not easily deducible by a person skilled in the art.

In this sense, the development of an exoskeleton begins with the search for the state of the art in patent sites such as Google Patents, Lens, Espacenet, USPTO, Patentscope, and sites of the different patent offices. Technological surveillance is also carried out to obtain statistical information that allows deciding the exoskeleton design approach based on technological trends and prospective studies.

With the help of these patent search tools, the key companies that develop exoskeletons are defined, among which are Fourier Intelligence (China), Axosuits (Romania), Free Bionics (Taiwan), Innophys Company (Japan), Noonee (Germany), Walkbot (South Korea), Ekso Bionics Holdings, Inc. (USA), ReWalk Robotics (USA), ReWalk Robotics (Israel), Ottobock (Germany), Lockheed Martin Corporation (USA), Parker Hannifin Corp. (USA), Cyberdyne, Inc. (Japan), DIH Technologies Corporation (China), Rex Bionics Ltd. (UK), Hyundai Motor Company (South Korea), US Bionics (USA), Gogoa.eu (Spain), ATOUN, Inc. (Japan), RB3D (France), BIONIK (Canada), Honda Motor Co. Ltd (Japan), Sarcos Corp. (USA), Technaid SL (Spain), Hocoma (Switzerland), Focal Meditech (Netherlands), Wearable Robotics SRL (Italy), B-TEMIA, Inc. (Canada), Bioventus (USA), ExoAtlet (Luxembourg), Meditouch (Israel), Suit X (USA), MarsiBionics (Spain), Rehab-Robotics Company Limited (China), Myomo, Inc. (USA), Wandercraft (France), Medexo Robotics (China).

The main pathologies that appear in the invention patents analyzed include the following pathologies: spinal cord injury, multiple sclerosis, cerebral palsy, and stroke. The systems that make up an exoskeleton are hardware, sensors, actuators, control systems, power sources, and software.

9.3 PATENTOMETRIC STUDY

This patentometric study is a systematic review using several tools such as Google Patents, Epacenet, Lens, USPTO, Patentscope, and WIPO statics. Figure 9.1 shows the production of industrial designs, invention patents or only patents, trademarks, and utility models between 2012 and 2021 [1].

Worldwide, more patents have been applied for using the Patent Cooperation Treaty (PCT) than directly in the regional patent offices (direct patents) in the period from 2012 to 2021, as can be seen in Figure 9.2 [2].

When analyzing patent applications and granted patents, it can be seen that China is the leader in this market, followed by the United States. It is interesting to see which Chinese companies have the most patent applications via PCT [3], which is shown in Table 9.1.

The Madrid System is a solution for registering and managing trademarks worldwide using one centralized system [4]. Table 9.2 shows the top applicants from China.

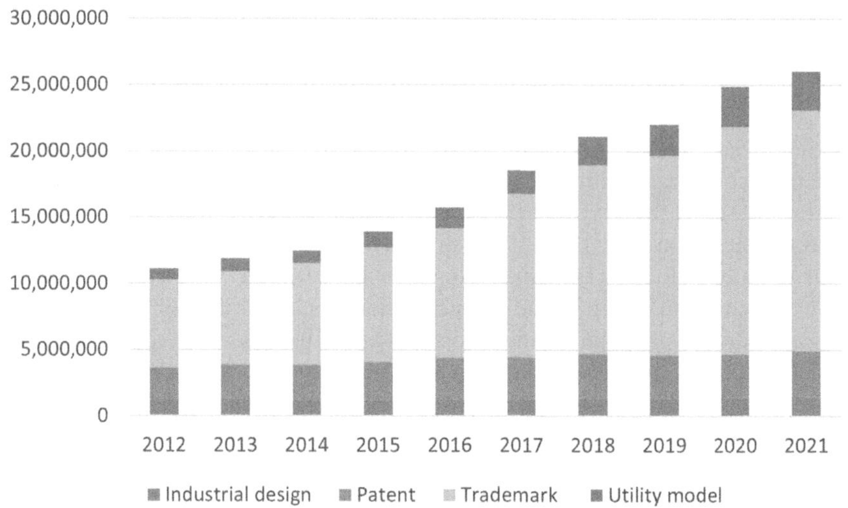

FIGURE 9.1   Industrial property between 2012 and 2021.

(*Credit*: WIPO)

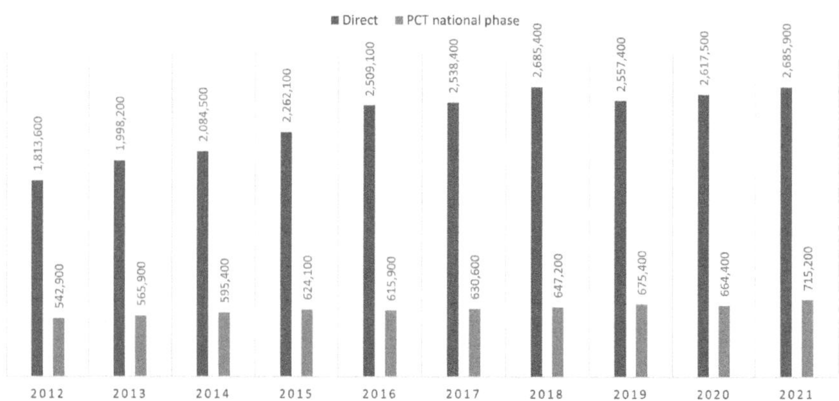

FIGURE 9.2   PCT patents and direct patents.

(*Credit*: WIPO)

The Hague System for the International Registration of Industrial Designs provides a solution for registering up to 100 designs in 95 countries by filing a single international application [5]. Table 9.3 shows the top applicants from China.

In the case of the USA, the main companies that use the PCT systems are shown in Table 9.4. Although it appears that these companies do not develop exoskeletons, many of them supply technological systems that deal with the development of these skeletons, such as materials companies as well as actuator and sensor manufacturers [6].

TABLE 9.1
PCT Top Applicants from China

Applicant	2019	2020	2021
Huawei Technologies Co., Ltd.	4,411	5,464	6,952
Guang Dong Oppo Mobile Telecommunications Corp., Ltd	1,927	1,801	2,208
Boe Technology Group Co., Ltd	1,864	1,892	1,980
Ping and Technology (Shenzhen) Co., Ltd.	1,691	1,304	1,564
Zte Corporation	1,085	1,316	1,493
Vivo Mobile Communication Co., Ltd.	603	955	1,336
Sz Dji Technology Co., Ltd	874	1,073	1,042
Aac Acoustic Technologies (Shenzhen) Co., Ltd.	1	298	679
Wuhan China Star Optoelectronics Semiconductor	506	872	648
Shenzhen China Star Optoelectronics Semiconductor	654	872	647

TABLE 9.2
Top Applicants from China

Applicant	2019	2020	2021
Huawei Technologies Co., Ltd.	164	197	98
Honor Device Co., Ltd.			38
Xiaomi, Inc.	22	25	21
Bestway Inflatables & Material Corp.	4	2	17
Hashkey Digital Asset Group Limited			15
Shengli Oilfield Shengji; Petroleum Equipment Co., Ltd.			15
Third Pole of the Earth; Industrial Development Cor. Ltd.			13
Midea Group Co., Ltd.	13	4	12
Shenzhen Smoore Technology Limited	4	1	12
Dongguan Yueke; Enterprise Management Serv. Co., Ltd.			11

TABLE 9.3
Top Applicants from China

Applicant	2019	2020	2021
Beijing Xiaomi Mobile Software Co., Ltd.	172	516	227
Midea Group Co., Ltd.	26	56	104
Ninebot Tech. Co., Ltd.	26	90	98
Citic Dicastal Co., Ltd.	92	36	78
Gree Electric Appliances, Inc. of Zhuhai	25	38	15
Beijing Rockrobo Technology Co., Ltd.		1	14
Shenzhen Tcl New Technology Co., Ltd.			12
Beijing Jingdong Qianshi Technology Co., Ltd.			8
Ecoflow, Inc.			8
Shenzhen Breo Technology Co., Ltd.			7

TABLE 9.4

PCT Top Applicants from the USA

Applicant	2019	2020	2021
Qualcomm Incorporated	2,127	2,173	3,931
Hewlett-Packard Development Company, L. P.	1,507	1,595	1,485
Microsoft Technology Licensing, LLC	1,370	1,529	1,303
Google, Inc.	777	781	763
3m Innovative Properties Company	662	789	660
International Business Machines Corporation	477	359	576
Applied Materials, Inc.	467	635	571
University of California	470	559	551
Micron Technology, Inc.	451	524	504
Halliburton Energy Services, Inc.	371	558	449

TABLE 9.5

Top Applicants from the USA

Applicant	2019	2020	2021
Apple, Inc.	104	80	92
Bath & Body Works Brand Management, Inc.	27	6	57
Gobrands, Inc.	2		43
Applied Materials, Inc.	20	36	41
Microsoft Corporation	63	52	40
Liberty Procurement Co., Inc.	4	24	38
Upper Deck Company		1	37
Dr. Seuss Enterprises, LP	1		32
Spectrum Brands, Inc.		5	31
Fk Irons, Inc.		1	28

Table 9.5 shows the Madrid System top applicants from the USA. These companies have applied for modification, renewal, or expansion in the issue of trademarks [6].

Table 9.6 shows the Hague System top applicants from the USA. These companies have applied to protect their industrial designs internationally [6].

9.3.1 TRENDS IN ROBOTICS PATENTS

Trends analysis in the development of robotic technology, which has been consolidated in invention patents, shows how China has grown in this field. Between 2005 and 2019, China led the granting of robotics patents, representing almost 35% of the world's total robotics patents. Japan reached 20.8%, South Korea 15.4%, and the United States approximately 13% of the total production of robotics patents in the

TABLE 9.6

Top Applicants from the USA

Applicant	2019	2020	2021
Procter & Gamble Co.	405	623	665
Gillette Company LLC	199	144	135
Microsoft Corporation	29	96	109
Gavrieli Brands LLC			92
Rh Us, LLC			78
Abbott Diabetes Care, Inc.			70
Magic Leap, Inc.	63	320	37
Spectrum Brands, Inc.	6	7	34
Paccar, Inc.			30
Ideal Industries Lighting LLC			

world during this period. The development of exoskeletons has an impact on industrial, medical and military categories [7].

The United States leads robotics patents in areas such as aerospace, medical, military/security, and telepresence, as well as robotics patents with artificial intelligence functions. China leads patents for industrial robotics, transportation, exoskeleton, agriculture, underwater applications, and education. [7].

9.3.2 INTERNATIONAL PATENT CLASSIFICATION (IPC)

The International Patent Classification (IPC), established by the Strasbourg Agreement of 1971, provides a hierarchical system of language-independent symbols for the classification of patents and utility models according to the different areas of technology to which they belong [8]. Exoskeletons have various IPC classifications depending on components and applications.

The Locarno Classification, established by the Locarno Agreement in 1968, is an international classification system used for the registration of industrial designs [9]. Industrial exoskeleton designs according to the Locarno classification are classes 24, 12, and 13. Class 24 is medical and laboratory equipment. The term "medical equipment" also covers surgical, dental, and veterinary equipment. In this context, subclassification 24-05 is walking aids, and subclassification 105129 groups robotic exoskeleton suits [9].

Class 12 refers to means of transport or hoisting, including all vehicles (land, sea, air, space) and others, including parts, components, and accessories which exist only in connection with a vehicle and cannot be placed in another class. These parts, components, and accessories of vehicles are to be placed in the subclass of the vehicle in question, not including scale models of vehicles (Cl. 21-01). Class 12 is placed in classification 105130 – Robotic exoskeleton suits for lifting loads [9].

Class 13 refers to equipment for production, distribution, or transformation of electricity, including only apparatuses that produce, distribute, or transform electric current, including electric motors [9].

The Nice Classification (NCL), established by the Nice Agreement (1957), is an international classification of goods and services that have applied for trademark registration [10]. In the Nice classification, the trademarks of exoskeletons are classified in class 7 or 10. Class 7 refers to machines, machine tools, power-operated tools; motors and engines: 070582 robotic exoskeleton suits, other than for medical purposes. Class 10 refers to surgical, medical, dental, and veterinary apparatus, and instruments; artificial limbs, eyes, and teeth; orthopedic articles; suture materials; therapeutic and assistive devices adapted for persons with disabilities; massage apparatus; apparatus, devices, and articles for nursing infants; and sexual activity apparatus, devices, and articles: 100264 robotic exoskeleton suits for medical purposes [10]. Table 9.7 shows the IPC classification using exoskeleton patents.

The IPC class A61H refers to physical therapy apparatus, e.g., devices for locating or stimulating reflex points in the body; artificial respiration; massage; and bathing devices for special therapeutic or hygienic purposes or specific parts of the body, A61H1/00: apparatus for passive exercising; vibrating apparatus; chiropractic devices, and A61H1/02: stretching or bending apparatus for exercising [11]. Figure 9.3 shows the top 20 countries for IPC class A61H1/02.

TABLE 9.7

IPC Classification for Exoskeletons

IPC	Description
A61H1/0244	Hip.
A61H1/02	Stretching or bending or torsional apparatus for exercising. Stretching or bending
A61H1/0237	apparatus for exercising the lower limbs.
A61H1/0262	Walking movement; appliances for aiding disabled users to walk.
A61H3/00	Appliances for aiding patients or disabled persons to walk about.
B25J13/088	Controls for manipulators employing sensing devices.
B25J9/0006	Exoskeletons, i.e., resembling a human figure.
A61H2201/0173	This means preventing injuries.
A61H2201/0196	Automatically adjusted according to the anthropometric user data. Driving means
A61H2201/1207	electric or magnetic drive.
A61H2201/1623	Back.
A61H2201/1626	Holding and means used in fastening or support.
A61H2201/1642	Holding.
A61H2201/165	Wearable interfaces. Movement of interface, i.e., force application means
A61H2201/1671	rotational.
A61H2201/50	Control.
A61H2201/5058	Sensors or detectors.
A61H2201/5061	Force sensors.
A61H2201/5084	Acceleration sensors.
A61H2203/0406	Standing on the feet.
A61H2205/088	Hip.
A61H2205/10	Leg.

Figure 9.4 shows the top assignees for IPC class A61H1/02. It is interesting to highlight that Toyota appears two times as Toyota Jidosha and Toyota Motor Corp in patent applications of exoskeletons.

Figure 9.5 shows the applications by year for IPC class A61H1/02. It is interesting to highlight the growth of patent applications for exoskeletons between 2012 and 2023.

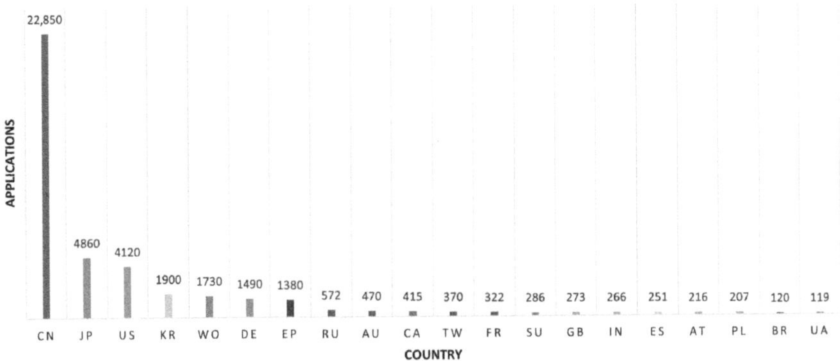

FIGURE 9.3 Top 20 countries for IPC class: A61H1/02.

(*Credit*: PatBase Analytics)

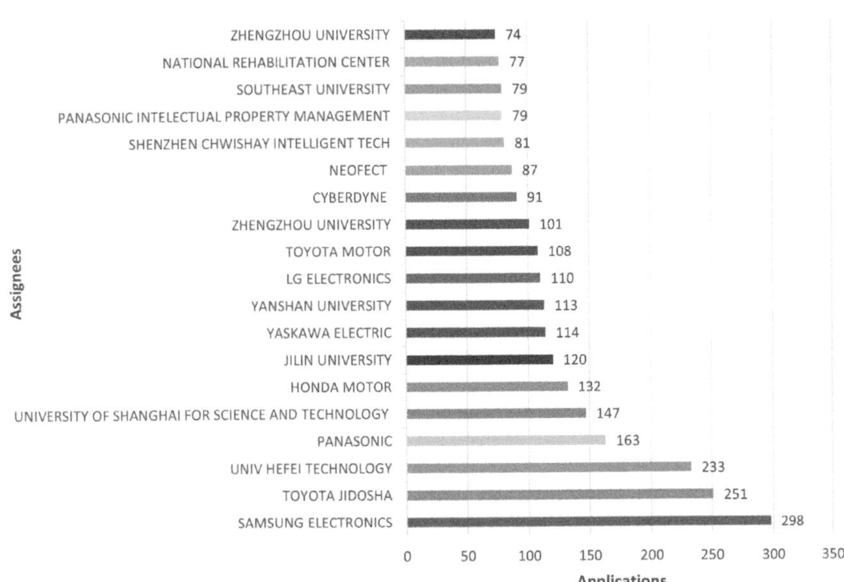

FIGURE 9.4 Top assignees for IPC class A61H1/02.

(*Credit*: PatBase Analytics)

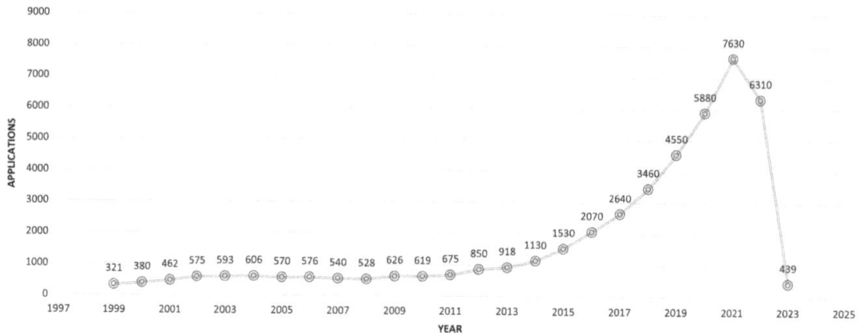

FIGURE 9.5   Applications by year for IPC class A61H1/02.

(*Credit*: PatBase Analytics)

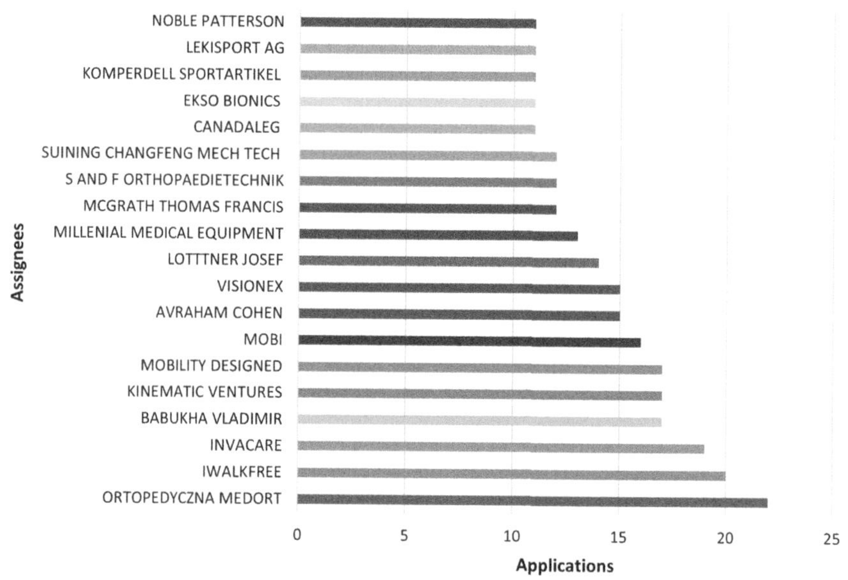

FIGURE 9.6   Top assignees for IPC class A61H3/02.

(*Credit*: PatBase Analytics)

The IPC class A61H3/00 refers to appliances for aiding patients or disabled persons to walk about, and A61H3/02 refers to the use of crutches [12]. Figure 9.6 shows the top 20 assignees for IPC class A61H3/02.

Figure 9.7 shows the top 20 countries for IPC class A61H3/02. It is possible to observe China in the lead in this IPC class.

Figure 9.8 shows the applications by year for IPC class A61H3/02. It is interesting to highlight the growth of patent applications for exoskeletons between 2012 and 2023.

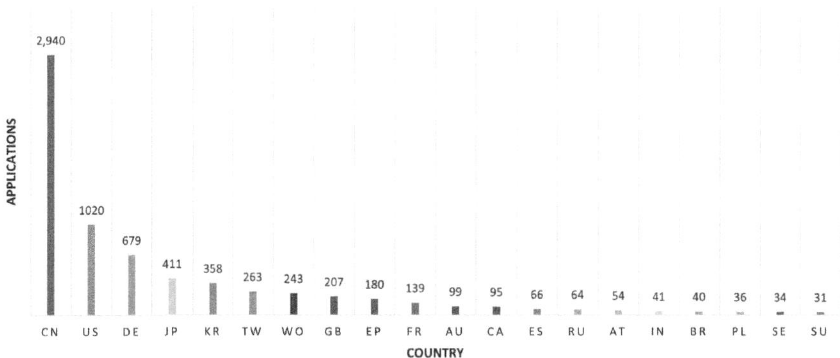

FIGURE 9.7   Top 20 countries for IPC class A61H3/02.

(*Credit*: PatBase Analytics)

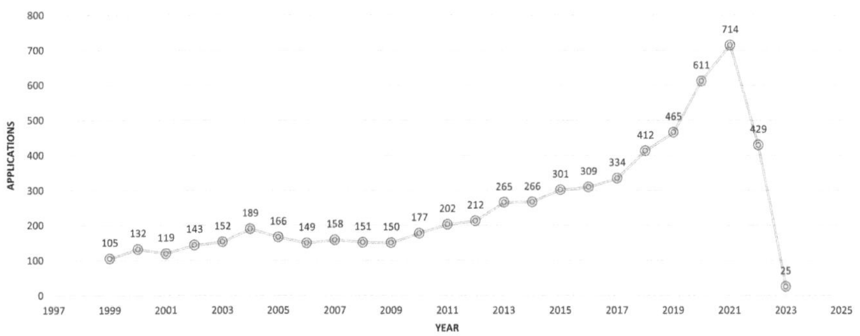

FIGURE 9.8   Applications by year for IPC class A61H3/02.

(*Credit*: PatBase Analytics)

The IPC class B25 refers to hand tools, portable power-driven tools, handles for hand implements, workshop equipment, and manipulators [13], including B25J: Manipulators, chambers provided with manipulation devices, and B25J13/00: Controls for manipulators. Figure 9.9 shows the top 20 assignees for IPC class B25J13/00.

Figure 9.10 shows the top 20 countries for IPC class B25J13/00 [13]. It is possible to observe Japan in the lead in this IPC class.

Figure 9.11 shows the applications by year for IPC class B25J13/00 [13]. It is interesting to highlight the growth of patent applications for exoskeletons since 2011.

The IPC class B25J refers to manipulators and chambers provided with manipulation devices, including B25J9/00: Programmed-controlled manipulators and B25J9/16: Programmed controls [14]. Figure 9.12 shows the top 20 assignees for IPC class B25J9/16.

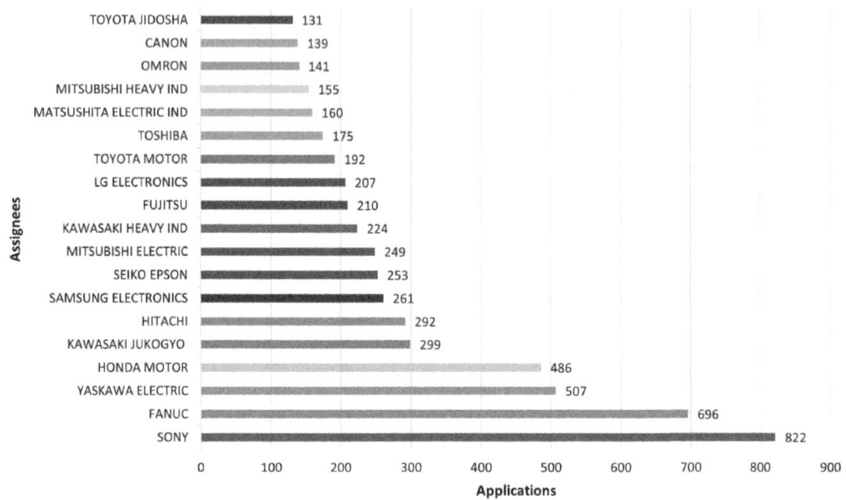

FIGURE 9.9   Top assignees for IPC class B25J13/00.

(*Credit*: PatBase Analytics)

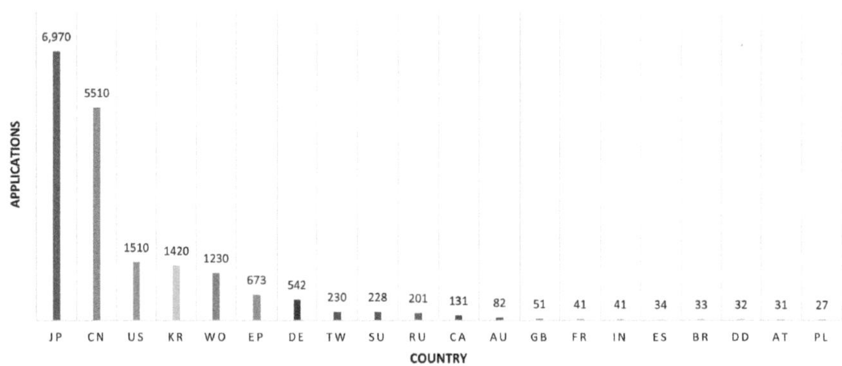

FIGURE 9.10   Top 20 countries for IPC class B25J13/00.

(*Credit*: PatBase Analytics)

Figure 9.13 shows the top 20 countries for IPC class B25J9/16. It is possible to observe China in the lead in this IPC class [14].

Figure 9.14 shows the applications by year for IPC class B25J9/16. It is interesting to highlight the growth of patent applications for exoskeletons since 2013 [14].

The evolution of exoskeletons has explored several alternatives, depending on the application. In the case of the structure, the soft exoskeleton suits for assistance with human movement have the IPC classifications shown in Table 9.8.

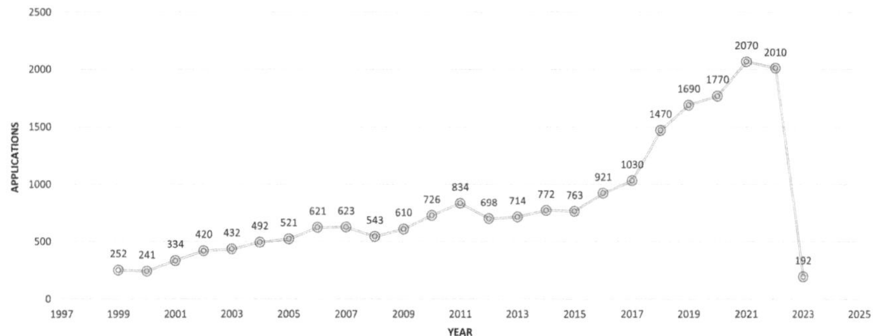

FIGURE 9.11   Applications by year for IPC class B25J13/00.

(*Credit*: PatBase Analytics)

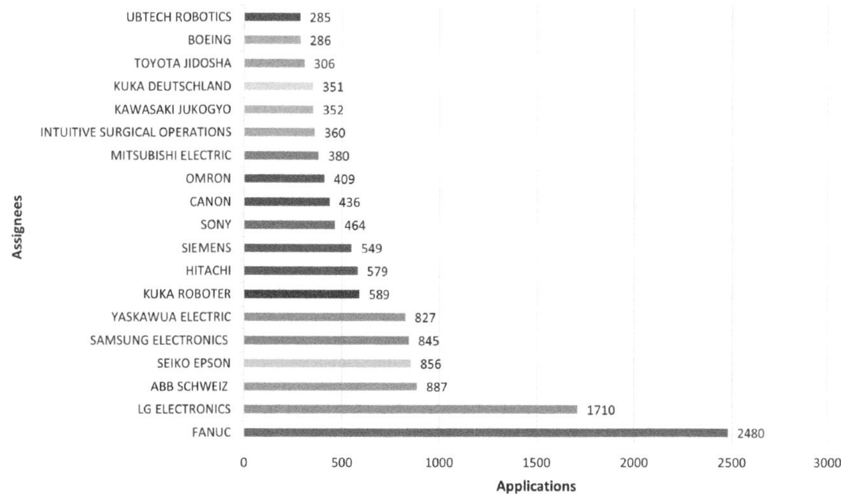

FIGURE 9.12   Top assignees for IPC class B25J9/16.

(*Credit*: PatBase Analytics)

9.4   EXOSKELETON CLAIMS

A patent document for an invention includes the invention's title, the patent history statement, the invention's field, the background, the summary of the invention in general terms, the drawings, a brief description, the detailed description of the invention, and the claims. The title of the detailed description of the invention constitutes the technical specification or description, and the Claims section is where the inventive activity is detailed. The claims define the limits of patent protection, a statement of what the inventor claims are his or her exclusive property. The information specified as protected by the claims cannot be freely used (copied, manufactured, or sold) by

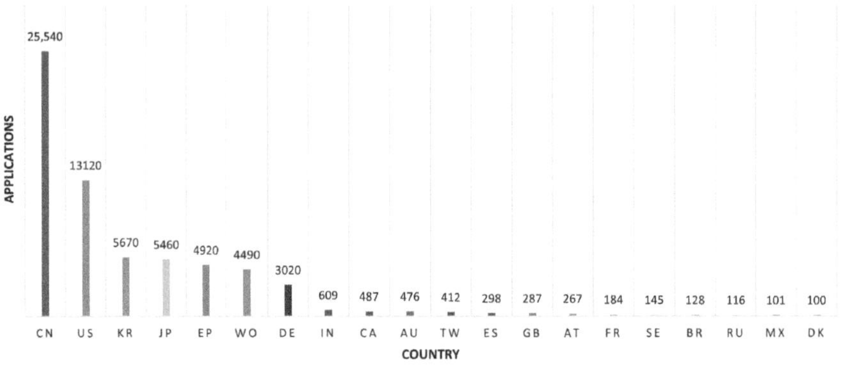

FIGURE 9.13   Top 20 countries for IPC class B25J9/16.

(*Credit*: PatBase Analytics)

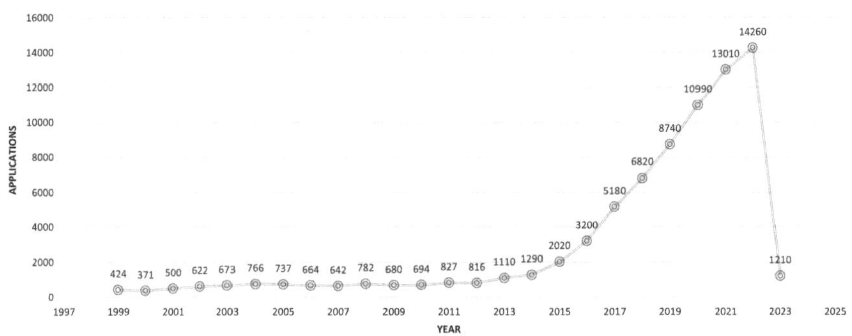

FIGURE 9.14   Applications by year for IPC class B25J9/16.

(*Credit*: PatBase Analytics)

others until the patent expires and the information is not protected [15]. This section presents some abstracts and claims for exoskeletons as an example of inventor/inventors' claims in a patent document.

9.4.1   EXOSKELETON FOR ASSISTING HUMAN MOVEMENT US 11,324,653 B2

The invention relates to an exoskeleton for assisting human movement, which can be fitted to the user in terms of dimensions, tension, and ranges of joint motion, either manually or automatically. The exoskeleton can be fitted to the user in the anteroposterior direction in the sagittal plane, with the user in a horizontal or sitting position, without requiring a functional transfer. The exoskeleton has a modular design that is compatible with human biomechanics and reproduces a natural and physiological movement in the user, with up to seven actuated and controlled degrees of movement

TABLE 9.8
IPC Classifications for Soft Exoskeletons

IPC	Description
A61H3/00	Appliances for aiding patients or disabled persons to walk about. Operating
A61F2/68	or control means.
A63B23/03508	For a single arm or leg.
A63B23/0355	A single apparatus is used for either the upper or lower limbs.
A61F2/70	Operating or control means electrical.
A61H1/024	Knee.
A61H1/0244	Hip.
A61H1/0266	Foot.
A61H2201/1215	Rotary drive.
A61H2201/1238	Driving means hydraulic or pneumatic drive.
A61H2201/1246	Driving means hydraulic or pneumatic drive by piston-cylinder.
A61H2201/1261	Driving means being driven by a human being, e.g., hand driven.
A61H2201/1481	Special movement conversion means.
A61H2201/149	Special movement conversion means rotation-linear or vice versa.
A61H2201/1628	Pelvis.
A61H2201/164	Feet or leg, e.g., pedal.
A61H2201/165	Wearable interfaces.
A61H2201/1652	Harness.
A61H2201/1664	Movement of interface, i.e., force application means linear.
A61H2201/1671	Movement of interface, i.e., force application means rotational.
A61H2201/5002	This means controlling a set of similar massage devices.
A61H2201/5007	Computer controlled.
A61H2201/501	Computer control connected externally.
A61H2201/5061	Force sensors.
A61H2201/5064	Position sensors.
A61H2201/5069	Angle sensors.
A61H2201/5079	Velocity sensors.
A61H2201/5084	Acceleration sensors.
A61H2201/5097	Control means thereof wireless.
A61H2230/60	Muscle strain, i.e., measured on the user, electromyography (EMG).
A61H2230/605	Muscle strain, i.e., measured on the user, EMG used as a control parameter
B25J9/0006	for the apparatus.
	Exoskeletons, i.e., resembling a human figure.

per limb, ensuring that the user maintains equilibrium during locomotion. There are 14 claims and 18 drawing sheets [16]. This is a granted patent where the claims are protected by the modular design.

9.4.2 Exoskeleton Comprising a Plurality of Autonomously Operable Modules US 2022/0354730 A1

An exoskeleton has a plurality of autonomously operable modules, each having a dedicated controller connected to an actuated joint. The exoskeleton further has a multimaster electrical communicator between the controllers of the modules. The controller of each module is configured for collecting information from sensors; sharing information with the remaining modules through the multimaster electrical communicator; determining which other modules are present; and autonomously calculating and commanding a desired trajectory of the actuated joint of the module for assisting the movement of the corresponding biological joint in coordination with the kinematic condition of other biological joints [17]. This is an application patent where the claims have been protected by the controller in interaction with several modules and functionalities.

9.4.3 JOINT TORQUE AUGMENTATION SYSTEM AND METHOD FOR GAIT ASSISTANCE US 9,662.262 B2

A joint torque augmentation system includes a linkage assembly configured to couple to a user. The linkage assembly includes a unidirectional link and a device joint. The linkage assembly is worn by a user or is configured to be joined to footwear. An actuator is coupled to the linkage assembly to provide torque at a joint of the user. A sensor is coupled to the user to measure the position of the user. A control system is coupled to the sensor and actuator. A phase of gait for the user is determined by the control system based on the position measured by the sensor. The actuator produces a tension force on the linkage assembly during the first phase of gait. A compliant element is coupled between the actuator and linkage assembly. The compliant element is tuned based on a load carried by the user. There are 24 claims and 26 drawing sheets [18]. This is a granted patent where the modular design protects the claims and the control system protects the claims in interaction with a compliant element.

9.4.4 SHOULDER MODULE FOR AN EXOSKELETON STRUCTURE US 10,589,435 B2

A shoulder module for an exoskeleton structure that connects to an elbow module attached to an arm of the user to a back module attached to the back of the user. The shoulder module has a plurality of connecting parts and a first pivot connecting two of the connecting parts while allowing rotation of one of the connecting parts concerning the other connecting part according to a first axis of rotation, during a rotation of the elbow module concerning the back module corresponding to an abduction or adduction movement of the shoulder of the user. The connecting parts include a connecting part comprising two parts that slide to allow the shortening or lengthening of the connecting part of the elbow module. There are 15 claims and 18 drawing sheets [19]. This is a granted patent where the claims have been protected by a mechanism.

9.4.5 EXOSKELETON STRUCTURE THAT PROVIDES FORCE ASSISTANCE TO THE USER US 10,639,784 B2

The invention relates to an exoskeleton structure that provides force assistance to a user. Said exoskeleton comprises a first module capable of joining to the first portion of a user's body, a second module capable of joining to a second portion of the user's body, and the second module is connected to the first module by means of a joint.

An actuator allows the rotation of the second module with respect to the first module, which comprises a stator and a rotor. This rotor can be driven in rotation with respect to the stator to move the second module in rotation with respect to the first module and an elastic return element. This element is arranged in a first range of angular movement of the rotor with respect to the stator so as not to exert any return force on the rotor and, in a second range of angular movement of the rotor with respect to the stator, to exert a return force. This tends to oppose the rotation of the rotor with respect to the stator. This occurs in a first direction of rotation and assists the rotation of the rotor with respect to the stator in a second direction of rotation opposite to the first direction of rotation. There are six claims and 18 drawing sheets [20]. This is a granted patent where the claims have been protected by a mechanism.

9.4.6 MODULAR EXOSKELETON STRUCTURE THAT PROVIDES FORCE ASSISTANCE US 2021/0069890 A1

A modular exoskeleton structure provides force assistance to a user. The structure includes a base module including a lumbar belt capable of surrounding the waist of the user, a battery and a control unit attached to the lumber belt, a first attachment part attached to the belt and capable of cooperating with a second complementary attachment part of a hip module to attach the hip module to the base module by snapping the second attachment part into the first attachment part, and a third attachment part attached to the belt and capable of cooperating with a complementary fourth attachment part of a back module for attaching the back module to the base module [21]. This is an application patent where the claims are protected by the modular design and its configurations.

9.4.7 ANKLE BRACE OR ANKLE EXOSKELETON US 2020/0253774 A1

The invention relates to the field of human necessities and can be used in medicine for treating patients with loss or impairment of the locomotor function of the lower extremities. An ankle link of orthosis or exoskeleton contains the base element and the first lever pivotally mounted on the base element. The first strut is hinged at the upper end of the first lever, and the second strut is hinged at the upper end of the base element. The foot support is connected by the first lateral side to the lower end of the first strut and the second lateral side to the lower end of the second strut by means of hinges having at least two degrees of freedom [22]. This is an application patent where the claims have been protected by a mechanism.

9.4.8 EXOSKELETON US 11,148,278 B2

This is a method for setting desired trajectories of movement of an exoskeleton for enabling movement in a user with a musculoskeletal disorder, a device for assisting walking in the user, and a method for controlling said device. Walking in the user can be enabled in predetermined modes of movement. The device has a part worn by the user, including a motorized lower limb exoskeleton equipped with a control device, embodied in an on-board controller of the exoskeleton, and a non-worn part which includes an external computer for a specialized assistant and a system for determining the parameters of desired trajectories of movement of the exoskeleton in a cartesian coordinate system. Control signals for exoskeleton actuators are generated, taking into consideration the mass and inertial properties of body segments of the user and elements of the exoskeleton, as well as requirements regarding the quality of control. There are eight claims and seven drawing sheets [23]. This is a granted patent where the claims are protected by the control system, modes of movement, and user interface.

9.4.9 Claims of Continuous Passive Mobilizing Robot for Rehabilitation of Upper Limbs MX 388107 B

This is a robot that mobilizes the left and right upper limb, aimed at medical rehabilitation and, in particular, to be used as a multi-articulated structure with four therapy modalities in such a way that the robot, the object of the invention, allows selecting the mobilization modes for the paretic limb, apparent load, circumferential, and follow-up. Figures 9.15 to 9.24 show the assembly and components of the exoskeleton [24].

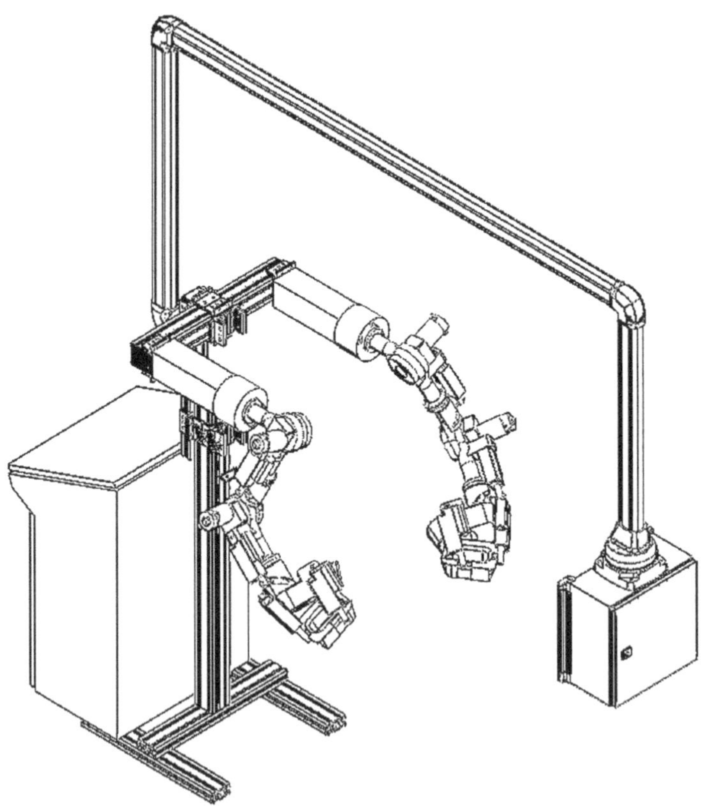

FIGURE 9.15   Front and top perspective view of a continuous passive mobilizing robot.

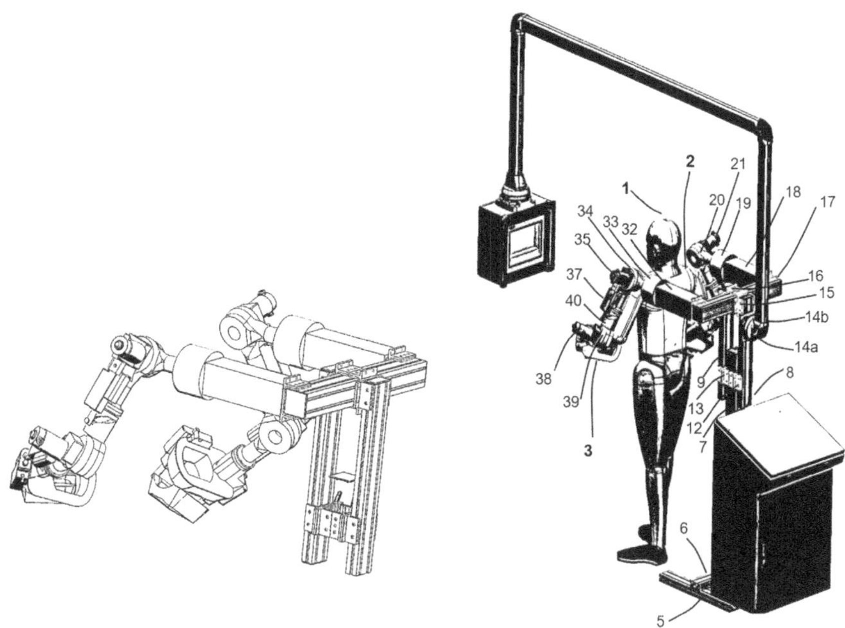

FIGURE 9.16 Top and rear perspective view of a continuous passive mobilizing robot.

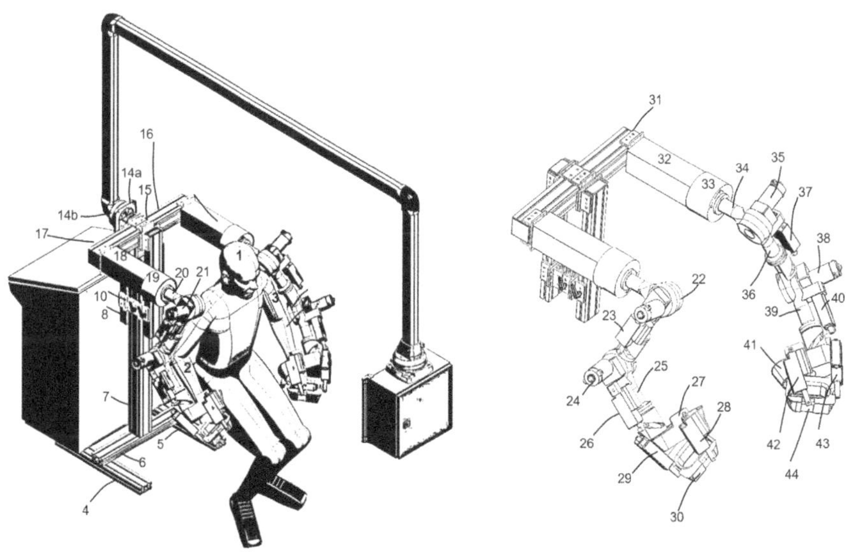

FIGURE 9.17 Front and top perspective view of a continuous passive mobilizing robot.

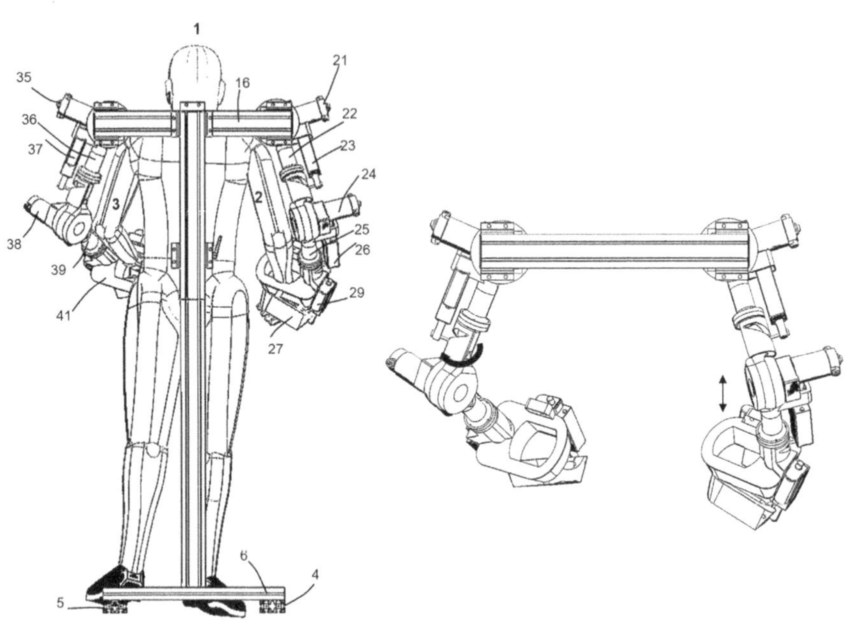

FIGURE 9.18 Rear view of a continuous passive mobilizing robot.

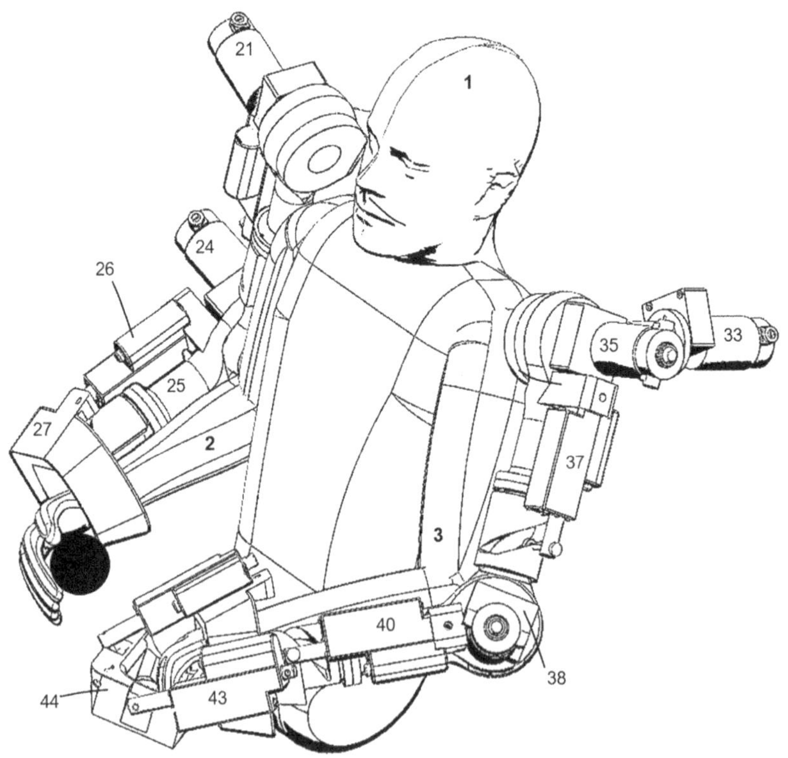

FIGURE 9.19 Left side view of a continuous passive mobilizing robot.

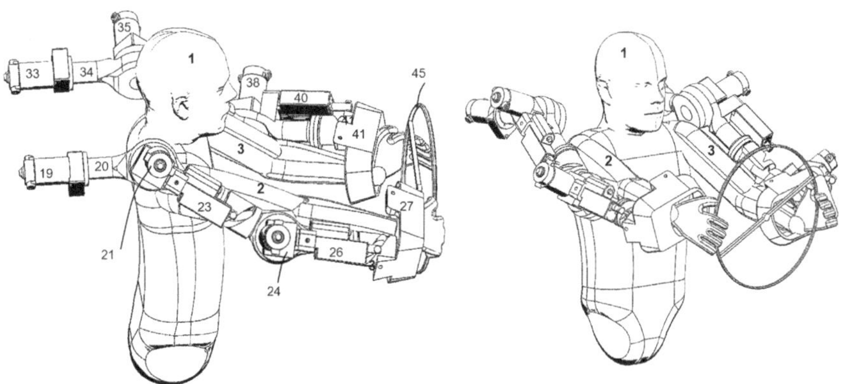

FIGURE 9.20   Side view and front perspective view of a continuous passive mobilizing robot.

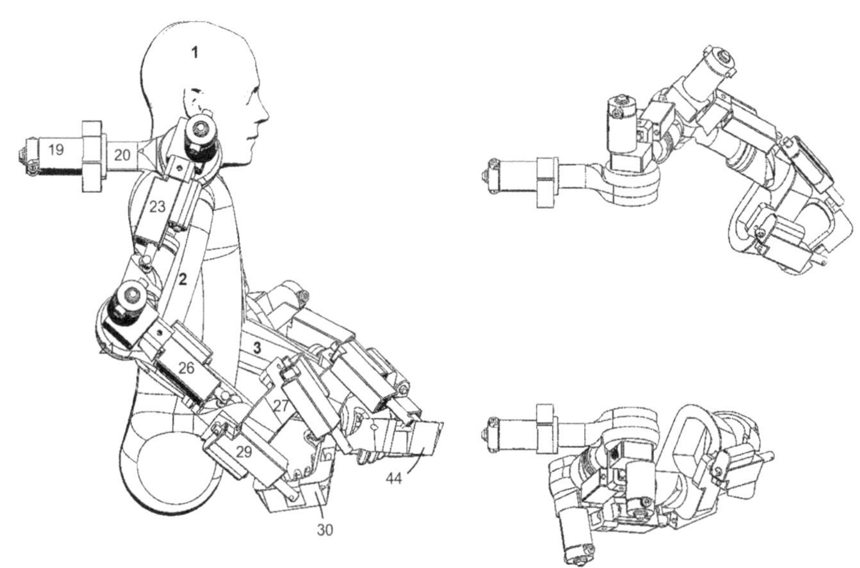

FIGURE 9.21   Right-side view of a continuous passive mobilizing robot.

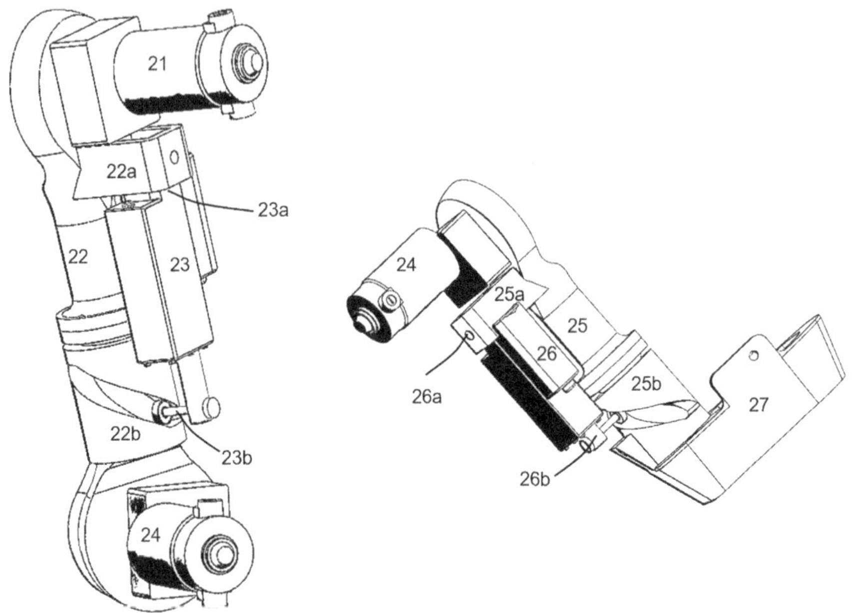

FIGURE 9.22 Front perspective view of an arm rotation mechanism (A) and a forearm rotation mechanism (B).

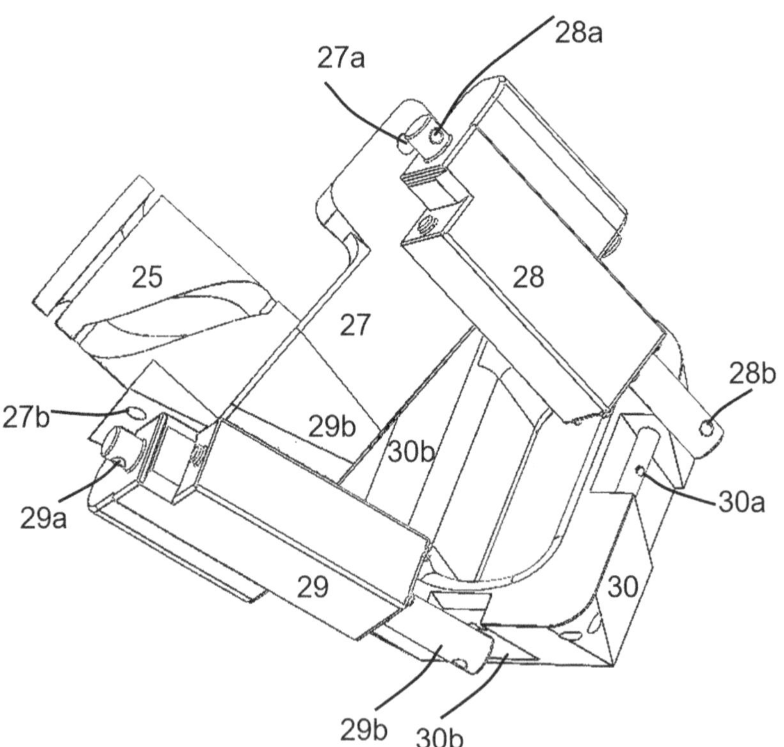

FIGURE 9.23 Top perspective view of wrist multi-orientation mechanism.

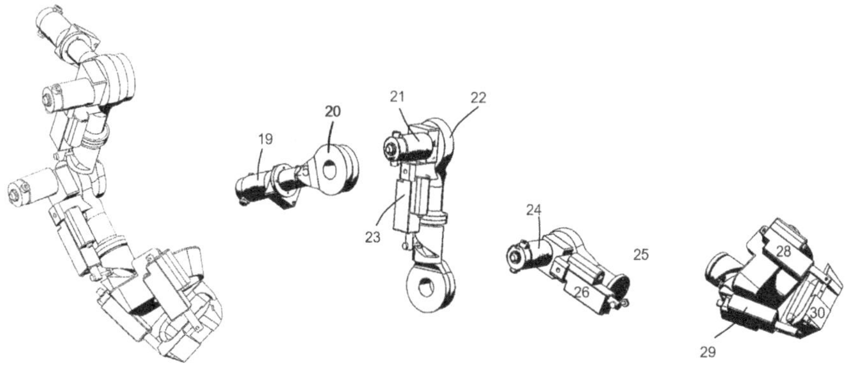

FIGURE 9.24 Exploded view of the right mobilizing unit.

Claims:

Having sufficiently described the invention, the following is considered a novelty, and therefore, the following is claimed as exclusive property:

1. A system of configurable mechanisms that constitutes a continuous passive mobilizing robot for the mobilization of an upper limb (2 or 3) and of the two upper limbs (2 and 3). This system comprises a control and power equipment (I) that supplies electrical power and control signals through the column group (II).

   This group is arranged as a central base to provide support and stability to the human-machine interface group (III), which is mounted on the upper part in front of a patient (1). The components and articulations of this group allow for adjusting their height and orientation manually in relation to mobilization.

   In a first case of operation, the right upper limb (2), by actuating the right mobilizing assembly (IV) ensures the right upper limb (2), limiting and directing it by the action of the motor (19) from its position at rest to its position of increase in angles when it rotates counterclockwise. A link (20) transmits the movement that continues perpendicularly by the action of a motor (21), and another link (22) transmits the rotational displacement in increasing angles when it rotates counterclockwise, raising the arm of the right upper limb (2). This is followed by the action of the motor (23), which transmits linear displacement through the section (23b) that follows a cam (22b) capable of limiting and generating abduction-adduction movements of the arm of the right upper limb (1).

   The link (22) forms part of the axis of rotation, where a motor (24) transmits flexion-extension movements of the elbow of the right upper limb (2). This is followed by the action of the motor (26), which transmits linear displacement through the section (26b) that follows a cam (25b) capable of limiting and generating pronation-supination movements of the forearm of the right upper limb (2). The section (25b) is attached to the wrist support (27), which by the action of the motor (29), limits and directs adduction-abduction movements (radial deviation-ulnar deviation) of the wrist.

Significantly, the action of the motor (28) limits and directs flexion-extension movements of the wrist. When action of the motors (28) and (29) both work synchronously according to the control signals, they manage to generate rotational movements of the wrist in a clockwise direction and vice versa.

This exoskeleton is characterized by the mechanisms of the right mobilizing set (IV) and can be configured for their ranges of movement, position, and speed from point-to-point references (set point) or trajectory tracking from the man-machine interface. Likewise, the mechanisms of the right mobilizing set (IV), separately or together, can be exchanged to the left mobilized set (V) and vice versa for the mobilization of the right upper limb (2) or the left upper limb (3). The column group (II) is integrated by a right base profile (4), a left base profile (5), a central base profile (6), a profile (7), a vertical adjustment device, and a horizontal adjustment device.

A system of configurable mechanisms, characterized in that the control and power equipment (I) is made up of a group of electrical power supply cables and a group of control cables. These groups start from the cabinet and are distributed through a harness through the column group (II) to the human-machine interface group (III), continuing to the right mobilizing assembly (IV) and the left mobilizing assembly (V).

A system of configurable mechanisms is characterized in that the human-machine interface group (III) includes a monitor and a support arm, which is coupled to the column group (II) and guides the distribution of the cables of the control and power equipment (I).

A system of configurable mechanisms is characterized in that the right mobilizer assembly (IV) is made up of a rotation mechanism A, a rotation mechanism B, and a wrist multi-orientation mechanism.

A system of configurable mechanisms is characterized in that the left mobilizer assembly (V) is made up of a rotation mechanism A, a rotation mechanism B, and a wrist multi-orientation mechanism.

2. A system of configurable mechanisms, according to claim 1, in which a column group (II) characterized in that the vertical adjustment device is made up of a profile (8); a profile (9); a right frontal closure section (11); a right rear closure section (10); a left front connection section (13) and a left rear connection section (12). Said vertical adjustment device allows the height to be varied by sliding on the profile column (7).

3. A system of configurable mechanisms, according to claim 1, in which a column group (II) is characterized in that the horizontal adjustment device is made up of a component (31); a coupling (15); a fixing element (16) and two adjustable couplings (17), one for the right mobilizer assembly and another for the left mobilizer assembly. Said couplings (17) allow the horizontal length to be varied when sliding on the component (31).

4. A system of configurable mechanisms, according to claim 1, in which a right mobilizing assembly (IV) is characterized in that the rotation mechanism

A is made up of an actuator for angular displacement A (21), a link (22) and an actuator (23), which is connected employing a prominent portion (23a) to a section (22a) and using a bearing placed at the end (23b), which always moves in contact with the walls of a shaped groove. The cam (22b) is duly calculated to provide the necessary angular travel to mobilize the shoulder. Said rotation mechanism A is coupled both to the right mobilizer assembly (IV) and the left mobilized assembly (V) through the coupling sections of the link (22), which allow the right and left coupling configuration.

5. A system of configurable mechanisms, according to claim 1, in which a right mobilizing set (IV) is characterized in that the rotation mechanism B is made up of an actuator for angular displacement B (24), a link (25) and an actuator (26), which is connected employing a prominent portion (25a) to a section (26a) and using a bearing placed at the end (25b), which always moves in contact with the walls of a shaped groove. A cam (26b) is duly calculated to provide the necessary angular path to mobilize the forearm. Said rotation mechanism is coupled both in the right mobilizing assembly and the left mobilizing assembly through the coupling sections of the link (25), which allow the right and left coupling configuration.

6. A system of configurable mechanisms, according to claim 1, in which a right mobilizing set (IV) characterized in that a wrist multi-orientation mechanism consists of a wrist support (27), an actuator (28), an actuator (29), a cam-shaped slot (25), and a hand rest (30).

7. A system of configurable mechanisms, according to claim 1, in which a left mobilizing set (V) characterized in that a multi-orientation wrist mechanism consists of a left wrist support, which is opposite to the wrist support (27), an actuator (28), an actuator (29), a cam-shaped slot (25), and a hand rest (30).

8. A system of configurable mechanisms, according to claim 1, in which a wrist multi-orientation mechanism is characterized in that it is exchanged from the right mobilizing assembly to the left mobilizing assembly by changing the wrist support (27) for the left wrist support.

9. A system of configurable mechanisms, according to claim 1, in which a control and power equipment (I) characterized in that a therapist executes the rehabilitation routines, which depend on speed, displacement limits, and positioning of 14 actuators (19, 21, 23, 24, 26, 28, 29, 33, 35, 37, 38, 40, 42, and 43).

10. A system of configurable mechanisms, according to claim 1, in which a right mobilizing set (IV) is characterized in that its operation is carried out from the operation of the actuator (19) to perform the adduction-abduction movements of the shoulder.

11. A system of configurable mechanisms, according to claim 1, in which a left mobilizing set (V) is characterized in that its operation is carried out from the operation of the actuator (33) to perform the adduction-abduction movements of the shoulder.

12. A system of configurable mechanisms, according to claim 1, in which a rotation mechanism A characterized in that its operation is carried out from

the operation of the actuator 21 to carry out the flexion-extension movements of the shoulder.

13. A system of configurable mechanisms, according to claim 1, in which a rotation mechanism A characterized in that its operation is carried out from the operation of the actuator (23) and the cam (22b) that guides the displacement of the bearing 23b, to perform internal and external rotation movements of the shoulder.

14. A system of configurable mechanisms, according to claim 1, in which a rotation mechanism B is characterized in that its operation is carried out from the operation of the actuator (24) to carry out the flexion-extension movements of the forearm.

15. A system of configurable mechanisms, according to claim 1, in which a multi-orientation mechanism characterized in that its operation is carried out from the operation of the actuator (26) and the cam (25b) that guides the displacement of the bearing (26b) to perform pronation supination movements.

16. A system of configurable mechanisms, according to claim 1, in which a multi-orientation mechanism characterized in that its operation is carried out from the operation of the actuator (28), coupled to wrist support (27), which through a hole practiced in section (27a) is mechanically connected to a prominent portion (28a) of the actuator (28) and through a section (28b), it is attached to an axis (30a) of the hand support (30) to carry out the flexion-extension movement of the wrist.

17. A system of configurable mechanisms, according to claim 1, in which a multi-orientation mechanism, characterized in that its operation is carried out from the operation of the actuator (29) employing a hole made in the section (27b), is mechanically connected to a prominent portion (29a) and using a section (29b) is attached to an axis (30b) of the hand support (30) to perform the movements of ulnar and radial deviation.

18. A system of configurable mechanisms, according to claim 1, is characterized in that it is capable of mobilizing the upper limb(s) in a standing and sitting position, using the vertical adjustment device (8, 9, 10, 11, 12, and 13) and the horizontal adjustment device (15, 16, 17, and 31).

19. A system of configurable mechanisms, according to claim 1, is characterized in that the mobilization in paretic mode is carried out by the selective movement of links, designated in the man-machine interface. First the upper limb and later the joints that will remain without movement (joint) (immobilized) and the joints that need to be mobilized (joints with controlled movement) are designated. The joints that are not designated will not have any electrical impulse, and due to the nature of the actuator and the decoupling of the motor-reducer, they will be able to move freely (free joint).

20. A system of configurable mechanisms, according to claim 1, is characterized in that the mobilization in the apparent load-lifting mode is carried out with one or both upper members (2 and 3), designated in the man-machine interface. First, the member(s) superior(s), and later the parameters of the

apparent load, in order to configure the repetitions of the lifting of apparent load with the force and degrees of freedom, are configured.

21. A system of configurable mechanisms, according to claim 1, is characterized in that the mobilization in shoulder-rudder mode is carried out with the right mobilizer set (IV) and the left mobilizer set (V), designating in the man-machine interface. First, the resistance parameters of the rudder (45) and later the routine for the circular movement of the rudder (45) by the right mobilizing set and the left mobilizing set, acting alternately one on the other, are designated.

22. A system of configurable mechanisms, according to claim 1, is characterized in that the mobilization in hemiplegia mode is carried out with the right mobilizer set (IV) and the left mobilizer set (V), designated in the man-machine interface. First, the mobilizer set without movement capacity (according to the member of the patient (1) with hemiplegia) and later the routine for the movement of the mobilizer set with movement capacity (patient member (1), driven according to the rehabilitation routine) are designated. This member is designated as the master, and the member with hemiplegia is designated as the slave.

9.4.10 CLAIMS OF CONTINUOUS PASSIVE MOBILIZING FOR KNEE REHABILITATION MX 393411 B

This is a mechanism that mobilizes the patient's knee, aimed at medical rehabilitation and, in particular, to be used as a multi-articulated structure with three therapy modalities in such a way that the mechanism, the object of the invention, allows selecting the lying, sitting, and standing therapy positions. Figures 9.25 to 9.32 show the components of the exoskeleton [25].

Claims:

Having sufficiently described the invention, it is considered a novelty, and therefore, the following is claimed as exclusive property:

1. A continuous passive mobilizing mechanism for knee rehabilitation of a lower limb comprises a main base consisting of a hip base (4), which contains a bolt in a right hole (4a) and a bolt in a left hole (4b) that are attached to a belt (5) that fits the patient's hip (1).

    This hip base (4) includes a prominent right section (4c) and a prominent left section (4d), both with a bolt to serve as an axis of rotation for a femur (6) linear actuator. The hip base (4) contains a right cut-out section (4e) and a left cut-out section (4f), which by means of a bolt, serve as a rotation axis and limit for angular displacement of a curved link A (7) and a fixing section (4g).

    A configurable mobilizing set (A, B) that consists of two configurations for the right lower limb and/or left lower limb is made up of the femur linear actuator (6) with an angular displacement bolt that joins the curved link A (7), which can be moved angularity from a front end (7a) using the cut-out left section (4f) of the hip base (4) as a turning point and delimiter.

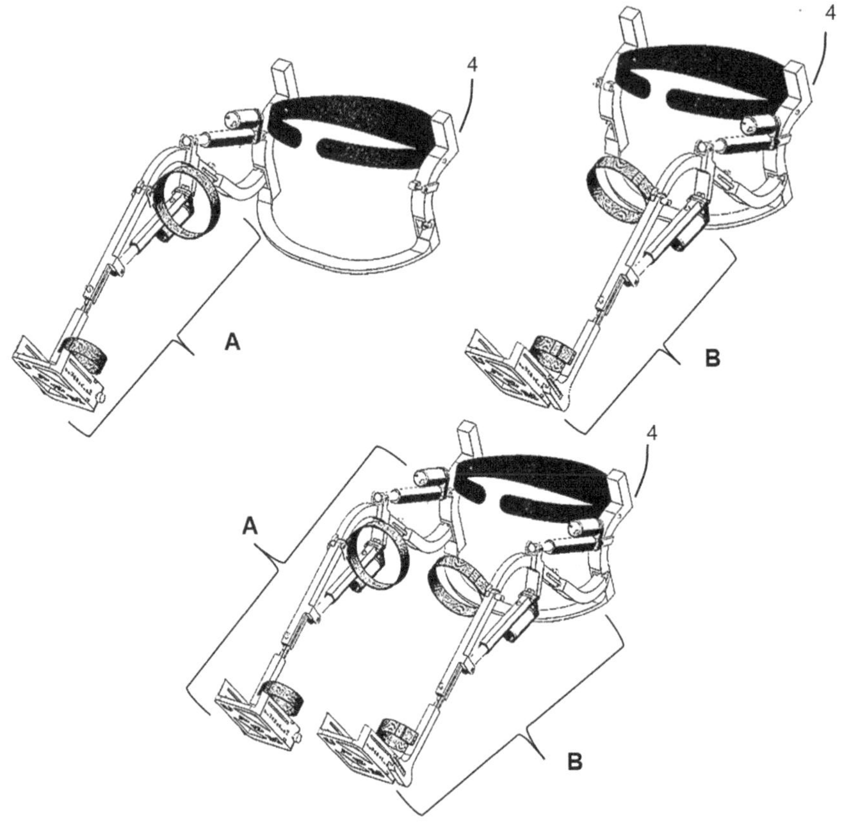

FIGURE 9.25   Front and top perspective view of a continuous passive knee mobilizer.

This curved link A (7) is connected to a curved link B (8) with a pin (18) and a slot (8a) made at its anterior end. A prominent portion (8b) and a prominent portion (8c) connect the femur linear actuator (6) and the tibial linear actuator (11). A straight link (10) with a prominent portion (10b), which by means of its front end (10a) is connected to the rear end (8d) of the curved link B (8) a knee adjustment band (9).

The straight link (10) that connects with a foot link (12) through a groove (10c) made at a rear end that houses and secures with a pin (19), the foot link (12) with a slot (12b) to support a tibia adjustment band (13).

A foot mobilizer support (15), which through a slot (15c) and a slot (5d) support a foot adjustment band (14), a support (20) to operate in lying mode and a conveyor belt (21) for standing mode; and an adaptive length mechanism for children and adults consisting of an adaptive length mechanism A and an adaptive length mechanism B.

The adaptive length mechanism A through the slot (8a) at the rear end of the curved link (8) accommodates, positions, and secures the appropriate

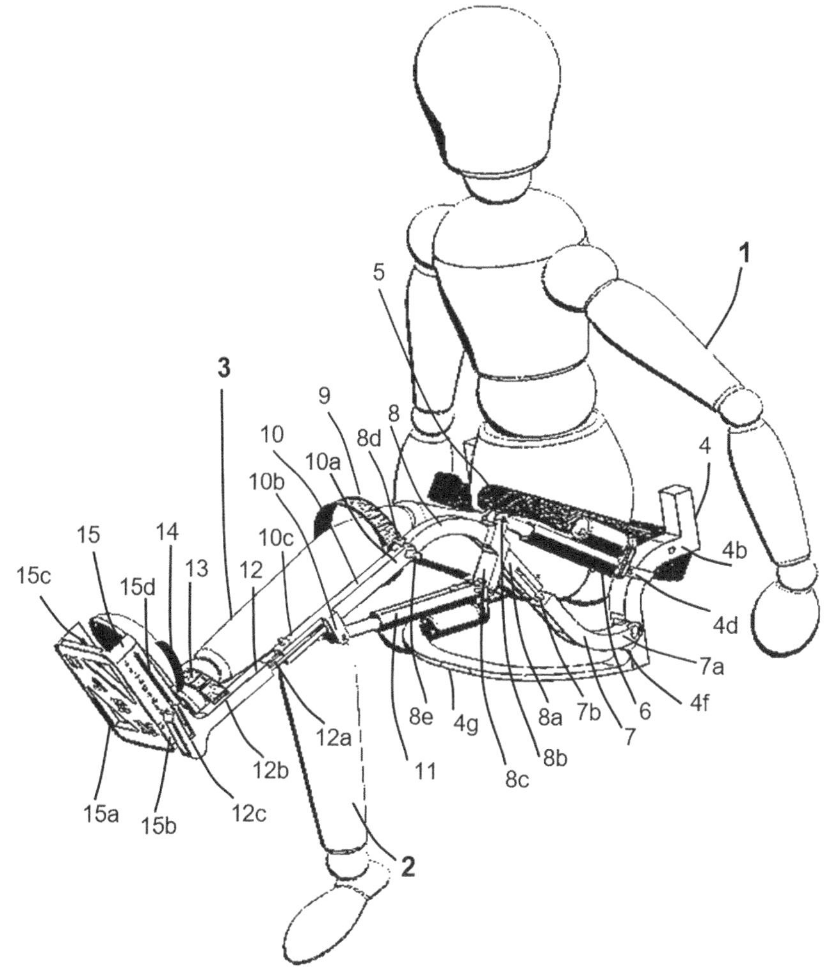

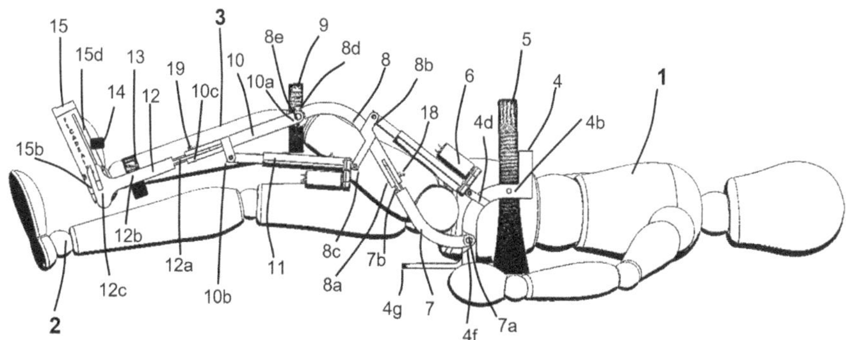

FIGURE 9.26 Side view of the mobilizer in seated mode.

FIGURE 9.27 Side view of the mobilizer in lying mode.

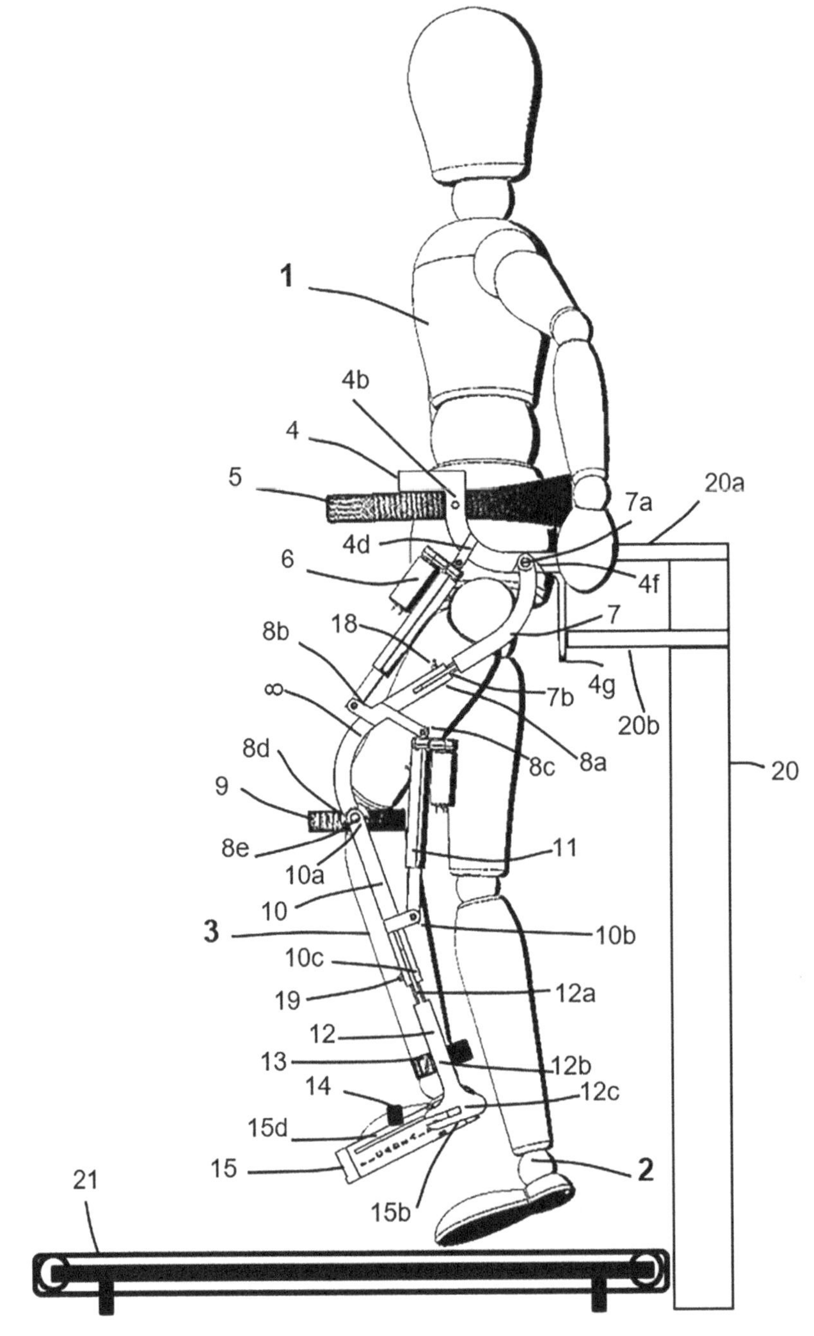

FIGURE 9.28 Side view of the mobilizer in standing mode.

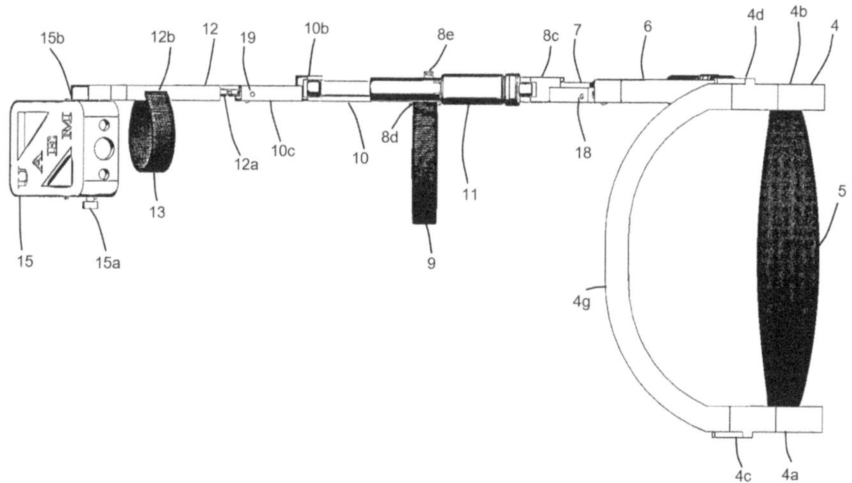

FIGURE 9.29 Bottom view of the mobilizer.

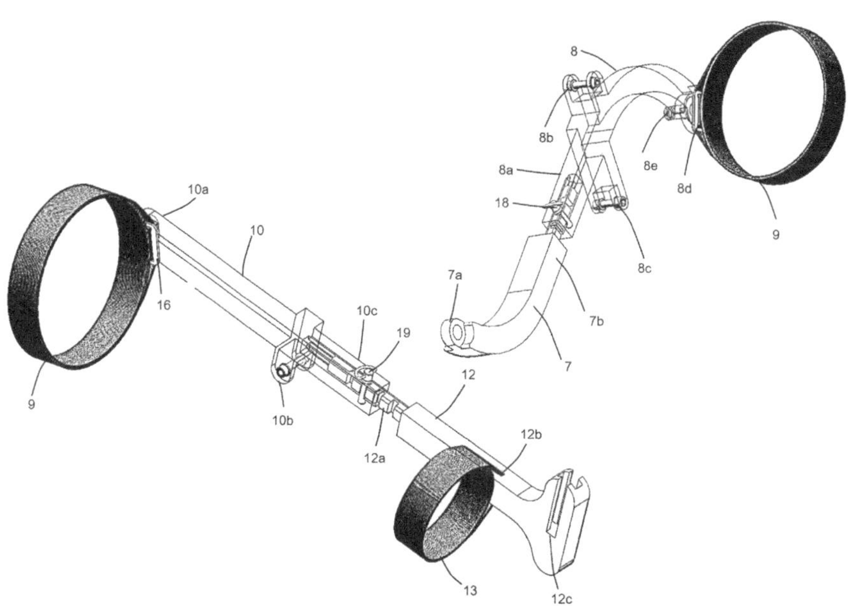

FIGURE 9.30 Perspective view of the adaptation mechanism.

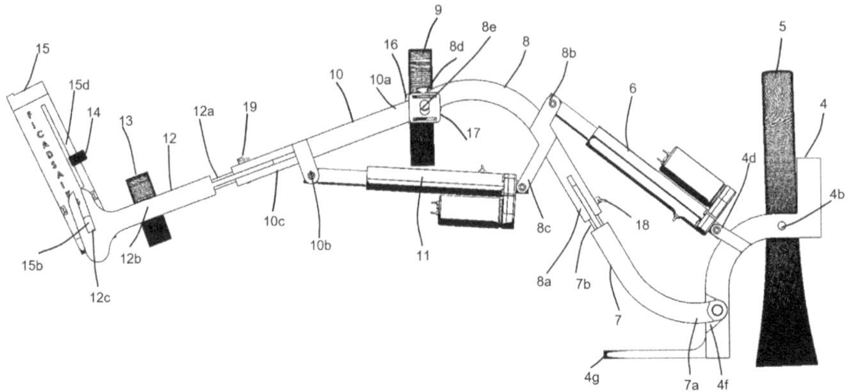

FIGURE 9.31 Side view of the main components of the assembled mobilizer.

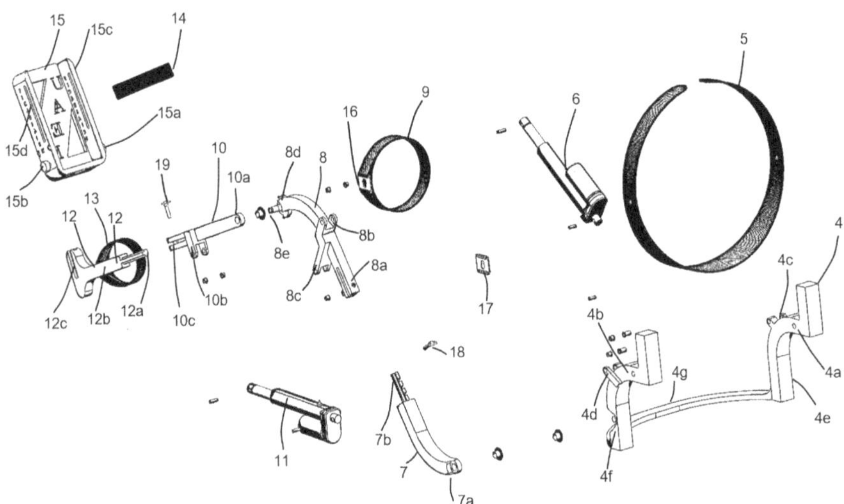

FIGURE 9.32 Exploded view of the mobilizer.

length for children, using the first two positions, and, for adults, using the third and fourth positions.

The adaptable length mechanism B through the slot (10c) at the rear end of the straight link (10) accommodates, positions, and secures, by itself or in combination with the adjustable length mechanism A, the appropriate length for children, using the first two positions, and for adults the third and fourth positions.

For the continuous passive mobilizing mechanism for knee rehabilitation of a lower limb to perform the mobilization routines, a group of electrical power supply cables and another group of control cables run through a harness through the configurable mobilizing set (set configurable mobilizer A/B) to the main base. The cable that connects the power supply is connected to an electrical power contact, and the group of control cables are connected to a panel. In this context, the therapist programs the rehabilitation routines to synchronously mobilize the femur actuator (6) and tibial linear actuator (11).

This exoskeleton is characterized in that the mechanisms of the configurable mobilizing set A/B can be configured for their ranges of movement, position, and speed from the panel. As well as the mechanisms of the configurable mobilizing set, A/B, separately or in a group, can be interchanged to work on the right or left side and mobilize the right lower limb (2) or the left lower limb (3), respectively.

The adaptable length mechanism can be configured for children and adults, which makes it possible to exchange and use the configurable mobilizer assembly on the left or right side.

The operation of the configurable mobilizer assembly A on the right lower limb (2) is made with the same components as for the configurable mobilizing set B, making it possible to connect without any adjustment to the front end (7a) of the curved link A (7), both in the right cut section (4e) and in the left cut section (4f). In the same way, the femur linear actuator (6) is connected both in the right prominent portion (4c) and in the prom portion. Inner left (4d). This is possible thanks to the fact that the femur linear actuator (6) and the tibial linear actuator (11) are positioned symmetrically to the links of the configurable mobilizing assembly. They allow operation in the same operating conditions in the right lower limb (2) and the left lower limb (3).

Likewise, the continuous passive mobilizer mechanism for knee rehabilitation has three modes of therapy (sitting, lying down, and standing) which are carried out by fixing the main base in a chair for sitting mode, in a bed for lying down mode and through the support (20), and the conveyor belt (21) for the standing mode, making the adjustments according to the required configuration.

2. The continuous passive mobilizing mechanism for knee rehabilitation, according to claim 1, in which the therapy in seated mode is performed by placing the belt (5) on the patient (1) at 45 degrees from the horizontal surface of the hip base (4) and adjusting the belt (5) as indicated by the therapist, resting the fixation section (4g) on the respective chair.

3. The continuous passive mobilizing mechanism for knee rehabilitation, according to claim 1, in which the therapy in lying mode is performed by placing the belt (5) on the patient (1) at 90 degrees from the horizontal surface of the hip base (4) and adjusting said belt (5), as indicated by the therapist, resting the fixing section (4g) on the respective bed.

4. The continuous passive mobilizer mechanism for knee rehabilitation, according to claim 1, in which the therapy in standing mode is performed by placing the belt (5) and the configurable mobilizing assembly (configurable mobilizing assembly A and B) in a vertical position, each time a fixing

section (4g) rests on the support (20) employing a connection section (20b) to said support.

5. The continuous passive mobilizing mechanism for knee rehabilitation, according to claim 1, in which the case of the knee adjustment band (9), is changed from the left knee band support (8d) to the knee band support right (8e); likewise, the tibia adjustment band (13) can be changed to be used on both sides, using the same slot (12b). In the case of the foot mobilizer support (15), it is possible to use it on both lower limbs, using the prominent circular portion (15a) for the right lower limb (2).

9.5 TECHNOLOGY TRANSFER

This section presents some case studies of technology transfer. The confidential data has been omitted. Precisely identifying which intellectual property will be the subject of the license is necessary to ensure both parties are on the same agreement and not exceeding their rights. A license agreement usually has six components: scope of the grant, exclusivity, territory, term, compensation, termination, and conclusion. The licensor is the holder of the right to the exclusive use of the trademark and grants its use to the licensee. There are four considerations to carry out a technology transfer: 1. Purchase of a patent or obtain a license where the patented technology is allowed to be used for certain acts in specific markets and for a specific period of time; 2. Cross licenses, where two companies usually exchange licenses to be able to exploit certain patents that are property of the other to carry out co-participation in the license agreement; 3. Inventing based on the invention, which involves modifying the product or process to avoid infringing the rights of other patent holders; 4. Patent grouping, where it is agreed that two or more companies group their respective patents in order to establish a patent rights management center to gain competitiveness in a certain technological sector.

9.5.1 Ekso Bionics and Lockheed Martin

Both companies signed the government field cross-license agreement and medical license agreement [26]. The details of license agreements can be consulted in the following links: https://www.sec.gov/Archives/edgar/data/1549084/0001144 20414019450/v373064_ex10-25.htm

9.5.2 Ekso Bionics Licenses Intellectual Property to Ottobock

Ekso Bionics, a robotic exoskeleton company, formalized a licensing agreement providing intellectual property to Ottobock. Ekso Bionics agrees to receive a combination of license and royalty payments in return for licensing two of its patents to Ottobock. Ekso is a wearable bionic suit that enables individuals with any amount of lower extremity weakness to stand up and walk over the ground. Ekso is forging a new frontier in rehabilitation for people living with the consequences of stroke, spinal cord injury, and other neurological conditions affecting gait [27]. The details of the license agreements can be consulted in the following link: https://ir.eksobionics.com/press-releases/detail/394/ekso-bionics-licences-intellectual-property-to-ottobock

9.5.3 Berkeley ExoWorks and the Regents of the University of California

Agreements cover the exclusive license agreement for lower extremity exoskeleton technology, a mechanism to enable normal gait despite leg injuries, decreasing oxygen consumption by use of a load-carrying exoskeleton, under-actuated transfemoral prosthetic knee, and controlling the swinging leg of an exoskeleton. These agreements include several U.S. patents and U.S. patent applications, being licensees of Berkeley ExoWorks [28].

9.5.4 ReWalk Robotics and Harvard

In July 2018, the ReWalk Robotics company signed a series of changes to its exclusive licensing and joint-research agreement with Harvard University that are relevant to the creation of its soft suit exoskeleton. Through the initial agreement for collaboration, both parties will work together to further the creation of soft-suit exoskeleton technology for the treatment of lower limb problems. The suit is designed to cure conditions including multiple sclerosis, stroke, and older people's mobility issues, among other medical issues. The new changes reorganize the way Harvard will receive payments from ReWalk Robotics and make minor modifications to the licensing agreement. The amendments also change the length and plan of the research agreement. The licensing agreement grants ReWalk Robotics an exclusive, worldwide royalty-bearing license for certain patents related to lightweight soft-suit exoskeleton technologies [29].

9.5.5 Exoskeleton and Method of Increasing the Flexibility of an Exoskeleton Joint

Ekso Bionics developed a tensegrity exoskeleton with government support. An exoskeleton configured to be coupled to a user includes a plurality of interconnected support elements constituted by rigid compression members interconnected through a tensegrity joint. The joint includes a tensile member having a first end and a second end coupled to the first and second ones of the support elements, respectively. This application represents a National Stage application of PCT/US2015/027523 entitled "Exoskeleton and Method of Increasing the Flexibility of an Exoskeleton Joint" filed April 24, 2015, pending, which claims the benefit of U.S. Provisional Patent Application Ser. No. 61/987,696, which was filed on May 2, 2014, and titled "Exoskeleton Joints Incorporating a Tensile Member". This invention was made with government support under Contract H92222-14-9-0001 awarded by the United States Special Operations Command. The government has certain rights in the invention [30].

9.5.6 Parker Hannifin Corp. (Licensee) and Vanderbilt University

Parker Hannifin Corp., a global leader in motion and control technologies, announced that it had signed an exclusive licensing agreement with Vanderbilt University for its exoskeleton technology, which allows individuals with severe spinal cord injury to walk and enhances rehabilitation of people who have suffered a stroke. The agreement gives Parker exclusive rights to develop, manufacture, and sell the device. Parker intends to invest in further development of the technology and establish a business unit targeting the commercial launch of the exoskeleton in 2014. This agreement offers Parker an exciting growth opportunity in the area of biomechanics. The Parker exoskeleton offers numerous advantages over existing technologies being tested in rehabilitation clinics. The exoskeleton is 40–50% lighter than competing devices and provides a modular design that can be assembled and disassembled for ease of use and transportation. The device is also smaller, with a slim profile and no bulky backpack components or footplates. A proprietary control interface allows for smooth operation that works in harmony with natural human movement and body position. The Parker exoskeleton is the only wearable device that incorporates a proven rehabilitation technology called functional electrical stimulation. The exoskeleton is currently being tested and refined through clinical research at the Shepherd Center in Atlanta, Georgia. [31]. In 2012, Parker Hannifin and Vanderbilt reached an agreement to license the technology, and soon after, the company began working to commercialize a robotic exoskeleton called Indego. Dr. Ryan Farris was a coinventor in the development of the technology as part of his doctoral work at Vanderbilt, and Parker Hannifin brought him on as the technical lead for the business unit tasked with bringing Indego to market [32].

9.5.7 Lockheed Martin (Licensee) with B-Temia

Lockheed Martin has licensed the Dermoskeleton technology from B-Temia, Inc. This is the same technology that runs the Keeogo lower body exoskeleton. Lockheed Martin will integrate the powered exoskeleton technology and apply it to its current product, such as the FORTIS, and as-of-yet unreleased products. The FORTIS takes the weight of heavy tools and directs it directly into the ground, bypassing the user. However, walking in it can be hindered since it is an entirely passive device. B-Temia Technology now has been applied only to a powered knee exoskeleton, such as the Keeogo [33].

9.5.8 Myomo and Ottobock Global Distribution Agreement

The maker of the mobile assistive arm exoskeleton MyomoPro has entered into an exclusive global distribution agreement with Ottobock. Ottobock is a giant in the world of prosthetics and orthotics with over 90 years of experience in the business. Without a doubt, this is a smart move for both companies. The Myomo and Ottobock global distribution agreement will allow exclusive sales of the patented MyoPro orthosis technology. Initially, with select markets in North America and Germany and then globally. In return, Ottobock gets to complete its portfolio of wearable technology. Ottobock's focus is on augmentative technology designed to improve its customers' quality of life. Myomo was recently awarded seed funds to develop pediatric medical devices [34].

9.5.9 BIOSERVO ENTERS LICENSE AGREEMENT WITH NASA AND GENERAL MOTORS

NASA, General Motors (GM), and Bioservo entered into the ultimate alliance to bring power gloves to the workplace. This is the greatest alliance between theoretical science and commercial engineering for an industrial application. The NASA-GM power glove is a power assist device that augments the user's muscle strength. Traditionally, similar gloves have been used in the medical rehabilitation field. Bioservo has been one of the earliest pioneers of power gloves for work and industry. The goal is to create a power glove that can provide force assistance to healthy people. Even healthy workers can tire out and repeatedly experience pain in the fingers after performing the same task. Reducing fatigue in the fingers and wrist could lead to improved productivity and a decrease in faults and injury rates. GM assembly plants will be used as a test bed to gauge the success of the project. Bioservo is the premier expert in remotely driven soft power gloves. The Soft Extra Muscle (SEM) Glove by Bioservo combines the best of classical rigid robots and soft wearable robotics. The SEM Glove itself is made out of light fabric. The batteries, motors, and controller are combined in a single casing that can be clipped on a belt or placed in a backpack and weighs about 600 g (1.3 pounds). This reduces the metabolic cost of carrying them. The force of the motors is transmitted to the SEM Glove through the equivalent of Bowden cables. The glove provides actuation for three fingers. The applied force is measured by circular sensors at the tip of the glove [35].

9.5.10 WYSS INSTITUTE AND REWALK ROBOTICS FORM COLLABORATION

In 2016, the Wyss Institute at Harvard University and ReWalk Robotics entered into a collaboration agreement to develop an exosuit for patients with limited mobility. The soft exoskeleton is dedicated to patients undergoing rehabilitation due to stroke or multiple sclerosis. The Wyss Institute at Harvard University has been developing soft exoskeletons. The force generated by the motors is transmitted to the legs using a variety of soft materials that pull specifically designed flexible textile straps. The collaboration includes an intellectual property license and funding for future research at the Institute. The Wyss Institute also gains access to ReWalk's business knowledge on bringing an exoskeleton product to market. ReWalk currently has offices in the United States, Germany, and Israel. In addition, ReWalk has a significant network of training centers around the world [36].

9.5.11 STRONGARM TECHNOLOGIES V22 AND FLx ARE SOLD ON 3M'S WEBSITE

3M is a distributor and manufacturer with over 55,000 products, predominantly in technology. StrongArm Technologies sells ErgoSkeletons, or ergonomic exoskeletons. These body posture devices prevent the spine from bending downwards during a lift, picking up heavy objects, or lift and carry, as it is most commonly referred to, and which is considered to be the primary activity for construction, factory, and other blue-collared workers. The V22 and FLx ErgoSkeletons are passive devices. They have no motors or sensors. The V22 weighs only 2.95 lb (1.33 kg). The V22, or Version 22, was followed up by a device that lacks arm cables with a clutch mechanism, FLx. The simplicity of the V22 and FLx is also why they are now the first exoskeletons to see mass distribution. In September 2015, 3M acquired a stake in StrongArm Technologies and invested $2.91 million in the development of more devices [37].

9.5.12 BIONIK LABORATORIES MERGER AGREEMENT WITH INTERACTIVE MOTION TECHNOLOGIES (IMT)

Bionik Laboratories, maker of the ARKE lower body exoskeleton, in 2016 entered into a merger agreement to acquire Interactive Motion Technologies, a spin-off from Massachusetts Institute of Technology. Interactive Motion Technologies specializes in wearables and exoskeletons for neurorehabilitation of the upper body. Their main product line is the InMotion series arm, wrist, and hand rehabilitation devices in addition to a knee exoskeleton. Interactive Motion Technologies was founded in 1998 in Watertown, Massachusetts, making it one of the oldest companies in the field. Bionik Laboratories (BNKL) is a Canadian-based company [38].

9.5.13 EKSO BIONICS ACQUIRES ZEROG TECHNOLOGY FROM EQUIPOIS

In 2015, Ekso Bionics acquired the zeroG and X-Are spring-loaded mechanical arms. The zeroG is currently used in all exoskeleton prototypes for industrial use. Ekso Bionics has been an innovation company, developing exoskeletons for the military, industry, and rehabilitation, both motorized and passive. Ekso Bionics, however, has never been a technology reseller [39].

Currently, most exoskeleton prototypes for holding heavy tools in an industrial environment share a similar design. Ekso Bionics and Lockheed Martin collaborated on the HULC, a hydraulically powered exoskeleton for military applications. The project was a failure, but a simplified HULC structure was used to create a passive exoskeleton [30]. Realizing its mistake, Ekso Bionics created Ekso Works and the two companies have had some disputes over which entity owns the intellectual rights to both passive exoskeletons. Ekso Bionics claims that their initial work created FORTIS, while Lockheed Martin maintains that they developed FORTIS independently without infringing any Ekso Bionics patents. US Bionics and Falltech have also launched their passive exoskeletons for industrial use that rely on zeroGv. Meanwhile, several European Union (EU) countries funded the RoboMate research project, which uses a very similar spring system to hold heavy objects in an industrial environment [39].

9.6 CLOSING REMARKS

The leading companies in the development of exoskeletons guide the technological trend, which can be seen in the statistics. China currently represents the largest market in the design and manufacture of the exoskeleton, followed by the United States. The main exoskeletons are Ekso Works by Ekso Bionics, FORTIS by Lockheed Martin, Modular Agile exoskeleton (MAX) by US Bionics, and OLAD by Falltech

The growth of patent applications and the generation of companies represent the transformation of invention patents into incremental and disruptive innovations, which influences the acceptability of exoskeletons for rehabilitation and assistance from the therapist's perspective. Also, the data on the production of intellectual property allows for consolidated confidence and approval of the users toward the exoskeletons, which is crucial to improve the quality of the human robot.

It is important to mention that universities and research centers generate many scientific communications on the development of exoskeletons. These developments do not manage to become products or come to market. In contrast, the statistical data of patents, together with information from the other eight chapters, allow us to visualize and infer factors that influence the acceptability of exoskeletons in clinical environments, perceived level of usefulness, and level of satisfaction toward the functionalities of rehabilitation technology. In the future, a new generation of physiotherapists will continuously use modern intellectual property tools to design exoskeletons based on information from user requirements, user experience, licensing agreements, and technologies such as actuators, methodologies, hardware, software, and controllers.

Evaluation activity. Please answer the next quiz
https://forms.office.com/r/kzzT8pUBB4

1. Industrial property includes patents, trademarks, and trade secrets.
   A. True
   B. False

2. Utility models are objects, utensils, devices, or tools that, because of a change in their arrangement, configuration, structure, or shape, present a different function with respect to the parts that make it up or provides an advantage in terms of their utility.
   A. True
   B. False

3. An invention patent is an original product or process that can be manufactured at an industrial level and that contains an inventive step.
   A. True
   B. False

4. The International Patent Classification (IPC), established by the Strasbourg Agreement 1971, provides for a hierarchical system of language independent symbols for the classification of patents and utility models according to the different areas of technology to which they pertain.
   A. True
   B. False

5. A license agreement usually has six components: scope of the grant, exclusivity, territory, term, compensation, termination, and conclusion.
   A. True
   B. False

REFERENCES

1. Industrial property between 2012 and 2021. January 4, 2023; Available from: https://www3.wipo.int/ipstats/.
2. PCT patents and direct patents. January 4, 2023; Available from: https://www3.wipo.int/ipstats/.
3. PCT top applicants from China. January 4, 2023; Available from: www.wipo.int/ipstats/en/statistics/country_profile/profile.jsp?code=CN.
4. Madrid system: The international trademark system. January 4, 2023; Available from: www.wipo.int/madrid/en/index.html.
5. Hague system: The international design system. January 4, 2023; Available from: www.wipo.int/hague/en/index.html.
6. Statistical country profiles: United States of America. January 4, 2023; Available from: www.wipo.int/ipstats/en/statistics/country_profile/profile.jsp?code=US.
7. Konaev, M. and S.M. Abdulla, Trends in robotics patents: A global overview and an assessment of Russia. In CSET Data Brief. Center for Security and Emerging Technology: Georgetown University's School, 2021. p. 37.
8. International Patent Classification (IPC). January 4, 2023; Available from: www.wipo.int/classifications/ipc/en/.
9. Locarno Classification. January 4, 2023; Available from: www.wipo.int/classifications/locarno/en/.
10. Nice Classification. January 4, 2023; Available from: www.wipo.int/classifications/nice/en/index.html.
11. IPC class: A61H1/02. January 4, 2023; Available from: www.patbase.com/stats/class.php?ipc=A61H1/02.
12. IPC class: A61H3/02. January 4, 2023; Available from: www.patbase.com/stats/class.php?ipc=A61H3/02.
13. IPC class: B25J13/00. January 4, 2023; Available from: www.patbase.com/stats/class.php?ipc=B25J13/00.
14. IPC class: B25J9/16. January 4, 2023; Available from: www.patbase.com/stats/class.php?ipc=B25J9/16.
15. Introduction to patents and patent searching. January 4, 2023; Available from: https://guides.library.utoronto.ca/c.php?g=250474&p=1670779.
16. Sanz Merodio, D., et al., Exoskeleton for assisting human movement, Patent No.: US 11,324,653 B2, in Google Patents. 2022, Marsi Bionics S.L. p. 29.
17. García Armada, E., et al., Exoskeleton for assisting human movement, Patent No.: US 2022/0354730 A1, in Google Patents. 2022, Marsi Bionics S.L. p. 27.
18. Hollander, K., et al., Joint torque augmentation system and method for gait assistance, Patent No.: US 9,662,262 B2, in Google Patents. 2017, Spring Active, Inc. p. 42.
19. Baptista, J., et al., Shoulder module for an exoskeleton structure, Patent No.: US 10,589,435 B2, in Google Patents. 2020, B Temia Inc, Safran Electronics and Defense SAS. p. 29.
20. Grenier, J., et al., Exoskeleton structure that provides force assistance to the user, Patent No.: US 10,639,784 B2, in Google Patents. 2020, B Temia Inc, Safran Electronics and Defense SAS. p. 29.
21. Grenier, J., et al., Modular exoskeleton structure that provides force assistance to the user, Patent No.: US 2021/0069890 A1, in Google Patents. 2022, B Temia Inc Safran Electronics and Defense SAS. p. 30.
22. Pismennaya, E. and K. Tolstov, Ankle Brace or Ankle Exoskeleton, Patent No.: US 2020/0253774 A1, in Google Patents. 2020, Exoatlet LLC. p. 20.
23. Bereziy, E.S., et al., Exoskeleton, Patent No.: US 11,148,278 B2, in Google Patents. 2021, Exoatlet LLC. p. 24.

24. Zuñiga Aviles, L.A., A.H. Vilchis Gonzalez, and J.C. Avila Vilchis, Continuous passive mobilizing robot for rehabilitation of upper limbs, Patent No.: MX 388107 B in Google Patents. 2022, UAEMex: Mexico. p. 30.
25. Zuñiga Aviles, L.A., A.H. Vilchis Gonzalez, and J.C. Avila Vilchis, Continuous passive mobilizing for knee rehabilitation, Patent No.: MX 393411 B in Google Patents. 2022, UAEMex: Mexico. p. 30.
26. License agreement: Ekso Bionics® and Lockheed Martin®. January 4, 2023; Available from: www.sec.gov/Archives/edgar/data/1549084/000114420414019450/v373064_ex10-25.htm.
27. Ekso Bionics® Licenses Intellectual Property to Ottobock®. January 4, 2023; Available from: https://ir.eksobionics.com/press-releases/detail/394/ekso-bionics-licences-intellectual-property-to-ottobock.
28. Berkeley ExoWorks and The Regents of the University of California. January 4, 2023; Available from: www.sec.gov/Archives/edgar/data/1549084/000114420414003452/v365778_ex10-19.htm.
29. ReWalk Robotics and Harvard. January 4, 2023; Available from: www.massdevice.com/rewalk-robotics-inks-soft-exoskeleton-research-licensing-deal-with-harvard/.
30. Ekso Bioinics exoskeleton. January 4, 2023; Available from: https://patents.justia.com/patent/9782892.
31. Parker Hannifin Corp (licensee) and Vanderbilt University. January 4, 2023; Available from: www.fierceelectronics.com/embedded/parker-acquires-exoskeleton-technology-rights.
32. Parker Hannifin Corp (licensee) and Vanderbilt University (manufacturing). January 4, 2023; Available from: www.protolabs.com/en-gb/resources/case-studies/parker-hannifin/.
33. Lockheed Martin Enters into a License Agreement with B-Temia. January 4, 2023; Available from: https://exoskeletonreport.com/2017/05/lockheed-martin-enters-license-agreement-b-temia-developer-keoogo/.
34. Myomo and Ottobock Global Distribution Agreement. January 4, 2023; Available from: https://exoskeletonreport.com/2017/01/myomo-ottobock-global-distribution-agreement/.
35. Bioservo Maker of the SEM Glove Enters License Agreement with NASA and GM. January 4, 2023; Available from: https://exoskeletonreport.com/2016/07/bioservo-maker-of-the-sem-glove-enters-license-agreement-with-nasa-and-gm/.
36. Wyss Institute and ReWalk Robotics Form Collaboration. January 4, 2023; Available from: https://exoskeletonreport.com/2016/06/wyss-institute-rewalk-robotics-form-collaboration-new-trend/.
37. StrongArm Technologies V22 and FLx Now Sold on 3M's Website. January 4, 2023; Available from: https://exoskeletonreport.com/2016/05/strongarm-technologies-v22-and-flx-now-sold-on-3ms-website/.
38. Bionik Laboratories Merger Agreement with IMT. January 4, 2023; Available from: https://exoskeletonreport.com/2016/03/bionik-laboratories-enters-merger-agreement-interactive-motion-technologies-inc-imt/.
39. Ekso Bionics Acquires zeroG™ Technology. January 4, 2023; Available from: https://exoskeletonreport.com/2015/12/in-an-aggressive-move-ekso-bionics-acquires-zerog-technology/.

Index

Note: Page numbers in *italics* indicate a figure and page numbers in **bold** indicate a table on the corresponding page. Page numbers followed by "n" with numbers refer to notes.